Connections between Parental Involvement and Treatment of Children with Autism Spectrum Disorders (ASD)

Connections between Parental Involvement and Treatment of Children with Autism Spectrum Disorders (ASD)

Editor

Sayyed Ali Samadi

MDPI • Basel • Beijing • Wuhan • Barcelona • Belgrade • Manchester • Tokyo • Cluj • Tianjin

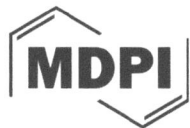

Editor
Sayyed Ali Samadi
Institute of Nursing and Health
Research
Ulster University
Newtownabbey
North Ireland
United Kingdom

Editorial Office
MDPI
St. Alban-Anlage 66
4052 Basel, Switzerland

This is a reprint of articles from the Special Issue published online in the open access journal *Brain Sciences* (ISSN 2076-3425) (available at: www.mdpi.com/journal/brainsci/special_issues/ASD_Parental).

For citation purposes, cite each article independently as indicated on the article page online and as indicated below:

LastName, A.A.; LastName, B.B.; LastName, C.C. Article Title. *Journal Name* **Year**, *Volume Number*, Page Range.

ISBN 978-3-0365-2042-1 (Hbk)
ISBN 978-3-0365-2041-4 (PDF)

© 2021 by the authors. Articles in this book are Open Access and distributed under the Creative Commons Attribution (CC BY) license, which allows users to download, copy and build upon published articles, as long as the author and publisher are properly credited, which ensures maximum dissemination and a wider impact of our publications.

The book as a whole is distributed by MDPI under the terms and conditions of the Creative Commons license CC BY-NC-ND.

Contents

About the Editor vii

Preface to "Connections between Parental Involvement and Treatment of Children with Autism Spectrum Disorders (ASD)" ix

Sayyed Ali Samadi
The Challenges of Bringing Up a Child with Autism Spectrum Disorders: Editorial for Brain Sciences Special Issue "Connections between Parental Involvement and Treatment of Children with Autism Spectrum Disorders (ASD)"
Reprinted from: *Brain Sciences* **2021**, *11*, 618, doi:10.3390/brainsci11050618 1

Shervin Assari, Shanika Boyce, Mohammed Saqib, Mohsen Bazargan and Cleopatra H. Caldwell
Parental Education and Left Lateral Orbitofrontal Cortical Activity during N-Back Task: An fMRI Study of American Adolescents
Reprinted from: *Brain Sciences* **2021**, *11*, 401, doi:10.3390/brainsci11030401 5

Noemí Carmona-Serrano, Antonio-José Moreno-Guerrero, José-Antonio Marín-Marín and Jesús López-Belmonte
Evolution of the Autism Literature and the Influence of Parents: A Scientific Mapping in Web of Science
Reprinted from: *Brain Sciences* **2021**, *11*, 74, doi:10.3390/brainsci11010074 19

Golnoush Akhlaghipour and Shervin Assari
Parental Education, Household Income, Race, and Children's Working Memory: Complexity of the Effects
Reprinted from: *Brain Sciences* **2020**, *10*, 950, doi:10.3390/brainsci10120950 35

Silvia Perzolli, Giulio Bertamini, Simona de Falco, Paola Venuti and Arianna Bentenuto
Emotional Availability and Play in Mother–Child Dyads with ASD: Changes during a Parental Based Intervention
Reprinted from: *Brain Sciences* **2020**, *10*, 904, doi:10.3390/brainsci10120904 55

Sayyed Ali Samadi, Shahnaz Bakhshalizadeh-Moradi, Fatemeh Khandani, Mehdi Foladgar, Maryam Poursaid-Mohammad and Roy McConkey
Using Hybrid Telepractice for Supporting Parents of Children with ASD during the COVID-19 Lockdown: A Feasibility Study in Iran
Reprinted from: *Brain Sciences* **2020**, *10*, 892, doi:10.3390/brainsci10110892 79

Hadi Samadi and Sayyed Ali Samadi
Understanding Different Aspects of Caregiving for Individuals with Autism Spectrum Disorders (ASDs) a Narrative Review of the Literature
Reprinted from: *Brain Sciences* **2020**, *10*, 557, doi:10.3390/brainsci10080557 93

Shervin Assari, Shanika Boyce, Golnoush Akhlaghipour, Mohsen Bazargan and Cleopatra H. Caldwell
Reward Responsiveness in the Adolescent Brain Cognitive Development (ABCD) Study: African Americans' Diminished Returns of Parental Education
Reprinted from: *Brain Sciences* **2020**, *10*, 391, doi:10.3390/brainsci10060391 109

Roy McConkey, Marie-Therese Cassin and Rosie McNaughton
Promoting the Social Inclusion of Children with ASD: A Family-Centred Intervention
Reprinted from: *Brain Sciences* **2020**, *10*, 318, doi:10.3390/brainsci10050318 . . . . **127**

Shervin Assari
Parental Education and Youth Inhibitory Control in the Adolescent Brain Cognitive Development (ABCD) Study: Blacks' Diminished Returns
Reprinted from: *Brain Sciences* **2020**, *10*, 312, doi:10.3390/brainsci10050312 . . . . **139**

About the Editor

Sayyed Ali Samadi

At the present, Dr. Samadi is the Senior Consultant for establishing rehabilitation and education services for children with developmental disabilities and their families at Bahoz center. The position started from September 2020 to the present time in the Kurdistan Region of Iraq - Erbil. He has acted as the Senior Consultant for Autism Spectrum Disorder Service Provision, at the Iranian State Welfare Organization (ISWO) from 2011 to 2019. Dr. Samadi received his Ph.D. in intellectual and developmental disabilities from the Ulster University, and he is also a Research Associate Fellow at the University of Ulster- Department of Nursing and Health Research - Centre for Intellectual and Developmental Disabilities.

Preface to "Connections between Parental Involvement and Treatment of Children with Autism Spectrum Disorders (ASD)"

Prevalence of autism spectrum disorders (ASD) is rising, and as a result, a greater level of training and treatment opportunities are required. The features of ASD impact both the family and the child. Parents, as the main caregivers, need to be considered in the provision of the services from the training to treatment providing. Findings suggest that parental involvement in the treatment process improves the generalizability of skills and increases the amount of intervention the child receives. Numerous benefits have been found in child and parent outcomes when parents are considered in the process as one of the main stakeholders. The purpose of this Special Issue is to discuss the impact of considering the parental role in training and intervention for ASD and undiagnosed similar conditions in different parts of the world. Different types of papers in the forms of reviews and original research from different researchers across the world were collected to review the impacts of parents in the training and treatment process. The different roles parents may play in the treatment and training process are also discussed, along with providing practical guidance on various ways of involving parents in the process of different service provisions for individuals with ASD.

Sayyed Ali Samadi
Editor

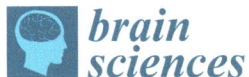

Editorial

The Challenges of Bringing Up a Child with Autism Spectrum Disorders: Editorial for Brain Sciences Special Issue "Connections between Parental Involvement and Treatment of Children with Autism Spectrum Disorders (ASD)"

Sayyed Ali Samadi

Centre for Intellectual and Developmental Disabilities-Institute of Nursing Research, University of Ulster, Newtownabbey BT37 0QB, Northern Ireland, UK; s.samadi@ulster.ac.uk

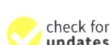

Citation: Samadi, S.A. The Challenges of Bringing Up a Child with Autism Spectrum Disorders: Editorial for Brain Sciences Special Issue "Connections between Parental Involvement and Treatment of Children with Autism Spectrum Disorders (ASD)". *Brain Sci.* 2021, 11, 618. https://doi.org/10.3390/brainsci11050618

Received: 8 April 2021
Accepted: 7 May 2021
Published: 12 May 2021

Publisher's Note: MDPI stays neutral with regard to jurisdictional claims in published maps and institutional affiliations.

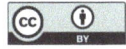

Copyright: © 2021 by the author. Licensee MDPI, Basel, Switzerland. This article is an open access article distributed under the terms and conditions of the Creative Commons Attribution (CC BY) license (https://creativecommons.org/licenses/by/4.0/).

There is no unique scientific method to guide parents in bringing up a child with autism spectrum disorders (ASD). Likewise, there are no distinctive interventions that can meet all the needs of individuals with ASD. Therefore, the aim of this Special Issue was not to focus on one particular model of intervention. Rather, the goal was to illustrate how the role of parents can be taken more seriously in whatever interventions are used or under development.

The papers in this Special Issue explore the transitioning and passing on of new styles of programs to parents and the community. This involves a conceptual shift where caregivers are considered equal members of the professional treatment team for the child. This means going beyond considering parents' opinions and receiving their support, enlisting the active participation of parents in training sessions and clinical decision-making in identifying goals and opportunities for the children, as well as in generalizing and maintaining newly acquired skills for themselves and other family members.

Underpinning this changed approach with parents is the adoption of new ways of thinking about ASD. In the main, ASD is broadly described as a medical diagnosis based on DSM or ICD definitions of behaviors and clinical symptoms. Hence, a medical model of service provision has been adopted in designing intervention goals. The medical model assumes that the curing or managing of a disability, either generally or completely, revolves around identifying the illness or disability from the in-depth clinical perspective of the individual. Yet, modern conceptions of disabilities—including ASD—acknowledge the impact of environmental influences on a child's development, such as the role of parents and family interactions as well as community and societal influences. Together, these can have strong influences on the levels of function of the individual with different types of disabilities [1].

This new perspective makes new space for parental engagement in the process of professional support for children with developmental disabilities in both assessment and intervention. The International Classification of Functioning, Disability and Health [2] describes a new assessment framework that considers the social and environmental impacts on medical and disabling conditions. This classification compares the person's current level of performance and the barriers they experience with the actions needed to enhance their functioning in their surrounding environments of the family and community. The adoption of social models may be particularly crucial in redefining the parental impacts on service provision and understanding their involvement in the intervention and treatment process for children with ASD. This has led to the creation of family-centered interventions for children with additional needs, be they through illness or disability.

Family-centered interventions is a general term that covers both a philosophy and a method of service delivery. It consists of a composition of elements such as values, skills, behaviors, and knowledge that recognizes the centrality of parents in the lives of their child with developmental disabilities. The main endeavor is to consider the unique position of every family member in supporting an individual with developmental disabilities to learn, grow, and thrive. It puts parental values, natural lifestyle, and the strengths, needs, and ideas of people with a disability and their parents and caregivers as the focal point of service provision, including the design of interventions and their implementation and evaluation.

Dunst et al. [3] demonstrated the efficacy of family-centered practice with all types of developmental programs. However, this approach was less developed in ASD at that time. While studies on parent-mediated ASD intervention have evolved gradually, available results indicate that more research is needed to understand the full impact of parent-mediated interventions on the child and family [4].

Parental efficacy plays a crucial role in family-centered practice, as it is also linked to family functioning in general. Family functioning theories emphasize the primary role of parents as the main component of the family unit, in that they provide the basis for the development and maintenance of all family members biologically, socially, and psychologically. Understanding parental and family members' needs for development in these different aspects is essential in order to facilitate the family's role in caregiving for a child with ASD. Enhancing parental awareness about their impacts, authorities, and roles can be obtained through different sources, such as training opportunities and listening to their voice when they talk about their ideas or explain issues from their perspective.

In this Special Issue, different contributing factors of parental involvement in the treatment of children with ASD have been considered. The coverage extends to the parental role in contributing to the general health and development of their offspring in other socially vulnerable groups as well as parents of children with ASD. Nevertheless, different aspects were not fully covered, and there is still much to learn. Paternal involvement in the treatment process of children with ASD is still in its early stages of progress. There is also a dearth of cross-cultural studies concerning parental involvement. A new area of research might be the impact of online diagnosis and intervention services that inevitably have to consider parents as the key person in creating these new styles of services. Profound changes due to the COVID-19 pandemic have impacted how intervention and assessment services are carried out by therapists, clinicians, and researchers. Research into parental satisfaction with these services and the effective provision of help and support to them could transform current provisions and usher in a new era of partnership working between professionals and parents [5].

In summation, it has been my privilege to work with the contributors, reviewers, and editors on this Special Issue. I appreciate their kind assistance, as it would not be possible to attain our goal without their time and consideration.

Funding: This research received no external funding.

Institutional Review Board Statement: Not applicable.

Informed Consent Statement: Not applicable.

Acknowledgments: I thank my colleagues and friends worldwide who participated in making this Special Issue a concrete success.

Conflicts of Interest: The author declares no conflict of interest.

References

1. Nevill, R.E.; Lecavalier, L.; Stratis, E.A. Meta-analysis of parent-mediated interventions for young children with autism spectrum disorder. *Autism* **2018**, *22*, 84–98. [CrossRef] [PubMed]
2. Corona, L.L.; Weitlauf, A.S.; Hine, J.; Berman, A.; Miceli, A.; Nicholson, A.; Stone, C.; Broderick, N.; Francis, S.; Juárez, A.P.; et al. Parent perceptions of caregiver-mediated telemedicine tools for assessing autism risk in toddlers. *J. Autism Dev. Disord.* **2020**, *51*, 476–486. [CrossRef] [PubMed]
3. Dunst, C.J.; Trivette, C.M.; Hamby, D.W. Meta-analysis of family-centered helpgiving practices research. *Ment. Retard. Dev. Disabil.* **2007**, *13*, 370–380. [CrossRef] [PubMed]

4. World Health Organisation (WHO). *International Classification of Functioning, Disability and Health (ICF) Short Version*; WHO: Geneva, Switzerland, 2001; Available online: https://apps.who.int/iris/bitstream/handle/10665/43737/9789241547321_eng.pdf?sequence=1 (accessed on 18 May 2020).
5. Samadi, S.A.; Samadi, H.; McConkey, R. A conceptual model for empowering families in less affluent countries who have a child with autism. In *Autism Spectrum Disorder-Recent Advances*; IntechOpen: London, UK, 2015.

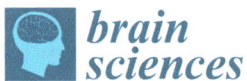

Article

Parental Education and Left Lateral Orbitofrontal Cortical Activity during N-Back Task: An fMRI Study of American Adolescents

Shervin Assari [1,2,*], Shanika Boyce [3], Mohammed Saqib [4], Mohsen Bazargan [1,5] and Cleopatra H. Caldwell [3,6]

1. Department of Urban Public Health, Charles R Drew University of Medicine and Science, Los Angeles, CA 90059, USA; Mohsenbazargan@cdrewu.edu
2. Department of Family Medicine, Charles R Drew University of Medicine and Science, Los Angeles, CA 90059, USA
3. Department of Pediatrics, Charles R Drew University of Medicine and Science, Los Angeles, CA 90059, USA; ShanikaBoyce@cdrewu.edu (S.B.); cleoc@umich.edu (C.H.C.)
4. Department of Health Behavior and Health Education, School of Public Health, University of Michigan, Ann Arbor, MI 48104, USA; saqimoha@umich.edu
5. Department of Family Medicine, University of California Los Angeles, Los Angeles, CA 90095, USA
6. Center for Research on Ethnicity, Culture, and Health (CRECH), School of Public Health, University of Michigan, Ann Arbor, MI 48104, USA
* Correspondence: assari@umich.edu; Tel.: +1-734-232-0445; Fax: +1-734-615-8739

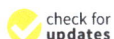

Citation: Assari, S.; Boyce, S.; Saqib, M.; Bazargan, M.; Caldwell, C.H. Parental Education and Left Lateral Orbitofrontal Cortical Activity during N-Back Task: An fMRI Study of American Adolescents. *Brain Sci.* **2021**, *11*, 401. https://doi.org/10.3390/brainsci11030401

Academic Editor: Valerio Santangelo

Received: 7 March 2021
Accepted: 19 March 2021
Published: 22 March 2021

Publisher's Note: MDPI stays neutral with regard to jurisdictional claims in published maps and institutional affiliations.

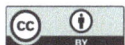

Copyright: © 2021 by the authors. Licensee MDPI, Basel, Switzerland. This article is an open access article distributed under the terms and conditions of the Creative Commons Attribution (CC BY) license (https://creativecommons.org/licenses/by/4.0/).

Abstract: *Introduction.* The Orbitofrontal Cortex (OFC) is a cortical structure that has implications in cognition, memory, reward anticipation, outcome evaluation, decision making, and learning. As such, OFC activity correlates with these cognitive brain abilities. Despite research suggesting race and socioeconomic status (SES) indicators such as parental education may be associated with OFC activity, limited knowledge exists on multiplicative effects of race and parental education on OFC activity and associated cognitive ability. *Purpose.* Using functional brain imaging data from the Adolescent Brain Cognitive Development (ABCD) study, we tested the multiplicative effects of race and parental education on left lateral OFC activity during an N-Back task. In our study, we used a sociological rather than biological theory that conceptualizes race and SES as proxies of access to the opportunity structure and exposure to social adversities rather than innate and non-modifiable brain differences. We explored racial variation in the effect of parental educational attainment, a primary indicator of SES, on left lateral OFC activity during an N-Back task between Black and White 9–10 years old adolescents. *Methods.* The ABCD study is a national, landmark, multi-center brain imaging investigation of American adolescents. The total sample was 4290 9–10 years old Black or White adolescents. The independent variables were SES indicators, namely family income, parental education, and neighborhood income. The primary outcome was the average beta weight for N-Back (2 back versus 0 back contrast) in ASEG ROI left OFC activity, measured by functional Magnetic Resonance Imaging (fMRI) during an N-Back task. Ethnicity, age, sex, subjective SES, and family structure were the study covariates. For data analysis, we used linear regression models. *Results.* In White but not Black adolescents, parental education was associated with higher left lateral OFC activity during the N-Back task. In the pooled sample, we found a significant interaction between race and parental education on the outcome, suggesting that high parental education is associated with a larger increase in left OFC activity of White than Black adolescents. *Conclusions.* For American adolescents, race and SES jointly influence left lateral OFC activity correlated with cognition, memory, decision making, and learning. Given the central role of left lateral OFC activity in learning and memory, our finding calls for additional research on contextual factors that reduce the gain of SES for Black adolescents. Cognitive inequalities are not merely due to the additive effects of race and SES but also its multiplicative effects.

Keywords: population groups; socioeconomic factors; adolescents; brain development; fMRI; cognitive; N-Back; memory; learning; orbitofrontal cortex

1. Introduction

Given that socioeconomic status (SES) indicators such as parental education [1] are closely associated with exposure to chronic stress [2] and social adversities, and given that stress and adversities jeopardize adolescents' brain development [3–6], it should be no surprise that there is a connection between SES indicators such as parental education and adolescents brain development [7–14]. Adolescents from low and high SES experience vastly different social and economic adversity levels, thus showing considerable brain function changes [15–17]. As a result of poor brain development, adolescents from low SES families become at risk of undesired cognitive, emotional, and behavioral outcomes such as poor school performance [18], depression [19], anxiety [20,21], antisocial behaviors [22], aggression [23], and sexual initiation [24–26], as well as the use of tobacco [27,28], alcohol [29,30], and other drugs [31].

The effects of SES and associated stress are not specific to a particular brain region, but their effects are shown for multiple brain regions, including the amygdala [15,32,33], hippocampus [34–36], as well as the cerebral cortex. However, due to the scarcity of research on SES's effects on brain regions, our understanding of brain regions that are affected by SES is inconsistent.

Among various brain regions and structures that carry the effect of SES is the Orbitofrontal Cortex (OFC), a cortical structure with major implications in cognition, memory, decision making, and learning. As such, OFC activity correlates with such cognitive brain abilities [37–40]. The OFC has been shown to be affected by stress and SES [41]. Individuals with low performance or shrinkage of the OFC may show poor learning ability and memory. Several studies have shown that race, SES, and stress impact OFC. Altered OFC structure and function are also shown to be a part of dementia [42], Alzheimer's disease [43,44], psychosis [45,46], post-traumatic stress disorder (PTSD) [47,48], depression [49–51], and drug use [52–54].

Most of the existing literature on the link between SES and adolescents' brain development has focused on various aspects of emotion regulation rather than domains of memory and cognition [15,32,33,55]. Similarly, most of the existing research on the effects of stress and SES is limited to amygdala structure and function [15,32,33,55]. For example, Javanbakht et al. have documented the effects of household SES and childhood stress on amygdala response to threatening stimuli [15,32,33]. However, less is known on the effect of SES and environment on the OFC [41,56].

Accurate knowledge regarding the nature of the undesired effect of low SES on brain development and function will help us better understand why low SES adolescents report worse developmental outcomes [57], school performance [57], mental health [58], emotion regulation [59,60], aggression [61], and substance use [58,62]. Such research-based knowledge on how SES operates as a social determinant of adolescents' brain development and function is core for breaking the vicious cycle between low family SES and poor child developmental outcomes across multiple emotional and behavioral domains.

Theoretically, the scarcity hypothesis explains why and how SES deteriorates healthy adolescents' brain development. According to this theoretical framework, low SES reflects the scarcity of resources that are essential for adolescents' brain development. In this view, food and home insecurity increase the risk for poor child development. As such, poor access to resources that are buffers against poor developmental outcomes is one of the many mechanisms that may explain the link between low SES and poor brain development [63]. Low family SES is also a proxy of poor parenting [64–68] and high parental risk behaviors [69,70] that can put child brain development in jeopardy [71]. Secondary to these cumulative risks, adolescents from low SES families remain at high level of risk of psychopathologies [72–74], problem behaviors [75–81], and poor school performance [82–84].

Multiple reasons suggest the association between SES and race/ethnicity are complex and interactive. First, race/ethnicity and SES have a major overlapping distribution [85,86]. Low SES may even mediate (explain) the racial and ethnic disparities in adolescents' brain development [87]. In addition, SES may have differential impacts on adolescent brain development across diverse racial and ethnic groups [55]. One study suggested that family income has stronger effects on brain function for the most disadvantaged than the least disadvantaged groups in the society [55].

In contrast, according to the Minorities' Diminished Returns (MDRs) framework [88], racial and ethnic minorities show weaker associations between SES and outcomes [89,90]. In several studies in children, youth, adults, and older adults, family SES shows weaker effects for Blacks than Whites [87,91–95]. As a result of MDRs, while White youth from high SES backgrounds show the lowest level of risk, Black adolescents remain at high risk regardless of SES, a pattern similarly relevant to behavioral, developmental, and health outcomes [89,96]. These patterns are shown across emotional, behavioral, and cognitive domains such as high-risk behaviors [96], aggression [96] and tobacco use [97], anxiety [98], depression [99], poor health [87], chronic disease, obesity, poor school attachment, impulsivity, and poor school performance [83]. These indicate a novel mechanism of health inequalities which is systematically overlooked by researchers and policymakers and suggest health disparities are not just due to lack of access to SES but also societal inequalities that slow, hinder, and block the process of translation of an SES resource (e.g., parental education) to an outcome (e.g., youth brain development).

Aims

To understand the social patterning of American adolescents' brain development, we conducted this study with two aims: First, to study the effect of SES on left lateral OFC activity measured during an N-Back task. Using the Adolescent Brain Cognitive Development (ABCD) data, which are from the state-of-the-art study of adolescents' brain development [100–113], we hypothesized that high parental education, as a major SES indicator, would be associated with a higher left lateral OFC activity. We also hypothesized that when comparing White and Black adolescents, the positive association between SES (parental education) and the left lateral OFC activity measured during an N-Back task would be weaker in Black than White adolescents, in line with the MDRs framework [88,96].

2. Methods

2.1. Study Design

We conducted a secondary analysis of the data from the Adolescent Brain Cognitive Development (ABCD) study [102,103,109,114,115]. This study applied a cross-sectional design and only used wave one of the ABCD data [100–113]. ABCD study is the largest brain imaging studies of adolescents in the US [109,116].

2.2. Sample and Sampling

Participants were recruited from school systems in 21 study sites, which were distributed across multiple states. The recruitment was limited to 9–10-year-old children. To increase the generalizability of the sample, schools were selected based on their distribution of race, ethnicity, SES, sex, and urbanicity. For more information, please consult a fully detailed description of the ABCD sample and sampling [112]. The current analysis was performed in 4290 9–10-year-old White or Black adolescents. Participants were included in this analysis if they had complete data on all study variables.

2.3. Variables

The study variables included demographic factors (age and sex), SES indicators (parental educational attainment, subjective SES), and left lateral OFC activity (mean beta weight for N-Back run 1 2 back conditions in APARC ROI left lateral orbitofrontal: tfmri_nback_r1_349). Left lateral OFC activity was measured using a task-based functional MRI measure during N-Back. Details of the procedures for harmonization of the fMRIs and imaging are explained elsewhere [102].

2.3.1. Outcome

The outcome was left lateral OFC activity measured as mean beta weight for N-Back run 1 2 back conditions in APARC ROI left lateral orbitofrontal: tfmri_nback_r1_349. We selected the left lateral OFC because it is shown to be impacted by poverty, trauma, and adversity [56,117–120].

2.3.2. Moderator

Race. Race was self-identified and treated as a dichotomous variable: Black = 1, White = 0 (reference group).

2.3.3. Independent Variables

Parental Educational Attainment. Participants were asked, "What is the highest grade or level of school you have completed or the highest degree you have received?" Responses ranged from 0 (Never attended/Kindergarten) to 21 (doctoral degree). This variable ranged from 1 to 21.

Financial Status. This study measured financial status using the following seven items: "In the past 12 months, has there been a time when you and your immediate family experienced any of the following:" (1)"Needed food but couldn't afford to buy it or couldn't afford to go out to get it?", (2) "Were without telephone service because you could not afford it?" (3)" Didn't pay the full amount of the rent or mortgage because you could not afford it?", (4) "Were evicted from your home for not paying the rent or mortgage?", (5)"Had services turned off by the gas or electric company, or the oil company wouldn't deliver oil because payments were not made?", (6) "Had someone who needed to see a doctor or go to the hospital but didn't go because you could not afford it?" and (7) "Had someone who needed a dentist but couldn't go because you could not afford it?" [121–127]. Subjective financial status predicts health beyond objective SES [121,123,124,128–130].

2.3.4. Confounders

Age, sex, ethnicity, and marital status were the confounders. Parents reported adolescents' age. Age was calculated as the distance of the date of birth to the date of enrollment to the study. Age was measured in years. Sex was a dichotomous variable with males as 1 and females as 0. Parental marital status was a dichotomous variable: Married = 1, unmarried = 0 (reference category). Parents reported their ethnicity. Participants' ethnicity was coded as 1 for Hispanic and 0 for non-Hispanic.

2.4. Data Analysis

We used Statistical Package for the Social Sciences (SPSS) for our data analysis. Frequency (%) and mean (standard deviation [SD]) were described overall and by race. We used Pearson Chi-square and independent samples *t*-test to compare Blacks and White adolescents. To perform our multivariable analyses, we ran four multivariable linear regressions. The independent variable was the SES indicator (parental education). The outcome was left lateral OFC activity during the N-Back task. All these models controlled for age, sex, financial difficulties, and marital status. *Model 1* was performed in Whites. *Model 2* was performed in Blacks. *Model 3* was performed in the pooled sample without the interaction term. *Model 4* was performed in the pooled sample with the interaction term. We reported unstandardized regression coefficients (b), standard errors (SE), 95% confidence interval (CI), *t* value, and their *p*-values. Any *p*-value of less than 0.05 was considered statistically significant. We did not adjust for multiple comparisons because, despite extensive fMRI data in the ABCD study, other brain regions' available data were not analyzed. As we only analyzed data on lateral OFC function, we kept our *p*-value threshold as 0.05.

2.5. Ethics

The study protocol of the ABCD study received approval from the Institutional Review Board (IRB) of the University of California, San Diego. Adolescent participants gave assent.

Adult participants (parents) signed informed consent [116]. As our analysis applied fully de-identified data, our study was exempt from a full IRB review by our institution.

3. Results

3.1. Descriptives

Table 1 shows the descriptive characteristics of the 4290 8–11 years old participating adolescents who were either White (n = 3436; 80.1%) or Blacks (n = 854; 19.9%). This table also describes the descriptive characteristics of the pooled sample overall and by race. Black and White adolescents differed in family SES but not age or gender or the left lateral OFC activity. Compared to White adolescents, Black adolescents were less likely to be from married families, had lower parental education, and had more financial stress.

Table 1. Descriptive data overall and by race (n = 4290).

	All (n = 4290)		Whites (n = 3436)		Blacks (n = 854)	
	n	%	n	%	n	%
Ethnicity * [a]						
Non-Hispanic	3582	83.5	2811	81.8	771	90.3
Hispanic	708	16.5	625	18.2	83	9.7
Sex * [a]						
Male	1985	46.3	1581	46	404	47.3
Female	2305	53.7	1855	54	450	52.7
Family Structure * [a]						
Not-Married	1258	29.3	707	20.6	551	64.5
Married	3032	70.7	2729	79.4	303	35.5
	Mean	SD	Mean	SD	Mean	SD
Age (Year) * [b]	9.49	0.51	9.50	0.50	9.49	0.51
Parental Education * [b]	0.94	0.15	0.96	0.12	0.87	0.20
Subjective Financial Status * [b]	16.89	2.48	17.22	2.36	15.56	2.53
the left lateral OFC Function * [b]	0.50	0.86	0.46	0.69	0.66	1.34

* p < 0.05 for a comparison of Whites and Blacks. [a] Chi-Square test, [b] independent samples t-test; OFC: Orbito-Frontal Cortex.

3.2. Race-Specific Associations

Table 2 reports the results of two race-specific models for the N-Back task results in White and Black children. *Model 1* was performed in White adolescents, and *Model 2* was performed in Black adolescents. We found that parental education was associated with left lateral OFC function during the N-Back task in White but not Black adolescents.

Table 2. Linear regressions by racial group.

	Model 1 White						Model 2 Black					
	b	SE	95% CI		t	p	b	SE	95% CI		t	p
Ethnicity	0.04	0.03	0.02	−0.03	0.10	1.11	0.266	−0.06	0.16	−0.01	−0.36	0.25	−0.37	0.708
Sex (Male)	0.06	0.02	0.04	0.01	0.11	2.52	0.012	−0.02	0.09	−0.01	−0.20	0.17	−0.17	0.864
Age	−0.09	0.02	−0.06	−0.13	−0.04	−3.73	<0.001	−0.10	0.09	−0.04	−0.27	0.08	−1.06	0.291
Married	−0.01	0.03	−0.01	−0.07	0.05	−0.43	0.666	−0.14	0.10	−0.05	−0.34	0.07	−1.32	0.187
Subjective Financial Status	−0.06	0.10	−0.01	−0.25	0.14	−0.59	0.557	0.04	0.23	0.01	−0.42	0.49	0.17	0.867
Parental education	0.01	0.01	0.04	0.00	0.02	2.22	0.026	−0.03	0.02	−0.06	−0.07	0.01	−1.62	0.105
Constant	1.10	0.25		0.61	1.59	4.38	<0.001	2.08	0.91		0.29	3.87	2.28	0.023

3.3. Overall Associations

Table 3 reports the results of regressions overall. In *Model 3*, parental education was not correlated with left lateral OFC activity during the N-Back task. In *Model 4*, a significant interaction was found, suggesting that parental education and left lateral

OFC activity during the N-Back task show a stronger positive association in White than Black adolescents.

Table 3. Linear regressions overall.

	Model 3 Main Effects							Model 4 Main Effects + Interaction						
	B	SE		95% CI		t	p	b	SE		95% CI		t	p
Race (Blacks)	0.04	0.03	0.02	−0.03	0.10	1.11	0.266	0.04	0.03	0.02	−0.03	0.10	1.11	0.266
Ethnicity	−0.01	0.04	0.00	−0.08	0.07	−0.16	0.875	0.02	0.04	0.01	−0.05	0.09	0.51	0.613
Sex (Male)	0.04	0.03	0.02	−0.01	0.09	1.63	0.103	0.04	0.03	0.03	−0.01	0.10	1.68	0.093
Age	−0.09	0.03	−0.05	−0.14	−0.04	−3.54	<0.001	−0.09	0.03	−0.05	−0.14	−0.04	−3.45	0.001
Married	−0.05	0.03	−0.03	−0.12	0.01	−1.64	0.102	−0.05	0.03	−0.02	−0.11	0.02	−1.40	0.162
Subjective Financial Status	−0.01	0.10	0.00	−0.19	0.18	−0.08	0.933	−0.04	0.12	−0.01	−0.29	0.20	−0.35	0.724
Parental education	0.00	0.01	0.00	−0.01	0.01	0.05	0.960	0.01	0.01	0.04	0.00	0.03	1.83	0.067
Race × Subjective Financial Status								0.07	0.19	0.03	−0.31	0.44	0.35	0.729
Race × Parental education								−0.05	0.01	−0.37	−0.08	−0.02	−3.70	<0.001
Constant	1.36	0.27		0.82	1.90	4.94	<0.001	1.14	0.29		0.58	1.71	3.99	<0.001

4. Discussion

Parental education was associated with White but not Black OFC activity during the N-Back task. We also found an interaction confirming the same results.

Several studies have explored separate, additive, or multiplicative effects of race and SES on brain function. Most of these studies, however, have investigated separate effects of SES and race. There are only a few, if any, on the multiplicative effects of SES and race on brain development [63,131]. In addition, across SES indicators, the most common indicator has been poverty status, followed by income [15,32,33]. Parental education attainment has not been commonly investigated. Regarding brain regions and structures, most research has studied the amygdala and limbic system [15,32,33], rather than the left lateral OFC. Finally, many scholars do not wish to explore racial differences in brain imaging and function to avoid conflict. This is an overly politicized area of research with significant policy implications. Political correctness has reduced the likelihood of researchers to study how race and SES interact on brain development.

A study explored the associations between family SES (childhood poverty) and functional connectivity between the following brain regions: The hippocampus, amygdala, superior frontal cortex, lingual gyrus, posterior cingulate, and putamen. The study showed that childhood poverty predicts a lower level of connectivity between these regions, and these reduced brain connectivities mediate the effect of childhood poverty on adolescents' depression [131]. In a series of fMRI publications, a group of researchers, including Javanbakht, established a link between low family SES and functional connectivities between PFC, amygdala, and other brain regions [15,32,33]. These altered connectivities may be why low SES is associated with hyperactivation of the reward network and hypoactivation of the executive network [63]. Thus, the effects of SES and poverty go beyond a particular brain structure and can be seen for connectivity between several brain structures that regulate memory, executive functioning, cognition, and emotion [132]. It is still unknown to what degree the effects of poverty on brain functions are mediated or moderated by positive parenting [133].

Our study findings suggested that Black adolescents face double jeopardy. While race is associated with some altered function of the hippocampus, low SES is also another risk factor for them. There is, however, racial variations in the effects of SES on hippocampus activation during an N-Back task. For Blacks, low SES may come with a higher impact on their hippocampus. The more salient effects of low SES on the hippocampus of Black than White adolescents may be due to the cumulative effects of adversities in the life of racial and ethnic minorities and underserved populations. Racial discrimination and race-related stress may also have some role. Racial discrimination has been shown to impact a wide array of brain regions such as the PFC, anterior insula, putamen, amygdala, caudate, hippocampus, anterior cingulate, and medial frontal gyrus [134].

However, our study is not in support of most previous epidemiological studies that have explored racial differences in the health effects of SES. Many studies have shown more significant effects of SES on outcomes for White than Black adolescents [87]. For example, family SES has shown larger effects on ADHD [90], anxiety [98], aggression [96], tobacco dependence [96], school bonding [135], school performance [83], and overall health [136] for White than Black adolescents. This epidemiological research introduces family SES as a more salient determinant of impulsivity for White than Black adolescents [137]. Thus, we observe poor mental health, physical health, and risk behaviors in high SES Black adolescents [89,90]. These patterns are described as MDRs and hold across age groups, SES indicators, and health outcomes [88].

Differential effects of SES for Black and White families contribute to the transgenerational transmission of inequalities [89,96,136]. Differential effects of SES mean that equal SES generates unequal outcomes for the next generation of adolescents, which means the reproduction of inequalities across generations for Blacks. However, most of the previous studies on MDRs have relied on self-reported outcomes and family SES. Thus, the evidence lacked biological and brain imaging studies that test differential effects of SES on adolescents' brain function. This paper extended the existing literature by testing such patterns on brain development.

4.1. Cautionary Note

In this study, we conceptualized and theorized race as a social factor (a proxy of poverty and SES) on how the brain is affected by low or high SES (parental education). Our approach is different from studies that explore racial variation in brain function or structure as such differences are innate and non-modifiable. We believe that the observed racial differences are more to do with living conditions than genetic predisposition. In this investigation, we studied the former rather than the latter.

4.2. Future Research Directions

There is a need for identification and elimination of structural causes of MDRs in Black adolescents and families. Some of the suspects that require future research include racial segregation, school segregation, stress, or exposure to toxins such as air pollutants and lead. These environmental factors may have a role in reducing the health effects of SES for Black families. Labor market discrimination, job availability, discrimination, and segregation may play a role in this regard. There is a need to compare other racial and ethnic groups such as Asian Americans, Native Americans, Hispanics, and immigrants for the effects of SES on the left lateral OFC. Research should also go beyond the left lateral OFC and include other structures that have implications for emotion regulation, memory, cognition, learning, and behaviors.

4.3. Limitations

To list the study limitations, one is the cross-sectional design. Due to the design issue, findings should not and cannot be interpreted as causation but rather an association between race, SES, and brain development. SES and brain development have bidirectional associations; thus, future research should also address reverse causation. Second, we only had two SES indicators, namely parental education and financial difficulties. This is particularly important because neighborhood and contextual factors could be why parental education does not generate the same outcome for Black and White families. Third, N-Back provides insight regarding both emotion regulation as well as working memory. This study, however, exclusively focused on a brain mechanism that is involved in working memory.

5. Conclusions

In summary, high parental education is correlated with the left lateral OFC activation during the N-Back task in a national sample of White but not Black American adolescents. This observation is also supported by an interaction in the pooled sample suggesting that the magnitude of parental education's effect on the left lateral OFC function during the N-Back task is less pronounced for Black than White adolescents. More research is needed on the complexities between the effects of race, SES, and social environment on adolescents' brain development, including but not limited to the left lateral OFC function and other structures with the implication in decision making, learning, and memory.

Author Contributions: S.A.: Conceptual model, data analysis, write up, revision, approval of the paper. S.B., M.S., M.B., C.H.C.: Conceptual model, revision, approval of the paper. All authors have read and agreed to the published version of the manuscript.

Funding: Assari is supported by the NIH grants CA201415-02, 5S21MD000103, 54MD008149, R25 MD007610, 2U54MD007598, 4P60MD006923, and U54 TR001627. Multiple NIH funds ABCD study under awards.

Institutional Review Board Statement: The study protocol of the ABCD study received approval from the Institutional Re-view Board (IRB) of the University of California, San Diego.

Informed Consent Statement: Informed consent was obtained from all subjects involved in tthe study.

Data Availability Statement: Data are available at The National Institute of Mental Health Data Archive (NDA) accessible at https://nda.nih.gov/abcd (accessed on 22 March 2021).

Acknowledgments: Data used in the preparation of this article were obtained from the Adolescent Brain Cognitive Development (ABCD) Study. This is a multisite, longitudinal study designed to recruit more than 10,000 children aged 9–10 years and follow them over 10 years into early adulthood. The ABCD Study is supported by the National Institutes of Health and additional federal partners under award numbers U01DA041022, U01DA041028, U01DA041048, U01DA041089, U01DA041106, U01DA041117, U01DA041120, U01DA041134, U01DA041148, U01DA041156, U01DA041174, U24DA041123, and U24DA041147. A full list of supporters is available at https://abcdstudy.org/nih-collaborators (accessed on 1 March 2021). A listing of participating sites and a complete listing of the study investigators can be found at https://abcdstudy.org/principal-investigators.html (accessed on 1 March 2021). ABCD consortium investigators designed and implemented the study and/or provided data but did not necessarily participate in analysis or writing of this report. This manuscript reflects the views of the authors and may not reflect the opinions or views of the National Institutes of Health (NIH) or ABCD consortium investigators. The ABCD data repository grows and changes over time. The ABCD data used in this report came from [NIMH Data Archive Digital Object Identifier (http://dx.doi.org/10.15154/1504041) (accessed on 1 March 2021)]. This manuscript reflects the views of the authors and may not reflect the opinions or views of the NIH or ABCD consortium investigators. The author wishes to thank Gavin Wells for his edits to this paper.

Conflicts of Interest: The authors declare no conflict of interest.

References

1. Oshri, A.; Hallowell, E.; Liu, S.; MacKillop, J.; Galvan, A.; Kogan, S.M.; Sweet, L.H. Socioeconomic hardship and delayed reward discounting: Associations with working memory and emotional reactivity. *Dev. Cogn. Neurosci.* **2019**, *37*, 100642. [CrossRef]
2. Lantz, P.M.; House, J.S.; Mero, R.P.; Williams, D.R. Stress, life events, and socioeconomic disparities in health: Results from the Americans' Changing Lives Study. *J. Health Soc. Behav.* **2005**, *46*, 274–288. [CrossRef] [PubMed]
3. Herzog, J.I.; Schmahl, C. Adverse Childhood Experiences and the Consequences on Neurobiological, Psychosocial, and Somatic Conditions Across the Lifespan. *Front. Psychiatry* **2018**, *9*, 420. [CrossRef] [PubMed]
4. McCreary, J.K.; Truica, L.S.; Friesen, B.; Yao, Y.; Olson, D.M.; Kovalchuk, I.; Cross, A.R.; Metz, G.A. Altered brain morphology and functional connectivity reflect a vulnerable affective state after cumulative multigenerational stress in rats. *Neuroscience* **2016**, *330*, 79–89. [CrossRef]
5. Pagliaccio, D.; Luby, J.L.; Bogdan, R.; Agrawal, A.; Gaffrey, M.S.; Belden, A.C.; Botteron, K.N.; Harms, M.P.; Barch, D.M. Amygdala functional connectivity, HPA axis genetic variation, and life stress in children and relations to anxiety and emotion regulation. *J. Abnorm. Psychol.* **2015**, *124*, 817–833. [CrossRef] [PubMed]
6. Pegg, S.; Ethridge, P.; Shields, G.S.; Slavich, G.M.; Weinberg, A.; Kujawa, A. Blunted Social Reward Responsiveness Moderates the Effect of Lifetime Social Stress Exposure on Depressive Symptoms. *Front. Behav. Neurosci.* **2019**, *13*, 178. [CrossRef]
7. Hair, N.L.; Hanson, J.L.; Wolfe, B.L.; Pollak, S.D. Association of Child Poverty, Brain Development, and Academic Achievement. *JAMA Pediatr.* **2015**, *169*, 822–829. [CrossRef] [PubMed]

8. Benavente-Fernandez, I.; Synnes, A.; Grunau, R.E.; Chau, V.; Ramraj, C.; Glass, T.; Cayam-Rand, D.; Siddiqi, A.; Miller, S.P. Association of Socioeconomic Status and Brain Injury with Neurodevelopmental Outcomes of Very Preterm Children. *JAMA Netw. Open* **2019**, *2*, e192914. [CrossRef] [PubMed]
9. Machlin, L.; McLaughlin, K.A.; Sheridan, M.A. Brain structure mediates the association between socioeconomic status and attention-deficit/hyperactivity disorder. *Dev. Sci.* **2019**, e12844. [CrossRef]
10. Fotenos, A.F.; Mintun, M.A.; Snyder, A.Z.; Morris, J.C.; Buckner, R.L. Brain volume decline in aging: Evidence for a relation between socioeconomic status, preclinical Alzheimer disease, and reserve. *Arch. Neurol.* **2008**, *65*, 113–120. [CrossRef]
11. Lawson, G.M.; Camins, J.S.; Wisse, L.; Wu, J.; Duda, J.T.; Cook, P.A.; Gee, J.C.; Farah, M.J. Childhood socioeconomic status and childhood maltreatment: Distinct associations with brain structure. *PLoS ONE* **2017**, *12*, e0175690. [CrossRef] [PubMed]
12. Deuschle, M.; Hendlmeier, F.; Witt, S.; Rietschel, M.; Gilles, M.; Sanchez-Guijo, A.; Fananas, L.; Hentze, S.; Wudy, S.A.; Hellweg, R. Cortisol, cortisone, and BDNF in amniotic fluid in the second trimester of pregnancy: Effect of early life and current maternal stress and socioeconomic status. *Dev. Psychopathol.* **2018**, *30*, 971–980. [CrossRef] [PubMed]
13. Betancourt, L.M.; Avants, B.; Farah, M.J.; Brodsky, N.L.; Wu, J.; Ashtari, M.; Hurt, H. Effect of socioeconomic status (SES) disparity on neural development in female African-American infants at age 1 month. *Dev. Sci.* **2016**, *19*, 947–956. [CrossRef] [PubMed]
14. Raizada, R.D.; Kishiyama, M.M. Effects of socioeconomic status on brain development, and how cognitive neuroscience may contribute to levelling the playing field. *Front. Hum. Neurosci.* **2010**, *4*, 3. [CrossRef] [PubMed]
15. Javanbakht, A.; King, A.P.; Evans, G.W.; Swain, J.E.; Angstadt, M.; Phan, K.L.; Liberzon, I. Childhood Poverty Predicts Adult Amygdala and Frontal Activity and Connectivity in Response to Emotional Faces. *Front. Behav. Neurosci.* **2015**, *9*, 154. [CrossRef]
16. Masten, C.L.; Telzer, E.H.; Eisenberger, N.I. An FMRI investigation of attributing negative social treatment to racial discrimination. *J. Cogn. Neurosci.* **2011**, *23*, 1042–1051. [CrossRef]
17. Wu, X.; Zou, Q.; Hu, J.; Tang, W.; Mao, L.; Zhu, J.; Jin, Y.; Wu, X.; Lu, L.; et al. Intrinsic Functional Connectivity Patterns Predict Consciousness Level and Recovery Outcome in Acquired Brain Injury. *J. Neurosci.* **2015**, *35*, 12932–12946. [CrossRef]
18. Sirin, S.R. Socioeconomic status and academic achievement: A meta-analytic review of research. *Rev. Educ. Res.* **2005**, *75*, 417–453. [CrossRef]
19. Mendelson, T.; Kubzansky, L.D.; Datta, G.D.; Buka, S.L. Relation of female gender and low socioeconomic status to internalizing symptoms among adolescents: A case of double jeopardy? *Soc. Sci. Med.* **2008**, *66*, 1284–1296. [CrossRef]
20. Lee, J.O.; Herrenkohl, T.I.; Kosterman, R.; Small, C.M.; Hawkins, J.D. Educational inequalities in the co-occurrence of mental health and substance use problems, and its adult socio-economic consequences: A longitudinal study of young adults in a community sample. *Public Health* **2013**, *127*, 745–753. [CrossRef]
21. Silvernale, C.; Kuo, B.; Staller, K. Lower socioeconomic status is associated with an increased prevalence of comorbid anxiety and depression among patients with irritable bowel syndrome: Results from a multicenter cohort. *Scand. J. Gastroenterol.* **2019**, *54*, 1070–1074. [CrossRef] [PubMed]
22. Palma-Coca, O.; Hernandez-Serrato, M.I.; Villalobos-Hernandez, A.; Unikel-Santoncini, C.; Olaiz-Fernandez, G.; Bojorquez-Chapela, I. Association of socioeconomic status, problem behaviors, and disordered eating in Mexican adolescents: Results of the Mexican National Health and Nutrition Survey 2006. *J. Adolesc. Health* **2011**, *49*, 400–406. [CrossRef]
23. Heshmat, R.; Qorbani, M.; Ghoreshi, B.; Djalalinia, S.; Tabatabaie, O.R.; Safiri, S.; Noroozi, M.; Motlagh, M.E.; Ahadi, Z.; Asayesh, H.; et al. Association of socioeconomic status with psychiatric problems and violent behaviours in a nationally representative sample of Iranian children and adolescents: The CASPIAN-IV study. *BMJ Open* **2016**, *6*, e011615. [CrossRef]
24. Stanger-Hall, K.F.; Hall, D.W. Abstinence-only education and teen pregnancy rates: Why we need comprehensive sex education in the US. *PLoS ONE* **2011**, *6*, e24658. [CrossRef]
25. Pilgrim, N.A.; Ahmed, S.; Gray, R.H.; Sekasanvu, J.; Lutalo, T.; Nalugoda, F.; Serwadda, D.; Wawer, M.J. Multiple sexual partnerships among female adolescents in rural Uganda: The effects of family structure and school attendance. *Int. J. Adolesc. Med. Health* **2015**, *27*, 319–328. [CrossRef]
26. Gutierrez, J.P.; Atienzo, E.E. Socioeconomic status, urbanicity and risk behaviors in Mexican youth: An analysis of three cross-sectional surveys. *BMC Public Health* **2011**, *11*, 900. [CrossRef]
27. Kaleta, D.; Usidame, B.; Dziankowska-Zaborszczyk, E.; Makowiec-Dabrowska, T. Socioeconomic Disparities in Age of Initiation and Ever Tobacco Smoking: Findings from Romania. *Cent. Eur. J. Public Health* **2015**, *23*, 299–305. [CrossRef] [PubMed]
28. Barreto, S.M.; de Figueiredo, R.C.; Giatti, L. Socioeconomic inequalities in youth smoking in Brazil. *BMJ Open* **2013**, *3*, e003538. [CrossRef] [PubMed]
29. Moore, G.F.; Littlecott, H.J. School- and family-level socioeconomic status and health behaviors: Multilevel analysis of a national survey in wales, United Kingdom. *J. Sch. Health* **2015**, *85*, 267–275. [CrossRef] [PubMed]
30. Silveira, C.M.; Siu, E.R.; Anthony, J.C.; Saito, L.P.; de Andrade, A.G.; Kutschenko, A.; Viana, M.C.; Wang, Y.P.; Martins, S.S.; Andrade, L.H. Drinking patterns and alcohol use disorders in Sao Paulo, Brazil: The role of neighborhood social deprivation and socioeconomic status. *PLoS ONE* **2014**, *9*, e108355. [CrossRef] [PubMed]
31. Gerra, G.; Benedetti, E.; Resce, G.; Potente, R.; Cutilli, A.; Molinaro, S. Socioeconomic Status, Parental Education, School Connectedness and Individual Socio-Cultural Resources in Vulnerability for Drug Use among Students. *Int. J. Environ. Res. Public Health* **2020**, *17*, 1306. [CrossRef] [PubMed]
32. Evans, G.W.; Swain, J.E.; King, A.P.; Wang, X.; Javanbakht, A.; Ho, S.S.; Angstadt, M.; Phan, K.L.; Xie, H.; Liberzon, I. Childhood Cumulative Risk Exposure and Adult Amygdala Volume and Function. *J. Neurosci. Res.* **2016**, *94*, 535–543. [CrossRef]

33. Javanbakht, A.; Kim, P.; Swain, J.E.; Evans, G.W.; Phan, K.L.; Liberzon, I. Sex-Specific Effects of Childhood Poverty on Neurocircuitry of Processing of Emotional Cues: A Neuroimaging Study. *Behav. Sci.* **2016**, *6*, 28. [CrossRef]
34. Wang, Y.; Zhang, L.; Kong, X.; Hong, Y.; Cheon, B.; Liu, J. Pathway to neural resilience: Self-esteem buffers against deleterious effects of poverty on the hippocampus. *Hum. Brain Mapp.* **2016**, *37*, 3757–3766. [CrossRef] [PubMed]
35. Baxendale, S.; Heaney, D. Socioeconomic status, cognition, and hippocampal sclerosis. *Epilepsy Behav.* **2011**, *20*, 64–67. [CrossRef] [PubMed]
36. Jenkins, L.M.; Chiang, J.J.; Vause, K.; Hoffer, L.; Alpert, K.; Parrish, T.B.; Wang, L.; Miller, G.E. Subcortical structural variations associated with low socioeconomic status in adolescents. *Hum. Brain Mapp.* **2020**, *41*, 162–171. [CrossRef]
37. Cox, S.M.; Andrade, A.; Johnsrude, I.S. Learning to like: A role for human orbitofrontal cortex in conditioned reward. *J. Neurosci.* **2005**, *25*, 2733–2740. [CrossRef]
38. Frey, S.; Petrides, M. Orbitofrontal cortex and memory formation. *Neuron* **2002**, *36*, 171–176. [CrossRef]
39. Oscar-Berman, M. The effects of dorsolateral-frontal and ventrolateral-orbitofrontal lesions on spatial discrimination learning and delayed response in two modalities. *Neuropsychologia* **1975**, *13*, 237–246. [CrossRef]
40. Premkumar, P.; Fannon, D.; Sapara, A.; Peters, E.R.; Anilkumar, A.P.; Simmons, A.; Kuipers, E.; Kumari, V. Orbitofrontal cortex, emotional decision-making and response to cognitive behavioural therapy for psychosis. *Psychiatry Res.* **2015**, *231*, 298–307. [CrossRef]
41. Goodwill, H.L.; Manzano-Nieves, G.; LaChance, P.; Teramoto, S.; Lin, S.; Lopez, C.; Stevenson, R.J.; Theyel, B.B.; Moore, C.I.; Connors, B.W.; et al. Early Life Stress Drives Sex-Selective Impairment in Reversal Learning by Affecting Parvalbumin Interneurons in Orbitofrontal Cortex of Mice. *Cell Rep.* **2018**, *25*, 2299–2307.e2294. [CrossRef]
42. Viskontas, I.V.; Possin, K.L.; Miller, B.L. Symptoms of frontotemporal dementia provide insights into orbitofrontal cortex function and social behavior. *Ann. N. Y. Acad. Sci.* **2007**, *1121*, 528–545. [CrossRef]
43. Hornberger, M.; Savage, S.; Hsieh, S.; Mioshi, E.; Piguet, O.; Hodges, J.R. Orbitofrontal dysfunction discriminates behavioral variant frontotemporal dementia from Alzheimer's disease. *Dement. Geriatr. Cogn. Disord.* **2010**, *30*, 547–552. [CrossRef]
44. Van Hoesen, G.W.; Parvizi, J.; Chu, C.C. Orbitofrontal cortex pathology in Alzheimer's disease. *Cereb. Cortex* **2000**, *10*, 243–251. [CrossRef]
45. Bellani, M.; Cerruti, S.; Brambilla, P. Orbitofrontal cortex abnormalities in schizophrenia. *Epidemiol. Psichiatr. Soc.* **2010**, *19*, 23–25. [CrossRef]
46. Chakirova, G.; Welch, K.A.; Moorhead, T.W.; Stanfield, A.C.; Hall, J.; Skehel, P.; Brown, V.J.; Johnstone, E.C.; Owens, D.G.; Lawrie, S.M.; et al. Orbitofrontal morphology in people at high risk of developing schizophrenia. *Eur. Psychiatry* **2010**, *25*, 366–372. [CrossRef] [PubMed]
47. Jin, C.; Qi, R.; Yin, Y.; Hu, X.; Duan, L.; Xu, Q.; Zhang, Z.; Zhong, Y.; Feng, B.; Xiang, H.; et al. Abnormalities in whole-brain functional connectivity observed in treatment-naive post-traumatic stress disorder patients following an earthquake. *Psychol. Med.* **2014**, *44*, 1927–1936. [CrossRef] [PubMed]
48. Morey, R.A.; Haswell, C.C.; Hooper, S.R.; De Bellis, M.D. Amygdala, Hippocampus, and Ventral Medial Prefrontal Cortex Volumes Differ in Maltreated Youth with and without Chronic Posttraumatic Stress Disorder. *Neuropsychopharmacology* **2016**, *41*, 791–801. [CrossRef] [PubMed]
49. Cheng, W.; Rolls, E.T.; Qiu, J.; Xie, X.; Wei, D.; Huang, C.C.; Yang, A.C.; Tsai, S.J.; Li, Q.; Meng, J.; et al. Increased functional connectivity of the posterior cingulate cortex with the lateral orbitofrontal cortex in depression. *Transl. Psychiatry* **2018**, *8*, 90. [CrossRef] [PubMed]
50. Frodl, T.; Bokde, A.L.; Scheuerecker, J.; Lisiecka, D.; Schoepf, V.; Hampel, H.; Moller, H.J.; Bruckmann, H.; Wiesmann, M.; Meisenzahl, E. Functional connectivity bias of the orbitofrontal cortex in drug-free patients with major depression. *Biol. Psychiatry* **2010**, *67*, 161–167. [CrossRef] [PubMed]
51. Taylor, W.D.; Macfall, J.R.; Payne, M.E.; McQuoid, D.R.; Steffens, D.C.; Provenzale, J.M.; Krishnan, K.R. Orbitofrontal cortex volume in late life depression: Influence of hyperintense lesions and genetic polymorphisms. *Psychol. Med.* **2007**, *37*, 1763–1773. [CrossRef] [PubMed]
52. London, E.D.; Ernst, M.; Grant, S.; Bonson, K.; Weinstein, A. Orbitofrontal cortex and human drug abuse: Functional imaging. *Cereb. Cortex* **2000**, *10*, 334–342. [CrossRef]
53. Lopez-Larson, M.P.; Rogowska, J.; Yurgelun-Todd, D. Aberrant orbitofrontal connectivity in marijuana smoking adolescents. *Dev. Cogn. Neurosci.* **2015**, *16*, 54–62. [CrossRef]
54. Moorman, D.E. The role of the orbitofrontal cortex in alcohol use, abuse, and dependence. *Prog. Neuropsychopharmacol. Biol. Psychiatry* **2018**, *87*, 85–107. [CrossRef]
55. Noble, K.G.; Houston, S.M.; Brito, N.H.; Bartsch, H.; Kan, E.; Kuperman, J.M.; Akshoomoff, N.; Amaral, D.G.; Bloss, C.S.; Libiger, O. Family income, parental education and brain structure in children and adolescents. *Nat. Neurosci.* **2015**, *18*, 773. [CrossRef] [PubMed]
56. Holz, N.E.; Boecker, R.; Hohm, E.; Zohsel, K.; Buchmann, A.F.; Blomeyer, D.; Jennen-Steinmetz, C.; Baumeister, S.; Hohmann, S.; Wolf, I.; et al. The long-term impact of early life poverty on orbitofrontal cortex volume in adulthood: Results from a prospective study over 25 years. *Neuropsychopharmacology* **2015**, *40*, 996–1004. [CrossRef] [PubMed]

57. Spera, C.; Wentzel, K.R.; Matto, H.C. Parental aspirations for their children's educational attainment: Relations to ethnicity, parental education, children's academic performance, and parental perceptions of school climate. *J. Youth Adolesc.* 2009, *38*, 1140–1152. [CrossRef]
58. Goodman, E.; Slap, G.B.; Huang, B. The public health impact of socioeconomic status on adolescent depression and obesity. *Am. J. Public Health* 2003, *93*, 1844–1850. [CrossRef] [PubMed]
59. Morris, A.S.; Silk, J.S.; Steinberg, L.; Myers, S.S.; Robinson, L.R. The role of the family context in the development of emotion regulation. *Soc. Dev.* 2007, *16*, 361–388. [CrossRef]
60. Park, S.; Holloway, S.D. No parent left behind: Predicting parental involvement in adolescents' education within a sociodemographically diverse population. *J. Educ. Res.* 2013, *106*, 105–119. [CrossRef]
61. Pabayo, R.; Molnar, B.E.; Kawachi, I. The role of neighborhood income inequality in adolescent aggression and violence. *J. Adolesc. Health* 2014, *55*, 571–579. [CrossRef]
62. Wills, T.A.; McNamara, G.; Vaccaro, D. Parental education related to adolescent stress-coping and substance use: Development of a mediational model. *Health Psychol.* 1995, *14*, 464. [CrossRef]
63. Yaple, Z.A.; Yu, R. Functional and Structural Brain Correlates of Socioeconomic Status. *Cereb. Cortex* 2019. [CrossRef] [PubMed]
64. Aubuchon-Endsley, N.L.; Kennedy, T.S.; Gilchrist, M.; Thomas, D.G.; Grant, S. Relationships among Socioeconomic Status, Dietary Intake, and Stress in Breastfeeding Women. *J. Acad. Nutr. Diet.* 2015, *115*, 939–946 e931. [CrossRef] [PubMed]
65. Braren, S.H.; Perry, R.E.; Ursache, A.; Blair, C. Socioeconomic risk moderates the association between caregiver cortisol levels and infant cortisol reactivity to emotion induction at 24 months. *Dev. Psychobiol* 2019, *61*, 573–591. [CrossRef]
66. Emmen, R.A.; Malda, M.; Mesman, J.; van Ijzendoorn, M.H.; Prevoo, M.J.; Yeniad, N. Socioeconomic status and parenting in ethnic minority families: Testing a minority family stress model. *J. Fam. Psychol.* 2013, *27*, 896–904. [CrossRef] [PubMed]
67. Jackson, A.P.; Brooks-Gunn, J.; Huang, C.C.; Glassman, M. Single mothers in low-wage jobs: Financial strain, parenting, and preschoolers' outcomes. *Child Dev.* 2000, *71*, 1409–1423. [CrossRef] [PubMed]
68. Liu, Y.; Lachman, M.E. Socioeconomic Status and Parenting Style from Childhood: Long-Term Effects on Cognitive Function in Middle and Later Adulthood. *J. Gerontol. B Psychol. Sci. Soc. Sci.* 2019, *74*, e13–e24. [CrossRef]
69. Dutra, L.; Bureau, J.F.; Holmes, B.; Lyubchik, A.; Lyons-Ruth, K. Quality of early care and childhood trauma: A prospective study of developmental pathways to dissociation. *J. Nerv. Ment. Dis.* 2009, *197*, 383–390. [CrossRef] [PubMed]
70. Ladebauche, P. Childhood trauma—When to suspect abuse. *RN* 1997, *60*, 38–42; quiz 43. [PubMed]
71. Assari, S.; Bazargan, M. Unequal Associations between Educational Attainment and Occupational Stress across Racial and Ethnic Groups. *Int. J. Environ. Res. Public Health* 2019, *16*, 3539. [CrossRef] [PubMed]
72. Chassin, L.; Presson, C.C.; Sherman, S.J.; Edwards, D.A. Parent educational attainment and adolescent cigarette smoking. *J. Subst. Abus.* 1992, *4*, 219–234. [CrossRef]
73. Kocaoglu, B.; Moschonis, G.; Dimitriou, M.; Kolotourou, M.; Keskin, Y.; Sur, H.; Hayran, O.; Manios, Y. Parental educational level and cardiovascular disease risk factors in schoolchildren in large urban areas of Turkey: Directions for public health policy. *BMC Public Health* 2005, *5*, 13. [CrossRef]
74. Padilla-Moledo, C.; Ruiz, J.R.; Castro-Pinero, J. Parental educational level and psychological positive health and health complaints in Spanish children and adolescents. *Child Care Health Dev.* 2016, *42*, 534–543. [CrossRef] [PubMed]
75. Kauhanen, L.; Leino, J.; Lakka, H.M.; Lynch, J.W.; Kauhanen, J. Adverse childhood experiences and risk of binge drinking and drunkenness in middle-aged finnish men. *Adv. Prev. Med.* 2011, *2011*, 478741. [CrossRef]
76. Choi, J.K.; Wang, D.; Jackson, A.P. Adverse experiences in early childhood and their longitudinal impact on later behavioral problems of children living in poverty. *Child Abus. Negl.* 2019, *98*, 104181. [CrossRef]
77. Cuevas, A.G.; Chen, R.; Slopen, N.; Thurber, K.A.; Wilson, N.; Economos, C.; Williams, D.R. Assessing the Role of Health Behaviors, Socioeconomic Status, and Cumulative Stress for Racial/Ethnic Disparities in Obesity. *Obesity* 2020, *28*, 161–170. [CrossRef]
78. Frankenberger, D.J.; Clements-Nolle, K.; Yang, W. The Association between Adverse Childhood Experiences and Alcohol Use during Pregnancy in a Representative Sample of Adult Women. *Womens Health Issues* 2015, *25*, 688–695. [CrossRef] [PubMed]
79. Peyrot, W.J.; Lee, S.H.; Milaneschi, Y.; Abdellaoui, A.; Byrne, E.M.; Esko, T.; de Geus, E.J.; Hemani, G.; Hottenga, J.J.; Kloiber, S.; et al. The association between lower educational attainment and depression owing to shared genetic effects? Results in ~25,000 subjects. *Mol. Psychiatry* 2015, *20*, 735–743. [CrossRef]
80. DeCuir, J.; Lovasi, G.S.; El-Sayed, A.; Lewis, C.F. The association between neighborhood socioeconomic disadvantage and high-risk injection behavior among people who inject drugs. *Drug Alcohol Depend.* 2018, *183*, 184–191. [CrossRef] [PubMed]
81. Kuchibhatla, M.; Hunter, J.C.; Plassman, B.L.; Lutz, M.W.; Casanova, R.; Saldana, S.; Hayden, K.M. The association between neighborhood socioeconomic status, cardiovascular and cerebrovascular risk factors, and cognitive decline in the Health and Retirement Study (HRS). *Aging Ment. Health* 2019, *24*, 1479–1486. [CrossRef]
82. Assari, S. Parental Educational Attainment and Academic Performance of American College Students; Blacks' Diminished Returns. *J. Health Econ. Dev.* 2019, *1*, 21–31.
83. Assari, S.; Caldwell, C.H. Parental Educational Attainment Differentially Boosts School Performance of American Adolescents: Minorities' Diminished Returns. *J. Fam. Reprod. Health* 2019, *13*, 7–13. [CrossRef]
84. Kiang, L.; Andrews, K.; Stein, G.L.; Supple, A.J.; Gonzalez, L.M. Socioeconomic stress and academic adjustment among Asian American adolescents: The protective role of family obligation. *J. Youth Adolesc.* 2013, *42*, 837–847. [CrossRef] [PubMed]

85. Williams, D.R. Race, socioeconomic status, and health the added effects of racism and discrimination. *Ann. N. Y. Acad. Sci.* **1999**, *896*, 173–188. [CrossRef]
86. Kaufman, J.S.; Cooper, R.S.; McGee, D.L. Socioeconomic status and health in blacks and whites: The problem of residual confounding and the resiliency of race. *Epidemiology* **1997**, *8*, 621–628. [CrossRef]
87. Assari, S. Parental Educational Attainment and Mental Well-Being of College Students; Diminished Returns of Blacks. *Brain Sci.* **2018**, *8*, 193. [CrossRef]
88. Assari, S. Unequal Gain of Equal Resources across Racial Groups. *Int. J. Health Policy Manag.* **2017**, *7*, 1–9. [CrossRef] [PubMed]
89. Assari, S.; Thomas, A.; Caldwell, C.H.; Mincy, R.B. Blacks' Diminished Health Return of Family Structure and Socioeconomic Status; 15 Years of Follow-up of a National Urban Sample of Youth. *J. Urban Health* **2018**, *95*, 21–35. [CrossRef]
90. Assari, S.; Caldwell, C.H. Family Income at Birth and Risk of Attention Deficit Hyperactivity Disorder at Age 15: Racial Differences. *Children* **2019**, *6*, 10. [CrossRef]
91. Assari, S.; Lankarani, M.M.; Caldwell, C.H. Does Discrimination Explain High Risk of Depression among High-Income African American Men? *Behav. Sci.* **2018**, *8*, 40. [CrossRef]
92. Fuller-Rowell, T.E.; Doan, S.N. The social costs of academic success across ethnic groups. *Child. Dev.* **2010**, *81*, 1696–1713. [CrossRef] [PubMed]
93. Fuller-Rowell, T.E.; Curtis, D.S.; Doan, S.N.; Coe, C.L. Racial disparities in the health benefits of educational attainment: A study of inflammatory trajectories among African American and white adults. *Psychosom. Med.* **2015**, *77*, 33–40. [CrossRef] [PubMed]
94. Hudson, D.L.; Bullard, K.M.; Neighbors, H.W.; Geronimus, A.T.; Yang, J.; Jackson, J.S. Are benefits conferred with greater socioeconomic position undermined by racial discrimination among African American men? *J. Men's Health* **2012**, *9*, 127–136. [CrossRef] [PubMed]
95. Hudson, D.L.; Neighbors, H.W.; Geronimus, A.T.; Jackson, J.S. The relationship between socioeconomic position and depression among a US nationally representative sample of African Americans. *Soc. Psychiatry Psychiatr. Epidemiol.* **2012**, *47*, 373–381. [CrossRef]
96. Assari, S.; Caldwell, C.H.; Bazargan, M. Association Between Parental Educational Attainment and Youth Outcomes and Role of Race/Ethnicity. *JAMA Netw. Open* **2019**, *2*, e1916018. [CrossRef] [PubMed]
97. Assari, S.; Mistry, R. Educational Attainment and Smoking Status in a National Sample of American Adults; Evidence for the Blacks' Diminished Return. *Int. J. Environ. Res. Public Health* **2018**, *15*, 763. [CrossRef]
98. Assari, S.; Caldwell, C.H.; Zimmerman, M.A. Family Structure and Subsequent Anxiety Symptoms; Minorities' Diminished Return. *Brain Sci.* **2018**, *8*, 97. [CrossRef]
99. Assari, S.; Caldwell, C.H. High Risk of Depression in High-Income African American Boys. *J. Racial Ethn. Health Disparities* **2018**, *5*, 808–819. [CrossRef]
100. Asaad, S.K.; Bjarkam, C.R. The Aalborg Bolt-Connected Drain (ABCD) study: A prospective comparison of tunnelled and bolt-connected external ventricular drains. *Acta Neurochir.* **2019**, *161*, 33–39. [CrossRef] [PubMed]
101. Bjork, J.M.; Straub, L.K.; Provost, R.G.; Neale, M.C. The ABCD study of neurodevelopment: Identifying neurocircuit targets for prevention and treatment of adolescent substance abuse. *Curr. Treat. Options Psychiatry* **2017**, *4*, 196–209. [CrossRef]
102. Casey, B.J.; Cannonier, T.; Conley, M.I.; Cohen, A.O.; Barch, D.M.; Heitzeg, M.M.; Soules, M.E.; Teslovich, T.; Dellarco, D.V.; Garavan, H.; et al. The Adolescent Brain Cognitive Development (ABCD) study: Imaging acquisition across 21 sites. *Dev. Cogn. Neurosci.* **2018**, *32*, 43–54. [CrossRef]
103. Lisdahl, K.M.; Sher, K.J.; Conway, K.P.; Gonzalez, R.; Feldstein Ewing, S.W.; Nixon, S.J.; Tapert, S.; Bartsch, H.; Goldstein, R.Z.; Heitzeg, M. Adolescent brain cognitive development (ABCD) study: Overview of substance use assessment methods. *Dev. Cogn. Neurosci.* **2018**, *32*, 80–96. [CrossRef] [PubMed]
104. Feldstein Ewing, S.W.; Chang, L.; Cottler, L.B.; Tapert, S.F.; Dowling, G.J.; Brown, S.A. Approaching Retention within the ABCD Study. *Dev. Cogn. Neurosci.* **2018**, *32*, 130–137. [CrossRef] [PubMed]
105. Michelini, G.; Barch, D.M.; Tian, Y.; Watson, D.; Klein, D.N.; Kotov, R. Delineating and validating higher-order dimensions of psychopathology in the Adolescent Brain Cognitive Development (ABCD) study. *Transl. Psychiatry* **2019**, *9*, 261. [CrossRef] [PubMed]
106. Beauchaine, T.P. Editorial: Family History of Depression and Child Striatal Volumes in the ABCD Study: Promise and Perils of Neuroimaging Research with Large Samples. *J. Am. Acad. Child. Adolesc. Psychiatry* **2020**. [CrossRef]
107. Marek, S.; Tervo-Clemmens, B.; Nielsen, A.N.; Wheelock, M.D.; Miller, R.L.; Laumann, T.O.; Earl, E.; Foran, W.W.; Cordova, M.; Doyle, O.; et al. Identifying reproducible individual differences in childhood functional brain networks: An ABCD study. *Dev. Cogn. Neurosci.* **2019**, *40*, 100706. [CrossRef]
108. Feldstein Ewing, S.W.; Bjork, J.M.; Luciana, M. Implications of the ABCD study for developmental neuroscience. *Dev. Cogn. Neurosci.* **2018**, *32*, 161–164. [CrossRef]
109. Alcohol Research: Current Reviews Editorial, S. NIH's Adolescent Brain Cognitive Development (ABCD) Study. *Alcohol Res.* **2018**, *39*, 97.
110. Hoffman, E.A.; Howlett, K.D.; Breslin, F.; Dowling, G.J. Outreach and innovation: Communication strategies for the ABCD Study. *Dev. Cogn. Neurosci.* **2018**, *32*, 138–142. [CrossRef]
111. Rozzell, K.; Moon, D.Y.; Klimek, P.; Brown, T.; Blashill, A.J. Prevalence of Eating Disorders among US Children Aged 9 to 10 Years: Data from the Adolescent Brain Cognitive Development (ABCD) Study. *JAMA Pediatr.* **2019**, *173*, 100–101. [CrossRef]

112. Garavan, H.; Bartsch, H.; Conway, K.; Decastro, A.; Goldstein, R.Z.; Heeringa, S.; Jernigan, T.; Potter, A.; Thompson, W.; Zahs, D. Recruiting the ABCD sample: Design considerations and procedures. *Dev. Cogn. Neurosci.* **2018**, *32*, 16–22. [CrossRef] [PubMed]
113. Hoffman, E.A.; Clark, D.B.; Orendain, N.; Hudziak, J.; Squeglia, L.M.; Dowling, G.J. Stress exposures, neurodevelopment and health measures in the ABCD study. *Neurobiol. Stress* **2019**, *10*, 100157. [CrossRef] [PubMed]
114. Karcher, N.R.; O'Brien, K.J.; Kandala, S.; Barch, D.M. Resting-State Functional Connectivity and Psychotic-like Experiences in Childhood: Results from the Adolescent Brain Cognitive Development Study. *Biol. Psychiatry* **2019**, *86*, 7–15. [CrossRef]
115. Luciana, M.; Bjork, J.M.; Nagel, B.J.; Barch, D.M.; Gonzalez, R.; Nixon, S.J.; Banich, M.T. Adolescent neurocognitive development and impacts of substance use: Overview of the adolescent brain cognitive development (ABCD) baseline neurocognition battery. *Dev. Cogn. Neurosci.* **2018**, *32*, 67–79. [CrossRef]
116. Auchter, A.M.; Hernandez Mejia, M.; Heyser, C.J.; Shilling, P.D.; Jernigan, T.L.; Brown, S.A.; Tapert, S.F.; Dowling, G.J. A description of the ABCD organizational structure and communication framework. *Dev. Cogn. Neurosci.* **2018**, *32*, 8–15. [CrossRef] [PubMed]
117. Gutierrez-Rojas, C.; Pascual, R.; Bustamante, C. Prenatal stress alters the behavior and dendritic morphology of the medial orbitofrontal cortex in mouse offspring during lactation. *Int. J. Dev. Neurosci.* **2013**, *31*, 505–511. [CrossRef]
118. Mychasiuk, R.; Muhammad, A.; Kolb, B. Chronic stress induces persistent changes in global DNA methylation and gene expression in the medial prefrontal cortex, orbitofrontal cortex, and hippocampus. *Neuroscience* **2016**, *322*, 489–499. [CrossRef]
119. Poletti, S.; Vai, B.; Smeraldi, E.; Cavallaro, R.; Colombo, C.; Benedetti, F. Adverse childhood experiences influence the detrimental effect of bipolar disorder and schizophrenia on cortico-limbic grey matter volumes. *J. Affect. Disord.* **2016**, *189*, 290–297. [CrossRef] [PubMed]
120. Seidel, K.; Poeggel, G.; Holetschka, R.; Helmeke, C.; Braun, K. Paternal deprivation affects the development of corticotrophin-releasing factor-expressing neurones in prefrontal cortex, amygdala and hippocampus of the biparental Octodon degus. *J. Neuroendocrinol.* **2011**, *23*, 1166–1176. [CrossRef]
121. Assari, S.; Smith, J.; Mistry, R.; Farokhnia, M.; Bazargan, M. Substance Use among Economically Disadvantaged African American Older Adults; Objective and Subjective Socioeconomic Status. *Int. J. Environ. Res. Public Health* **2019**, *16*, 1826. [CrossRef] [PubMed]
122. Chen, E.; Paterson, L.Q. Neighborhood, family, and subjective socioeconomic status: How do they relate to adolescent health? *Health Psychol.* **2006**, *25*, 704–714. [CrossRef]
123. Moon, C. Subjective economic status, sex role attitudes, fertility, and mother's work. *Ingu Pogon Nonjip* **1987**, *7*, 177–196. [PubMed]
124. Assari, S.; Preiser, B.; Lankarani, M.M.; Caldwell, C.H. Subjective Socioeconomic Status Moderates the Association between Discrimination and Depression in African American Youth. *Brain Sci.* **2018**, *8*, 71. [CrossRef] [PubMed]
125. Boe, T.; Petrie, K.J.; Sivertsen, B.; Hysing, M. Interplay of subjective and objective economic well-being on the mental health of Norwegian adolescents. *SSM Popul. Health* **2019**, *9*, 100471. [CrossRef]
126. Wright, C.E.; Steptoe, A. Subjective socioeconomic position, gender and cortisol responses to waking in an elderly population. *Psychoneuroendocrinology* **2005**, *30*, 582–590. [CrossRef]
127. Ye, Z.; Wen, M.; Wang, W.; Lin, D. Subjective family socio-economic status, school social capital, and positive youth development among young adolescents in China: A multiple mediation model. *Int. J. Psychol.* **2020**, *55*, 173–181. [CrossRef]
128. Ursache, A.; Noble, K.G.; Blair, C. Socioeconomic Status, Subjective Social Status, and Perceived Stress: Associations with Stress Physiology and Executive Functioning. *Behav. Med.* **2015**, *41*, 145–154. [CrossRef]
129. Senn, T.E.; Walsh, J.L.; Carey, M.P. The mediating roles of perceived stress and health behaviors in the relation between objective, subjective, and neighborhood socioeconomic status and perceived health. *Ann. Behav. Med.* **2014**, *48*, 215–224. [CrossRef]
130. Manuck, S.B.; Phillips, J.E.; Gianaros, P.J.; Flory, J.D.; Muldoon, M.F. Subjective socioeconomic status and presence of the metabolic syndrome in midlife community volunteers. *Psychosom. Med.* **2010**, *72*, 35–45. [CrossRef]
131. Barch, D.; Pagliaccio, D.; Belden, A.; Harms, M.P.; Gaffrey, M.; Sylvester, C.M.; Tillman, R.; Luby, J. Effect of Hippocampal and Amygdala Connectivity on the Relationship Between Preschool Poverty and School-Age Depression. *Am. J. Psychiatry* **2016**, *173*, 625–634. [CrossRef]
132. Finn, A.S.; Minas, J.E.; Leonard, J.A.; Mackey, A.P.; Salvatore, J.; Goetz, C.; West, M.R.; Gabrieli, C.F.O.; Gabrieli, J.D.E. Functional brain organization of working memory in adolescents varies in relation to family income and academic achievement. *Dev. Sci.* **2017**, *20*. [CrossRef]
133. Brody, G.H.; Yu, T.; Nusslock, R.; Barton, A.W.; Miller, G.E.; Chen, E.; Holmes, C.; McCormick, M.; Sweet, L.H. The Protective Effects of Supportive Parenting on the Relationship between Adolescent Poverty and Resting-State Functional Brain Connectivity during Adulthood. *Psychol. Sci.* **2019**. [CrossRef]
134. Clark, U.S.; Miller, E.R.; Hegde, R.R. Experiences of Discrimination Are Associated With Greater Resting Amygdala Activity and Functional Connectivity. *Biol. Psychiatry Cogn. Neurosci. Neuroimaging* **2018**, *3*, 367–378. [CrossRef] [PubMed]
135. Assari, S. Family Socioeconomic Position at Birth and School Bonding at Age 15; Blacks' Diminished Returns. *Behav. Sci.* **2019**, *9*, 26. [CrossRef] [PubMed]
136. Assari, S.; Caldwell, C.H.; Mincy, R.B. Maternal Educational Attainment at Birth Promotes Future Self-Rated Health of White but Not Black Youth: A 15-Year Cohort of a National Sample. *J. Clin. Med.* **2018**, *7*, 93. [CrossRef] [PubMed]
137. Assari, S.; Caldwell, C.H.; Mincy, R. Family Socioeconomic Status at Birth and Youth Impulsivity at Age 15; Blacks' Diminished Return. *Children* **2018**, *5*, 58. [CrossRef] [PubMed]

Review

Evolution of the Autism Literature and the Influence of Parents: A Scientific Mapping in Web of Science

Noemí Carmona-Serrano [1], Antonio-José Moreno-Guerrero [2,*], José-Antonio Marín-Marín [3] and Jesús López-Belmonte [2]

1. Ceuta Autism Association, University of Granada, 51001 Ceuta, Spain; nhoe@correo.ugr.es
2. Department of Didactics and School Organization, University of Granada, 51001 Ceuta, Spain; jesuslopez@ugr.es
3. Department of Didactics and School Organization, University of Granada, 18071 Granada, Spain; jmarin@ugr.es
* Correspondence: ajmoreno@ugr.es

Abstract: Parents interventions are relevant to address autism spectrum disorder (ASD). The objective of this study is to analyze the importance and evolution of ASD and its relationship with the parents (ASD-PAR) in the publications indexed in Web of Science. For this, a bibliometric methodology has been used, based on a scientific mapping of the reported documents. We have worked with an analysis unit of 1381 documents. The results show that the beginnings of scientific production date back to 1971. There are two clearly differentiated moments in scientific production. A first moment (1971–2004), where the production volume is low. A second moment (2005–2019), where the volume of production increases considerably. Therefore, it can be said that the subject began to be relevant for the scientific community from 2005 to the present. The keyword match rate between set periods marks a high level of match between periods. It is concluded that the main focus of the research on ASD-PAR is on the stress that is generated in families with children with ASD, in addition to the family problems that the fact that these children also have behavior problems can cause.

Keywords: autism; parent-based intervention; bibliometric analysis; scientific mapping; scimat; web of science

1. Introduction

Autism spectrum disorder (ASD) is conceived as a series of neurodevelopmental disorders with a multifactorial nature that affects 1.5% of the world population [1]. This disorder has alterations in the social plane [2], in the communicative aspects and in turn presents repetitive and stereotyped behaviors [3]. However, ASD is not limited only to that, but also these people have other deficiencies such as limitations in executive functioning, sensory perception and attention. They may also present depression, aggressiveness, challenging actions, emotional problems [4–7]. In this symptomatological line, there are also people with high levels of anxiety, which is aggravated if the person has a low cognitive level [8,9].

All of the above can be combined with another problem, such as an intellectual disability and an altered sensory system [10]. In this regard, the sense of touch stands out as a relevant element in human relationships, the condition of which causes disorders in the social aspect [11,12]. At a sensory level, people with ASD also present alterations in the reception of the sound around them [13], as well as in processing the visual stimuli of the environment [14]. However, the limitations of these people are not only here, on the sensory level. Moreover, both at the motor level [15], the use of language [16], the use of writing [17], and at the planning and structuring level of the tasks and actions of daily life [18], present limitations and alterations. However, not all of its capabilities are affected.

People with ASD have greater precision in color processing [19] and greater processing of music than other typically developing people [20].

Expert literature reveals that the gender of these people can be an influencing factor in their conditions. In this sense, men reflect more restricted and repetitive behaviors and actions than women. This may be due to a disorder in brain structures, more specifically those related to social integration and cortico-striatum [21]. Despite these advances, there is currently no drug that contributes to improving all the disorders presented. Therefore, the intervention is postulated from a therapeutic perspective [22].

These interventions, if carried out early, can cause an important and significant improvement in the deficiencies of these people [23]. In addition, early intervention can enhance other types of unaffected skills [24,25]. This will contribute to a greater adaptation to the environment and to carrying out activities of daily life [26]. The nature of these interventions must be based on observation [27]. In all this, the family plays a fundamental role, as the agent or group of people closest to the person with ASD. Interventions carried out by the family can have a positive effect on these types of people [28]. Therefore, families value the fact of being involved in the therapeutic intervention process of their children [29]. This is currently being a focus under study [30]. However, family members' knowledge of effective intervention guidelines is limited compared to other experts in this field of knowledge [31]. This lack of training can trigger behavioral patterns of social isolation [32]. Likewise, families can not only focus their daily activity on caring for the member with ASD, but they also have to provide financial support, so the workload is considerable [33]. Along these lines, families that have children with ASD experience higher rates of negativity than any other family [34].

Family training is positioned as a primary factor to achieve direct intervention to improve various indicators related to stress, depression, behavior problems, as well as improve the mental health of all members of the family unit [25]. These interventions must pursue quality rather than quantity [35]. State-of-the-art research postulates that adequate family cohesion can be beneficial to improving the quality of life of family members of people with ASD [36]. Likewise, the literature also reveals how companion animals can cause good results in reducing stress, both in people with ASD and in other members of the family unit [37].

Justification and Objectives

This research analyzes the concept of "autism" in the parental environment (ASD-PAR) from a bibliometric perspective of the literature [38].

The Web of Science (WoS) has been taken as the database under study, as it is one of the largest databases in the world on social sciences. The novelty that this work assumes is the realization of an analysis of the documents published under an innovative technique of documentary study. In particular, in this research, a performance analysis and scientific mapping of the reported documents linked to the aforementioned terms has been carried out. In order to carry out bias-free research, the analytical structure of previous impact publications has been used to follow a study model validated by experts [39,40].

Specifically, this study is based on analyzing the significance and evolution of ASD-PAR in the publications indexed in WoS. It was started from an initial search in said database and no study was reported to the one presented in this work. Therefore, this research is raised under an exploratory nature in order to reveal to the scientific community and readers interested in the subject all the progress, evolution and upcoming trends [41]. This work will contribute to the reduction in the literary gap concerning the analyzed terms and will establish new knowledge bases on the state of the question, as well as start the path towards future works.

The objectives pursued by this study are: (a) to know the performance of the scientific production on ASD-PAR in WoS; (b) to determine the scientific evolution on ASD-PAR in WoS; (c) to discover the most relevant topics about ASD-PAR in WoS; (d) to locate the most representative authors on ASD-PAR in WoS.

2. Materials and Methods

2.1. Research Design

For the development of the study and the subsequent achievement of the objectives, a bibliometric research design was used. This methodology bases its potential in quantifying and comprehensively evaluating scientific documentation [42,43]. The design presented in this work will allow the efficient search, registration, analysis and prediction of the existing literature on the subject [44].

Specifically, the design has been based on a co-word analysis [45], as well as the study of various indices (h, g, hg and q2) [46]. The h index is an indicator that is used to measure the quality of the scientists' production according to the number of citations received in their publications. The g index allows us to delve into the productive analytics of researchers who have a similar value in the h index. The hg index is a combination of the previous indices. It allows us to obtain a result that takes into account the potentialities of the indices "h" and "g" and reduces their drawbacks. Finally, the q2 index is prepared from a quantitative measure (h index) and another based on the qualitative properties of the h nucleus [47,48].

The investigative actions carried out will allow the generation of maps with nodes to represent the performance, the location of the subdomains of the concepts and the development of the linked topics [49] on ASD-PAR in the WoS database.

2.2. Procedure

The research has been carried out in various phases following the considerations and protocols of the specialists to carry out a pertinent and methodical study [50–53]. The first action was to select the database (WoS). Then, the search concepts were specified (autism, parents, father and mother). Next, the search equation was created: "autism" (TITLE) AND "mother *" OR "father *" OR "parents" (TITLE). Next, the search process was carried out in the main WoS collection, in the indices SCI-EXPANDED, SSCI, A & HCI, CPCI-S, CPCI-SSH, BKCI-S, BKCI-SSH, ESCI, CCR-EXPANDED and IC. The starting date of the search is 1900, which is the time when the database starts to collect manuscripts.

Once the actions of each phase had been carried out, a total of 1572 publications were reported. This initial number of documents was refined through the establishment of various criteria [54,55]. The exclusion criteria were: 1—Documents published in 2020. This is because the year has not yet ended and new documents dated 2020 may be included in the coming months ($n = 130$); 2—Repeated or poorly indexed documents in WoS ($n = 61$). After applying these criteria, the final unit of analysis was established in 1381 publications. Figure 1 synthesizes in a flow diagram the actions deployed following the PRISMA protocol.

In order to present the results of scientific performance and production, a series of inclusion criteria have been established, which were delimited in: 1—Year of publication (all production except 2020). The search began in 1900. The first manuscript on this subject appeared in 1971; 2—Language ($x \geq 20$); 3—Publication area ($x \geq 100$); 4—Type of documents ($x \geq 100$); 5—Organizations ($x \geq 29$); 6—Authors ($x \geq 15$); 7—Sources of origin ($x \geq 40$); 8—Countries ($x \geq 100$); 9—The four most cited documents ($x \geq 350$).

2.3. Data Analysis

The tools used to perform the data analysis were Analyze Results, Creation Citation Report (programs to collect the year, authorship, country, type of document, institution, language, medium and most cited documents) and SciMAT (program to carry out the structural and dynamic development of the documents reported from a longitudinal perspective). For a correct performance of the tools, the considerations of other previous works were followed [56,57].

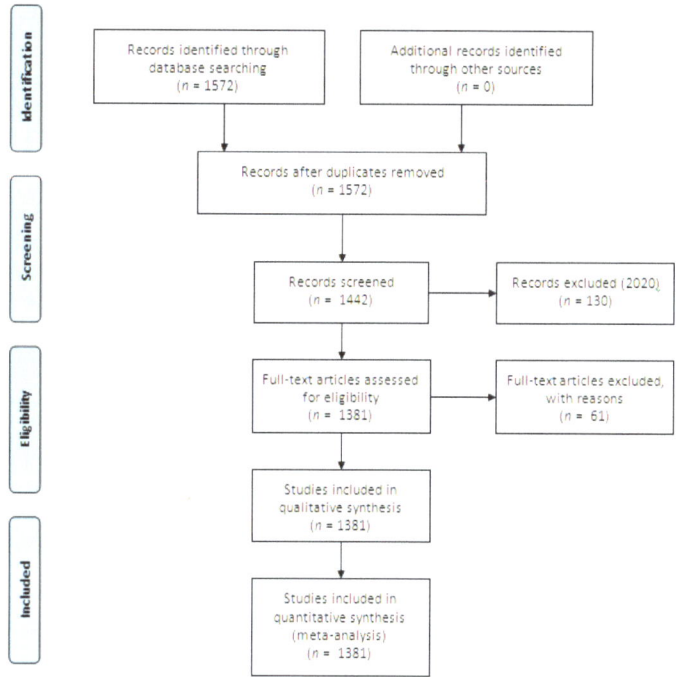

Figure 1. Flowchart according to the PRISMA Declaration.

With SciMAT, likewise, a co-word analysis was carried out that covered various processes [58]. In the recognition process, the keywords (n = 3080) of the entire document package of the unit of analysis were studied. Afterwards, the co-occurrence node maps were designed. Next, a normalized network of co-words was generated and the most significant keywords were selected (n = 2887). Moreover, the most relevant topics and concepts were compiled with a clustering algorithm. In the process of reproduction, different thematic networks and strategic diagrams articulated in four quadrants were created. Each quadrant, depending on its location, presents a different meaning (upper right = motor and relevant themes; upper left = deep-rooted and isolated themes; lower left = disappearing or projected themes; lower right = themes of little development and cross-cutting). The principles of density and centrality intervened in this process. Density measures the internal strength of the network. Centrality measures the level of connection of a network with others [59]. For the determination process, the literature reported in different periods was configured. All this to analyze the evolution of the nodes in different time intervals. In this work, three periods have been established (P_1 = 1971–2012; P_2 = 2013–2016; P_3 = 2017–2019). These intervals have been established under the criterion of documentary similarity between the different periods. To determine the associative strength between the periods, the number of keywords they contained in common was used as a reference. On the other hand, for the analysis of authorship, only an interval was established that covers the entire time period that has marked the publication report (P_X = 1971–2019). Finally, in the performance process, various production indicators connected to their corresponding inclusion criteria were defined [60]. The analysis unit determines the unit of valuation on the keywords established by the authors of the publications, as well as the keywords established by WoS. The frequency threshold reflects the minimum frequency threshold for keywords that are repeated in each time interval. The network type refers to the network to be configured (co-occurrence network). The threshold of the co-occurrence union value establishes the marked periods, according to authors and keywords. The normalization measure determines the connection threshold, determining the minimum relationship for co-occurrence. The normalization measure reveals the measure to normalize the network. For this, the equivalence index eij was used. This is calculated as follows: $eij = cij2/Root\ (ci-cj)$. In a disaggregated manner, cij is the number of coincidences of i and j in the set of documents, ci is the number of occurrences of i, and cj is the number of occurrences of j. On the other hand, the clustering algorithm is used to elaborate the map and its links. The evolutionary measure determines the degree of similarity necessary to elaborate the evolution map, which is established with the Jaccard index. Finally, for the transition map, the inclusion rate is used. All these parameters have served for the optimal configuration of SciMAT (Table 1).

Table 1. Production indicators and inclusion criteria.

Configuration	Values
Analysis unit	Keywords authors, keywords WoS
Frequency threshold	Keywords: $P_1 = (4), P_2 = (4), P_3 = (4)$ Authors: $P_X = (5)$
Network type	Co-occurrence
Co-occurrence union value threshold	Keywords: $P_1 = (2), P_2 = (2), P_3 = (2)$ Authors: $P_X = (3)$
Normalization measure	Equivalence index: $eij = cij2/Root\ (ci-cj)$
Clustering algorithm	Maximum size: 9; Minimum size: 3
Evolutionary measure	Jaccard index
Overlapping measure	Inclusion Rate

3. Results

3.1. Scientific Performance and Production

The evolution of manuscript production in the scientific field of ASD-PAR has two clearly differentiated moments. Although the search began in 1900, it was not until 1971 that the first manuscripts appeared under the theme of this study. From that date until 2004, the volume of production is relatively low, not exceeding 20 documents per year. In the second period, which runs from 2005 to 2019, the number of scientific productions increases gradually and considerably until the present day. Only one evolutionary anomaly is observed between 2015 and 2017, where there are downward and upward peaks in scientific production (Figure 2).

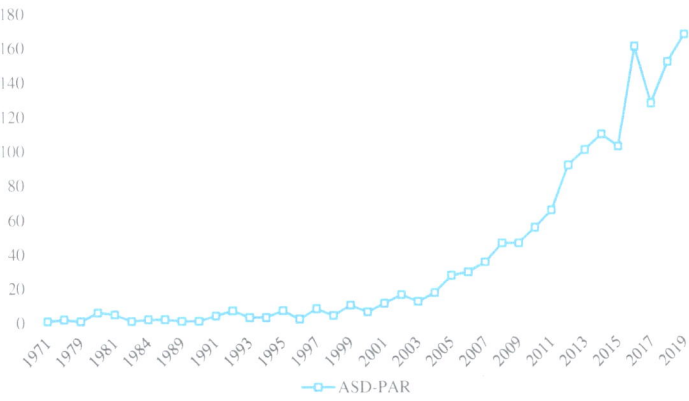

Figure 2. Evolution of scientific production. Note: Y-axis: number of manuscripts; X-axis: dates of publication.

The language used in manuscripts about ASD-PAR is mainly English. It is followed, by far, by French (Table 2).

Table 2. Scientific language of publications.

Languages	n
English	1380
French	22

The area of knowledge that houses research on ASD-PAR is developmental psychology, although it is closely followed by other areas of knowledge, such as psychiatry and rehabilitation (Table 3).

Table 3. Areas of knowledge.

Areas of Knowledge	n
Psychology developmental	496
Psychiatry	345
Rehabilitation	335
Education Special	289

The type of document used to present the research results are research articles. This type of document is far from the other typologies (Table 4).

Table 4. Type of document.

Type of Document	n
Article	1011
Meeting abstract	170
Book review	141

The main institution in this line of research is the University of California System, although it is closely followed by the Universities of Wisconsin (Table 5).

Table 5. Institutions.

Institutions	n
University of California System	53
University of Winconsin System	44
University of North Carolina	30

There are three authors who stand out in this line of research, namely Seltzer, M.M., Ekas, N.V. and Hastings, R.P., with regard to the volume of production (Table 6).

Table 6. Most prolific authors.

Authors	n
Seltzer, M.M.	17
Ekas, N.V.	16
Hastings, R.P.	16

Of all the journals compiling studies on ASD-PAR, the Journal of Autism and Developmental Disorders stands out very considerably in terms of volume of production (Table 7).

Table 7. Source of origin.

Source	n
Journal of Autism and Developmental Disorders	157
Autism	89
Research in Autism Spectrum Disorders	63
Journal of Intellectual Disability Research	47

The country with the highest production volume over ASD-PAR is the United States, being far away from the rest of the countries (Table 8).

Table 8. Most productive countries.

Countries	n
USA	606
England	143
Australia	127
Canada	111

The four most frequently cited manuscripts on ASD-PAR (Table 9) refer to parental stress in families with young children with ASD with an average age of 26.9 months [61], to the higher stress in families with students with ASD than other families with children with other symptoms [62], to the level of well-being in families with students with ASD, where it is higher in relation to disabilities such as Down's or Fragile X syndrome [63], or that those families with students with ASD who present behavioral problems show higher levels of stress than those families with children with ASD who do not show behavioral problems [64].

Table 9. Most cited articles on autism spectrum disorder and its relationship with parents (ASD-PAR).

References	Citations
[61]	505
[62]	448
[63]	420
[64]	350

3.2. Structural and Thematic Development

The evolution of keywords shows the development of research on a subject of study according to the keywords used by the authors. In this case, one can observe the keywords that have been used in a specific period, the keywords that are no longer used in a specific period, the new keywords that are used in a specific period and the keywords that coincide between contiguous periods. As can be seen in Figure 3, the percentage of coincidence between periods is high, being close to 40%. This indicates that research on ASD-PAR is based on similar lines of research, given that there is coincidence between researchers.

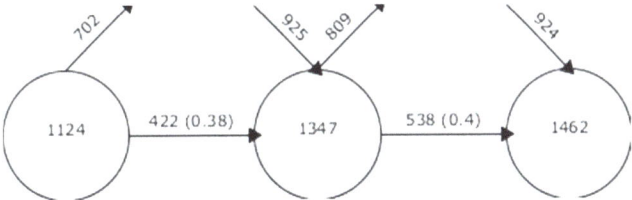

Figure 3. Continuity of keywords between contiguous intervals.

The study of the academic performance of a given field of study analyses the various bibliometric values shown by the research topics. In this case, in the first period (1971–2012) the subjects with the most bibliometric values are "Young-children" and "stress". In the second period (2013–2016), the themes with the most bibliometric values are "behavior-problems" and "families". In the third period, the theme with the most bibliometric values is "mothers" (Table 10).

Table 10. Thematic performance in ASD-PAR.

Interval 1971–2012						
Denomination	Works	Index h	Index g	Index hg	Index q2	Citations
Adolescents	15	12	15	13.42	23.75	582
Behavior-problems *	44	32	44	37.52	51.54	4423
Diagnosis	24	20	24	21.91	31.3	1145
Family-history	23	21	23	21.98	37.79	1966
Parent-training *	17	12	17	14.28	22.45	778
Patterns	5	5	5	5	13.96	341
Perceptions	11	10	11	10.49	18.44	521
Phenotype	22	18	22	19.9	30.59	1196
Population	4	4	4	4	14.83	209
Positive-perception	3	3	3	3	12.96	227
Predictors	4	4	4	4	25.69	547
Scale	3	3	3	3	6	32
Stress	106	49	84	54.16	69.3	7316
Support	6	5	5	5	20	385
Twin	25	20	25	22.36	41.95	1914
Young-children *	107	52	89	68.03	69.17	8102
Interval 2013–2016						
Denomination	Works	Index h	Index g	Index hg	Index q2	Citations
Access	5	4	5	4.47	13.71	140
Adults	44	17	28	21.82	22.2	878
Behavior	17	9	16	12	13.42	312
Behavior-problems *	127	30	52	39.5	40.62	3360
Broader-autism-phenotype	14	10	14	11.83	14.83	254
Depression	16	11	16	13.27	17.55	498
Developmental-disbilities	6	5	6	5.48	8.06	191
Disabilities	16	7	14	9.9	10.58	257
Education	13	9	13	10.82	11.62	198
Families	150	29	51	38.46	39.2	3369
High-functioning-autism	5	4	4	4	10.77	125
Model	5	4	5	4.47	9.38	71
Pervasive-develpmental-disorders	20	11	18	14.07	16.58	556
Program	19	12	19	15.1	18	460
Recognition	3	3	3	3	11.75	144
Toodlers	9	7	9	7.94	10.25	191
Young-children *	43	17	35	24.39	23.32	1309

Table 10. *Cont.*

	Interval 2017–2019					
Denomination	Works	Index h	Index g	Index hg	Index q2	Citations
Acceptance	5	4	5	4.47	6.63	44
Adjustment	8	3	6	4.24	5.74	59
Affiliate-stigma	20	6	10	7.75	8.12	122
Autism	47	9	13	10.82	12	276
Child	3	2	3	2.45	3.46	12
Children	70	7	11	8.77	10.58	267
Coping	9	4	5	4.47	5.66	36
Impairment	3	3	3	3	3	15
Intervention	66	9	12	10.39	10.39	300
Language	13	3	5	3.87	4.58	35
Mindfulness	30	9	13	10.82	10.82	229
Mothers	220	14	19	16.31	17.15	969
Multiple-incidence	6	3	4	3.46	7.75	49
Needs	4	3	3	3	3.46	13
Parent-training *	9	4	7	5.29	7.21	57
Psychiatric-disorders	16	5	8	6.32	5.92	76
Services	20	7	10	8.37	9.17	122
Social-support	72	9	13	10.82	10.39	363
Young-adults	7	4	7	5.29	8.94	70

Note: (*): Themes repeated in different periods.

Strategic diagrams provide information on the relevance of a theme in a given time period. Figure 4 shows the position of the different themes, showing the index h, and taking into account both the external connection force (centrality) and the internal connection force (density).

In the first period (1971–2012), the driving themes are "adolescents", which are related to "adults", "depressed-Mood", "expressed-emotion", "quality", "validity", "reliability", "schizophrenia" and "symptoms"; "phenotype, which relates to "brain", "deficits", "disorders", "personality-characteristics", "pervasive-developmental-disorders", "psychiatric-disorders", and "weak-central-coherence"; "twin", which relates to "broad-autism-phenotype", "children", "genetics", "history", "individuals""infantile-autism", "personality" and "traits"; "behavior-problems", which relates to "fathers", "family-stress", "intellectual-disability", "maternal-stress", "mental-health", "parenting-stress", "preschool-children" and "syndrome-specificity"; "stress", which relates to "adjustment", "coping", "depression", "families", "health", "mothers", "parents" and "social-support"; and "Young-children", which relates to "autism", "behavior", "communication", "disabilities", "Down-Syndrome", "intervention", "mental-retartion" and "spectrum-disorders". In this period, research is focused on the behavioral problems of children with ASD, stress in families, in young children and adolescents.

In the second period (2013–2016), the motor themes are "behavior-problems", which is related to "Down-Syndrome", "intellectual-disability", "mental-health", "mothers", "parenting-stress", "preschool-children", "stress" and "syndrome-specificity"; "families", which is related to "adjustment", "autism", "autism-spectrum-disorders", "fathers", "impact", "marital-satisfaction" and "parents"; "Young-children", which relates to "double-abcx-model", "intervention", "joint-attention", "meta-analysis", "school-age-children", "skills", "social-support" and "support"; "adults", which relates to "adolescents", "Asperger-syndrome", "children", "gender", "health", "positive-perceptions", "prevalence" and "validity"; and "pervasive-developmental-disorders", which relates to "coping-strategies", "diagnosis", "parental-stress", "population", "randomized-controlled-trial", "spectrum-disorders", "symptom-severity" and "traits". During this period, the focus is on behavioral problems, families, and people of various ages with ASD and generalized developmental disorders.

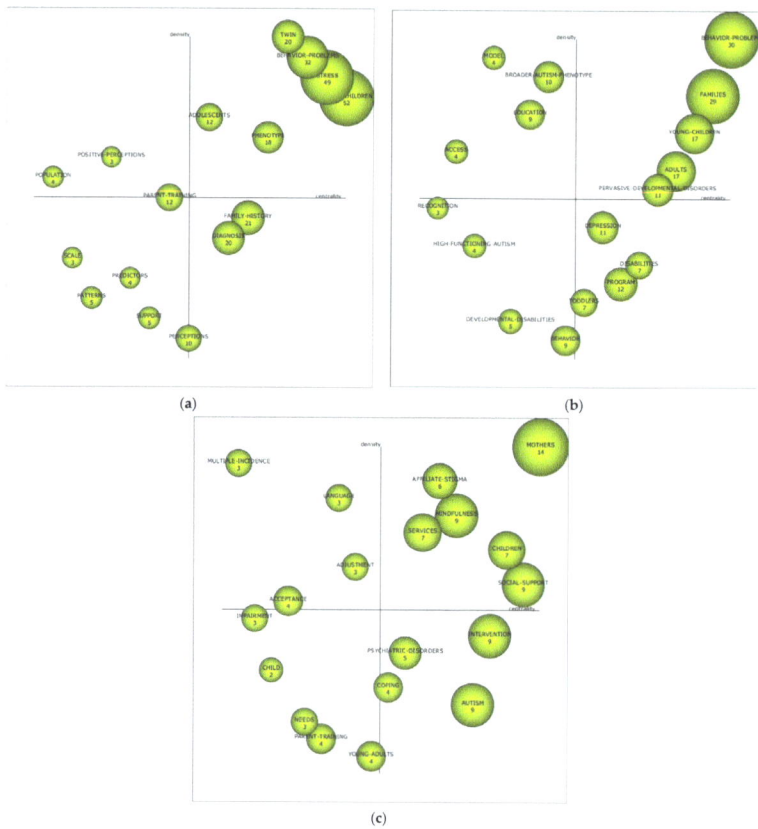

Figure 4. Strategic diagram per ASD-PAR index-h. Note: (**a**) Interval 1971–2012; (**b**) Interval 2013–2016; (**c**) Interval 2017–2019.

In the third period (2017–2019), the motor themes are "mothers", which is related to "autism-spectrum-disorder", "families", "fathers", "mental-health", "parents", "preschool-children", "quality-of-life" and "stress"; "affiliate-stigma", which relates to "stigma", "people", "caregivers", "family-caregivers", "intellectual-disability", "perceptions" and "psychological-distress"; "services", which relates to "advocacy", "anxiety", "awareness", "behaviour-problems", "care", "decreases-aggression", "depression", "disparities", "education", "health", "health-care" and "meta-synthesis"; "mindfulness", which relates to "parent-intervention", "program", "stress-reduction" and "therapy"; "children", which relates to "adolescents", "ASD", "diagnosis", "individual", "prevalence", "risk-factors", "transition" and "youth"; and "social-support", which relates to "ASD", "developmental-disabilities", "disabilities", "Down-Syndrome", "parenting-stress", "impact", "predictors" and "satisfaction". In other words, during this period, the focus is more on the care, services and social support that families and people with ASD can receive. In addition, the themes of "child", "needs", "parent-training" and "Young-adults" must be taken into account during this period, as they are considered to be unknown themes. In other words, they may disappear from the lines of research, or become the driving forces of the coming years in the field of research.

3.3. Thematic Evolution of Terms

The thematic evolution of a field of knowledge shows the relationship that is established between the different subjects in contiguous periods. This gives an idea of the different lines of research established in a specific research topic. The type of relationship that can be established between the topics can be conceptual and non-conceptual. The conceptual relationship occurs when two themes share common constructs. The non-conceptual relationship is generated when the two topics do not share keywords in common. The conceptual relationship is represented by a solid line. The non-conceptual relationship is shown with dashed lines. The size of the line indicates the number of relationships (the thicker the line, the greater the relationship).

In the field of study of ASD-PAR, it can be indicated that a conceptual gap exists. In other words, there is not one theme that is repeated in all three periods. This indicates a variety of themes in the fields of study undertaken. This does not mean that there are not diverse lines of research over time. In this case, two can be highlighted, on the one hand the line "behavior_problems-behavior_problems-mothers" and "stress-families-mothers". That is, the lines of research established over time focus mainly on behavioral problems and their repercussions on families, and on the stress generated in the family environment by living with a person with ASD. In addition, Figure 5 shows that there are more conceptual than non-conceptual relationships, which shows the strong relationship between the various topics. It can also be seen that between the second and third periods several lines of research are being established, which may set the trend for study in the coming years.

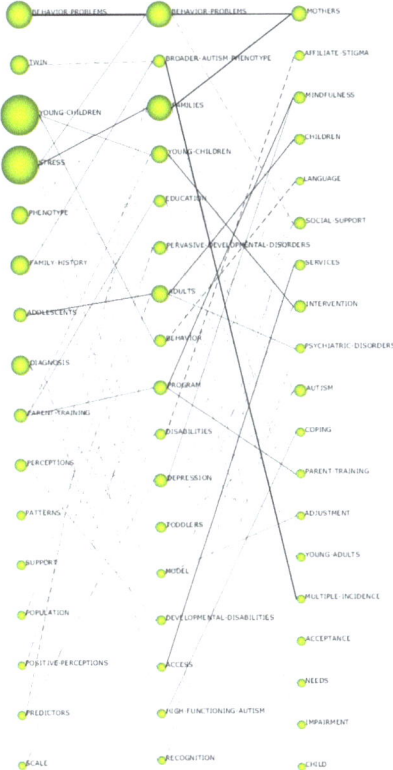

Figure 5. Thematic evolution by h-index.

3.4. Authors with the Highest Relevance Index

Taking into account the authors in the ASD-PAR field of study, it can be indicated that those considered as drivers are Estes, A., Toret, G. and González-Bono, E. Although, due to their location in the diagram, we must take into consideration Chen, L.S., Seltzer, M.M.

and Zwaigenbaum, L., because they may become the relevant authors in this field of study (Figure 6).

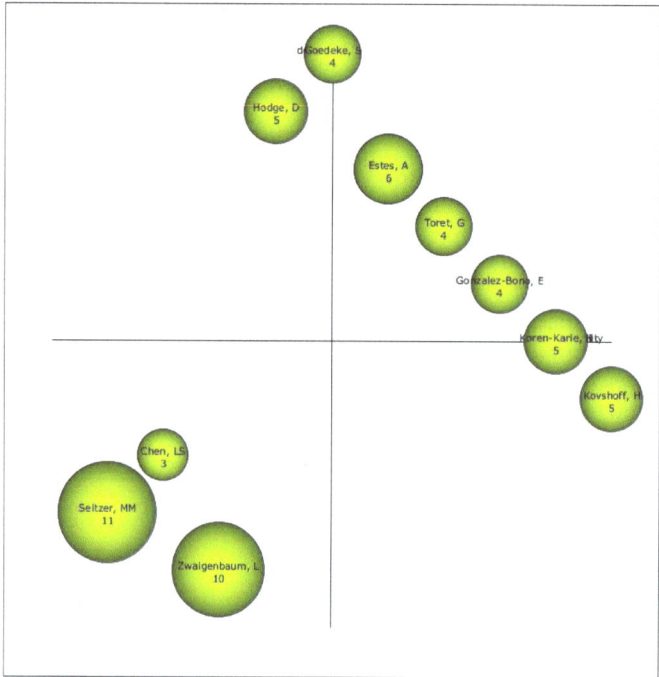

Figure 6. Strategic author diagram of the entire production.

4. Discussion

The actions of family members acquire a relevant value when it comes to intervening and treating people with ASD [28,29]. The literature shows a pronounced interest in carrying out studies that represent an advance in this field of knowledge [30]. In this sense, research reports effective mechanisms and actions to address this disorder in the best possible way [25,31–37]. With the completion of this study, we have tried to analyze all the literature concerning ASD and the family environment, in order to report the most significant and relevant findings that the scientific community has obtained on the state of the matter.

The performance and production analysis on ASD-PAR in WoS allows to establish a profile on this field of study. In this case, it can be indicated that the beginnings of scientific production in Wos date back to 1971. There are two clearly differentiated moments in scientific production: a first moment (1971–2004), where the volume of production is low, and a second moment (2005–2019), where the volume of production increases considerably. It can therefore be said that the subject matter began to be relevant for the scientific community from 2005 to the present day. The manuscripts are presented in the form of articles, which indicates that this field of study is well established in the scientific community, in English and in the Journal of Autism and Developmental Disorders. The area of knowledge where this type of study is compiled is developmental psychology. Analyzing the following areas of knowledge, it can be seen that studies on ASD-PAR are oriented towards the psychological and rehabilitative support of families who have children or relatives with ASD. The main institution conducting research on ASD-PAR is the University of California System. However, the volume of the University of Wisconsin System is noteworthy in this regard. In this case, the first places are occupied by universities in the

United States, which happens to be the country with the highest volume of production. In relation to the authors, it is necessary to bear in mind several premises. On the one hand, there are those with a higher rate of production, including Seltzer, M.M., Ekas, N.V. and Hastings, R.P. On the other hand, there are the most relevant within the scientific community, in this case Estes, A., Toret, G. and González-Bono, E. Finally, the authors Chen, L.S., Seltzer, M.M. and Zwaigenbaum, L., should be taken into consideration as they are probably the most relevant in the near future. The most cited article is by [56] and the lines of research of the most cited articles focus on the stress and well-being of families with children with ASD.

The index of key word coincidence between the established periods marks a high level of coincidence between periods, which shows a high degree of agreement on the existing lines of research on the subject of ASD-PAR. The academic performance indicates that there is no single subject that presents high bibliometric values in the three periods analyzed. In general, it is shown that stress, behavioral problems, families and mothers are the most relevant research topics in the field of study of ASD-PAR.

The study developed also indicates that there is no theme that is repeated, as a motor theme, in the three established time diagrams. However, similar themes of study are visualized, which focus on stress in the family, mothers, behavioral problems of people with ASD and the problems of people with ASD at different ages. This is specifically reflected in each of the established time periods. In the first period (1971–2012), motor issues were focused on "Twin", "behavior-problems", "stress", "young-children", "adolescents" and "phenotype". In other words, on the behavioral problems presented by children with ASD, the stress of families and on the children and adolescents themselves. In the second period (2013–2016), the motor themes were oriented towards "behavior-problems", "families", "young-children", "adults" and "pervasive-developmental-disorders". This means behavioral problems, families, people of various ages with ASD and generalized developmental disorders. In the last period (2017–2019) the driving themes are "mothers", "affiliate-stigma", "mindfulness", "services", "children" and "social support". In other words, in this period, the driving themes are more oriented towards the care, action services and social support that families and people with ASD can receive.

If we look at the thematic evolution of the studies on ASD-PAR, we can see that there is a conceptual gap, although two clearly defined and time-based lines of research can be observed, such as "behavior_problems-behavior_problems-mothers" and "stress-families-mothers". In this case, it can be said that the research is oriented towards behavioral problems and their impact on families, and the stress generated in the family environment by living with a person with ASD.

5. Conclusions

It is concluded that the field of study on ASD-PAR began in WoS in 1971, but it was not until 2005 that it began to be relevant and interesting for the scientific community. The main focus of research on ASD-PAR is on the stress that is generated in families that have children with ASD, in addition to the family problems that can result from the fact that these children also have behavioral problems.

The limitations of this study focus on the purification of the database, since the researchers of this manuscript have had to read each of the documents, in order to properly apply the PRISMA protocol. Another of the limitations focuses on the debugging of the database, given that badly written or badly expressed key words must be modified or eliminated. Finally, the inclusion criteria can be considered, which have been established from the perspective of the researchers themselves, from their experience and with the intention of showing the most relevant information on this field of study. The future line of research derived from this investigation focuses on developing studies focused on families who have children with ASD, broadening the field of knowledge.

6. Theoretical and Practical Implications

This study has a number of theoretical and practical implications. Among the theoretical implications are the broadening of the field of knowledge about ASD-PAR. Until now, no such research has been carried out. This research provides clear information on the lines of study established by the scientific community. In addition, it presents a specific profile of this type of research. Another of the theoretical implications is that the most recent research has been compiled in order to prepare the introduction to this manuscript, offering up-to-date and high-impact information on the research carried out in this field of study. Amongst the practical implications, this work allows those groups responsible for attending to families with children with ASD to provide information on where the lines of study are heading, as well as offering data on the most relevant authors in this field of knowledge. Likewise, in the development of the different analyses, information is offered on various methods and actions to attend to families with children with ASD.

Author Contributions: Conceptualization, N.C.-S. and J.-A.M.-M.; methodology, J.L.-B. and A.-J.M.-G.; software, A.-J.M.-G.; formal analysis, J.L.-B. and A.-J.M.-G.; investigation, N.C.-S., J.L.-B., A.-J.M.-G. and J.-A.M.-M.; data curation, A.-J.M.-G.; writing—original draft preparation, J.L.-B. and N.C.-S.; writing—review and editing, N.C.-S., J.L.-B. and A.-J.M.-G.; visualization, J.-A.M.-M.; supervision, J.L.-B. and J.-A.M.-M. All authors have read and agreed to the published version of the manuscript.

Funding: This research was funded by the project "Application of quality standards in the organization of educational institutions" (ISPRS-2017–2021).

Institutional Review Board Statement: Not applicable.

Informed Consent Statement: Not applicable.

Data Availability Statement: Data is contained within the article.

Acknowledgments: To the research group AREA (HUM-672) of the University of Granada (Spain).

Conflicts of Interest: The authors declare no conflict of interest.

References

1. Fusar-Poli, L.; Brondino, N.; Politi, P.; Aguglia, E. Missed diagnoses and misdiagnoses of adults with autism spectrum disorder. *Eur. Arch. Psychiatry Clin. Neurosci.* **2020**, 1–12. [CrossRef] [PubMed]
2. Lorah, E.R.; Karnes, A.; Miller, J.; Welch-Beardsley, J. Establishing Peer Manding in Young Children with Autism Using a Speech-Generating Device. *J. Dev. Phys. Disabil.* **2019**, *31*, 791–801. [CrossRef]
3. Vásquez, B.; del Sol, M. Neuronal Morphology in Autism Spectrum Disorder. *Int. J. Morphol.* **2020**, *38*, 1513–1518.
4. Fernandez-Prieto, M.; Moreira, C.; Cruz, S.; Campos, V.; Martínez-Regueiro, R.; Taboada, M.; Carracedo, A.; Sampaio, A. Executive Functioning: A Mediator Between Sensory Processing and Behaviour in Autism Spectrum Disorder. *J. Autism Dev. Disord.* **2020**, 1–13. [CrossRef] [PubMed]
5. Hofvander, B.; Bering, S.; Tärnhäll, A.; Wallinius, M.; Billstedt, E. Few differences in the externalizing and criminal history of young violent offenders with and without autism spectrum disorders. *Front. Psychiatry* **2019**, *10*, 1–8. [CrossRef] [PubMed]
6. Li, Y.; Zhou, Z.; Chang, C.; Qian, L.; Li, C.; Xiao, T.; Xiang, X.; Kangkang, C.; Fang, H.; Ke, X. Anomalies in uncinate fasciculus development and social defects in preschoolers with autism spectrum disorder. *BMC Psychiatry* **2019**, *19*, 399. [CrossRef]
7. Muskett, A.; Capriola-Hall, N.N.; Radtke, S.R.; Factor, R.; Scarpa, A. Repetitive behaviors in Autism Spectrum Disorder: Associations with depression and anxiety symptoms. *Res. Autism Spectr. Disord.* **2019**, *68*, 101449. [CrossRef]
8. Adams, D.; Emerson, L.M. The Impact of Anxiety in Children on the Autism Spectrum. *J. Autism Dev. Disord.* **2020**. [CrossRef]
9. Sadler, K.M. Video Self-Modeling to Treat Aggression in Students Significantly Impacted by Autism Spectrum Disorder. *J. Spec. Educ. Technol.* **2019**, *34*, 215–225. [CrossRef]
10. Scott, K.E.; Kazazian, K.; Mann, R.S.; Möhrle, D.; Schormans, A.L.; Schmid, S.; Allman, B.L. Loss of Cntnap2 in the Rat Causes Autism-Related Alterations in Social Interactions, Stereotypic Behavior, and Sensory Processing. *Autism Res.* **2020**, *13*, 1698–1717. [CrossRef]
11. Masson, H.L.; de Beeck, H.O.; Boets, B. Reduced task-dependent modulation of functional network architecture for positive versus negative affective touch processing in autism spectrum disorders. *NeuroImage* **2020**, *219*, 117009. [CrossRef]
12. Kovarski, K.; Malvy, J.; Khanna, R.K.; Arsène, S.; Batty, M.; Latinus, M. Reduced visual evoked potential amplitude in autism spectrum disorder, a variability effect? *Transl. Psychiatry* **2019**, *9*, 1–9. [CrossRef] [PubMed]

13. Schwartz, S.; Wang, L.; Shinn-Cunningham, B.G.; Tager-Flusberg, H. Atypical Perception of Sounds in Minimally and Low Verbal Children and Adolescents with Autism as Revealed by Behavioral and Neural Measures. *Autism Res.* **2020**, *13*, 1718–1729. [CrossRef] [PubMed]
14. Pereira, J.A.; Sepulveda, P.; Rana, M.; Montalba, C.; Tejos, C.; Torres, R.; Ranganatha, S.; Ruiz, S. Self-Regulation of the Fusiform Face Area in Autism Spectrum: A Feasibility Study with Real-Time fMRI Neurofeedback. *Front. Hum. Neurosci.* **2019**, *13*, 1–17. [CrossRef] [PubMed]
15. Ardalan, A.; Assadi, A.H.; Surgent, O.J.; Travers, B.G. Whole-Body Movement during Videogame Play Distinguishes Youth with Autism from Youth with Typical Development. *Sci. Rep.* **2019**, *9*, 1–11. [CrossRef]
16. Adams, C.; Gaile, J. Evaluation of a parent preference-based outcome measure after intensive communication intervention for children with social (pragmatic) communication disorder and high-functioning autism spectrum disorder. *Res. Dev. Disabil.* **2020**, *105*, 103752. [CrossRef]
17. Zajic, M.C.; Solari, E.J.; McIntyre, N.S.; Lerro, L.; Mundy, P.C. Observing Visual Attention and Writing Behaviors During a Writing Assessment: Comparing Children with Autism Spectrum Disorder to Peers with Attention-Deficit/Hyperactivity Disorder and Typically Developing Peers. *Autism Res.* **2020**, *61*, 1–13. [CrossRef]
18. Escolano-Pérez, E.; Acero-Ferrero, M.; Herrero-Nivela, M.L. Improvement of planning skills in children with Autism Spectrum Disorder after an educational intervention: A pilot study from a mixed methods approach. *Front. Psychol.* **2019**, *10*, 2824. [CrossRef]
19. Kopec, J.; Hagmann, C.; Shea, N.; Prawl, A.; Batkin, D.; Russo, N. Examining the Temporal Limits of Enhanced Visual Feature Detection in Children with Autism. *Autism Res.* **2020**, *13*, 1561–1572. [CrossRef]
20. Bacon, A.; Beaman, C.P.; Liu, F. An exploratory study of imagining sounds and "hearing" music in autism. *J. Autism Dev. Disord.* **2019**, *50*, 1123–1132. [CrossRef]
21. Van't Westeinde, A.; Cauvet, É.; Toro, R.; Kuja-Halkola, R.; Neufeld, J.; Mevel, K.; Bölte, S. Sex differences in brain structure: A twin study on restricted and repetitive behaviors in twin pairs with and without autism. *Mol. Autism* **2019**, *11*, 1–20. [CrossRef] [PubMed]
22. Schiavi, S.; Carbone, E.; Melancia, F.; Buzzelli, V.; Manduca, A.; Campolongo, P.; Pallotini, V.; Trezza, V. Perinatal supplementation with omega-3 fatty acids corrects the aberrant social and cognitive traits observed in a genetic model of autism based on FMR1 deletion in rats. *Nutr. Neurosci.* **2020**, 1–14. [CrossRef] [PubMed]
23. Tupou, J.; Waddington, H.; Sigafoos, J. Evaluation of a brief teacher coaching program for delivering an early intervention program to preschoolers with autism spectrum disorder. *Infants Young Child.* **2020**, *33*, 259–282. [CrossRef]
24. Kasilingam, N.; Waddington, H.; Van Der Meer, L. Early Intervention for Children with Autism Spectrum Disorder in New Zealand: What Children Get and What Parents Want. *Int. J. Disabil. Dev. Educ.* **2019**, 1–17. [CrossRef]
25. Shooshtari, M.H.; Zarafshan, H.; Mohamadian, M.; Zareee, J.; Karimi-Keisomi, I.; Hooshangi, H. The Effect of a Parental Education Program on the Mental Health of Parents and Behavioral Problems of Their Children with Autism Spectrum Disorder. *Iran. J. Psychiatry Clin. Psychol.* **2020**, *25*, 356–367. [CrossRef]
26. Pérez-Fuster, P.; Sevilla, J.; Herrera, G. Enhancing daily living skills in four adults with autism spectrum disorder through an embodied digital technology-mediated intervention. *Res. Autism Spectr. Disord.* **2019**, *58*, 54–67. [CrossRef]
27. Taheri-Torbati, H.; Sotoodeh, M.S. Using video and live modelling to teach motor skill to children with autism spectrum disorder. *Int. J. Incl. Educ.* **2019**, *23*, 405–418. [CrossRef]
28. Ratliff-Black, M.; Therrien, W. Parent-Mediated Interventions for School-Age Children with ASD: A Meta-Analysis. *Focus Autism Other Dev. Disabil.* **2020**. [CrossRef]
29. Rivard, M.; Millau, M.; Mello, C.; Clément, C.; Mejia-Cardenas, C.; Boulé, M.; Magnan, C. Immigrant Families of Children with Autism disorder's Perceptions of Early Intensive Behavioral Intervention Services. *J. Dev. Phys. Disabil.* **2020**, 1–19. [CrossRef]
30. Hu, X.; Han, Z.R.; Bai, L.; Gao, M.M. The mediating role of parenting stress in the relations between parental emotion regulation and parenting behaviors in Chinese families of children with autism spectrum disorders: A dyadic analysis. *J. Autism Dev. Disord.* **2019**, *49*, 3983–3998. [CrossRef]
31. Beverly, B.L.; Mathews, L.A. Speech-Language Pathologist and Parent Perspectives on Speech-Language Pathology Services for Children with Autism Spectrum Disorders. *Focus Autism Other Dev. Disabil.* **2020**, 1088357620954380. [CrossRef]
32. Dueñas, A.D.; Plavnick, J.B.; Goldstein, H. Effects of a Multicomponent Peer Mediated Intervention on Social Communication of Preschoolers with Autism Spectrum Disorder. *Except. Child.* **2020**. [CrossRef]
33. Lien, K.; Lashewicz, B.; Mitchell, J.; Boettcher, N. Blending Traditional and Nurturing Fathering: Fathers of Children with Autism Managing Work and Family. *Fam. Relat.* **2020**. [CrossRef]
34. Garrido, D.; Petrova, D.; Cokely, E.; Carballo, G.; Garcia-Retamero, R. Parental Risk Literacy is Related to Quality of Life in Spanish Families of Children with Autism Spectrum Disorder. *J. Autism Dev. Disord.* **2020**, 1–10. [CrossRef] [PubMed]
35. Walton, K.M. Leisure time and family functioning in families living with autism spectrum disorder. *Autism* **2019**, *23*, 1384–1397. [CrossRef] [PubMed]
36. Lei, X.; Kantor, J. Social support and family quality of life in Chinese families of children with autism spectrum disorder: The mediating role of family cohesion and adaptability. *Int. J. Dev. Disabil.* **2020**, 1–8. [CrossRef]
37. Carlisle, G.K.; Johnson, R.A.; Wang, Z.; Brosi, T.C.; Rife, E.M.; Hutchison, A. Exploring Human–Companion Animal Interaction in Families of Children with Autism. *J. Autism Dev. Disord.* **2020**, 1–13. [CrossRef]

38. Segura-Robles, A.; Moreno-Guerrero, A.J.; Parra-González, E.; López-Belmonte, J. Review of Research Trends in Learning and the Internet in Higher Education. *Soc. Sci.* **2020**, *9*, 101. [CrossRef]
39. Cobo, M.J.; López, A.G.; Herrera, E.; Herrera, F. Science mapping software tools: Review, analysis, and cooperative study among tools. *J. Am. Soc. Inf. Sci. Technol.* **2011**, *62*, 1382–1402. [CrossRef]
40. López-Belmonte, J.; Moreno-Guerrero, A.J.; López-Núñez, J.A.; Pozo-Sánchez, S. Analysis of the Productive, Structural, and Dynamic Development of Augmented Reality in Higher Education Research on the Web of Science. *Appl. Sci.* **2019**, *9*, 5306. [CrossRef]
41. Rodríguez-García, A.M.; López-Belmonte, J.; Agreda-Montoro, M.; Moreno-Guerrero, A.J. Productive, Structural and Dynamic Study of the Concept of Sustainability in the Educational Field. *Sustainability* **2019**, *11*, 5613. [CrossRef]
42. Leung, X.Y.; Sun, J.; Bai, B. Bibliometrics of social media research: A co-citation and co-word analysis. *Int. J. Hosp. Manag.* **2017**, *66*, 35–45. [CrossRef]
43. López-Belmonte, J.; Parra-González, M.E.; Segura-Robles, A.; Pozo-Sánchez, S. Scientific Mapping of Gamification in Web of Science. *Eur. J. Investig. Health Psychol. Educ.* **2020**, *10*, 832–847. [CrossRef]
44. Martínez, M.A.; Cobo, M.J.; Herrera, M.; Herrera, E. Analyzing the scientific evolution of social work using science mapping. *Res. Soc. Work Pr.* **2015**, *25*, 257–277. [CrossRef]
45. Hirsch, J.E. An index to quantify an individual's scientific research output. *Proc. Natl. Acad. Sci. USA* **2005**, *102*, 16569–16572. [CrossRef] [PubMed]
46. Moreno-Guerrero, A.J.; Gómez-García, G.; López-Belmonte, J.; Rodríguez-Jiménez, C. Internet Addiction in the Web of Science Database: A Review of the Literature with Scientific Mapping. *Int. J. Environ. Res. Public Health* **2020**, *17*, 2753. [CrossRef]
47. Alonso, S.; Cabrerizo, F.J.; Herrera-Viedma, E.; Herrera, F. hg-index: A new index to characterize the scientific output of researchers based on the h-and g-indices. *Scientometrics* **2010**, *82*, 391–400. [CrossRef]
48. Cabrerizo, F.J.; Alonso, S.; Herrera-Viedma, E.; Herrera, F. q2-Index: Quantitative and qualitative evaluation based on the number and impact of papers in the Hirsch core. *J. Informetr.* **2010**, *4*, 23–28. [CrossRef]
49. López-Robles, J.R.; Otegi-Olaso, J.R.; Porto, I.; Cobo, M.J. 30 years of intelligence models in management and business: A bibliometric review. *Int. J. Inf. Manag.* **2019**, *48*, 22–38. [CrossRef]
50. López-Belmonte, J.; Marín-Marín, J.A.; Soler-Costa, R.; Moreno-Guerrero, A.J. Arduino Advances in Web of Science. A Scientific Mapping of Literary Production. *IEEE Access* **2020**, *8*, 128674–128682. [CrossRef]
51. Carmona-Serrano, N.; López-Belmonte, J.; Cuesta-Gómez, J.-L.; Moreno-Guerrero, A.-J. Documentary Analysis of the Scientific Literature on Autism and Technology in Web of Science. *Brain Sci.* **2020**, *10*, 985. [CrossRef] [PubMed]
52. Carmona-Serrano, N.; López-Belmonte, J.; López-Núñez, J.-A.; Moreno-Guerrero, A.-J. Trends in autism research in the field of education in Web of Science: A bibliometric study. *Brain Sci.* **2020**, *10*, 1018. [CrossRef] [PubMed]
53. López-Belmonte, J.; Moreno-Guerrero, A.J.; López-Núñez, J.A.; Hinojo-Lucena, F.J. Augmented Reality in education. A scientific mapping in Web of Science. *Interact. Learn. Environ.* **2020**, 1–15. [CrossRef]
54. Moral-Muñoz, J.A.; Herrera-Viedma, E.; Santisteban-Espejo, A.; Cobo, M.J. Software tools for conducting bibliometric analysis in science: An up-to-date review. *Prof. Inf.* **2020**, *29*, 4. [CrossRef]
55. Moreno-Guerrero, A.J.; López-Belmonte, J.; Marín-Marín, J.A.; Soler-Costa, R. Scientific development of educational artificial intelligence in Web of Science. *Future Internet* **2020**, *12*, 124. [CrossRef]
56. López-Núñez, J.A.; López-Belmonte, J.; Moreno-Guerrero, A.J.; Ramos, M.; Hinojo-Lucena, F.J. Education and Diet in the Scientific Literature: A Study of the Productive, Structural, and Dynamic Development in Web of Science. *Sustainability* **2020**, *12*, 4838. [CrossRef]
57. Montero-Díaz, J.; Cobo, M.J.; Gutiérrez-Salcedo, M.; Segado-Boj, F.; Herrera-Viedma, E. Mapeo científico de la Categoría «Comunicación» en WoS (1980–2013). *Comunicar* **2018**, *26*, 81–91. [CrossRef]
58. Herrera-Viedma, E.; López-Robles, J.R.; Guallar, J.; Cobo, M.J. Global trends in coronavirus research at the time of Covid-19: A general bibliometric approach and content analysis using SciMAT. *Prof. Inf.* **2020**, *29*. [CrossRef]
59. Callon, M.; Courtial, J.P.; Laville, F. Co-word analysis as a tool for describing the network of interactions between basic and technological research: The case of polymer chemistry. *Scientometrics* **1991**, *22*, 155–205. [CrossRef]
60. López-Belmonte, J.; Segura-Robles, A.; Moreno-Guerrero, A.J.; Parra-González, E. Machine Learning and Big Data in the Impact Literature. A Bibliometric Review with Scientific Mapping in Web of Science. *Symmetry* **2020**, *12*, 495. [CrossRef]
61. Davis, N.O.; Carter, A.S. Parenting stress in mothers and fathers of toddlers with autism spectrum disorders: Associations with child characteristics. *J. Autism Dev. Disord.* **2008**, *38*, 1278–1291. [CrossRef] [PubMed]
62. Hayes, S.A.; Watson, S.L. The Impact of Parenting Stress: A Meta-analysis of Studies Comparing the Experience of Parenting Stress in Parents of Children With and Without Autism Spectrum Disorder. *J. Autism Dev. Disord.* **2012**, *43*, 629–642. [CrossRef] [PubMed]
63. Abbeduto, L.; Seltzar, M.M.; Shattuck, P.; Krauss, M.W.; Orsmond, G.; Murphy, M.M. Psychological well-being and coping in mothers of youths with autism, Down syndrome, or fragile X syndrome. *Am. J. Ment. Retard.* **2004**, *109*, 237–254. [CrossRef]
64. Estes, A.; Munson, J.; Dawson, G.; Koehler, E.; Zhou, X.H.; Abbott, R. Parenting stress and psychological functioning among mothers of preschool children with autism and developmental delay. *Autism* **2009**, *13*, 375–387. [CrossRef] [PubMed]

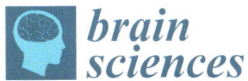

Article

Parental Education, Household Income, Race, and Children's Working Memory: Complexity of the Effects

Golnoush Akhlaghipour [1] and Shervin Assari [2,3,*]

[1] Department of Neurology, University of California Irvine, Irvine, CA 92697, USA; golnoush.akhlaghi@gmail.com
[2] Department of Family Medicine, Charles R Drew University of Medicine and Science, Los Angeles, CA 90059, USA
[3] Department of Urban Public Health, Charles R Drew University of Medicine and Science, Los Angeles, CA 90059, USA
* Correspondence: assari@umich.edu; Tel.: +1-734-232-0445; Fax: +1-734-615-8739

Received: 7 October 2020; Accepted: 4 December 2020; Published: 7 December 2020

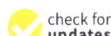

Abstract: *Background.* Considerable research has linked social determinants of health (SDoHs) such as race, parental education, and household income to school performance, and these effects may be in part due to working memory. However, a growing literature shows that these effects may be complex: while the effects of parental education may be diminished for Blacks than Whites, household income may explain such effects. *Purpose.* Considering race as sociological rather than a biological construct (race as a proxy of racism) and built on Minorities' Diminished Returns (MDRs), this study explored complexities of the effects of SDoHs on children's working memory. *Methods.* We borrowed data from the Adolescent Brain Cognitive Development (ABCD) study. The total sample was 10,418, 9- and 10-year-old children. The independent variables were race, parental education, and household income. The primary outcome was working memory measured by the NIH Toolbox Card Sorting Test. Age, sex, ethnicity, and parental marital status were the covariates. To analyze the data, we used mixed-effect regression models. *Results.* High parental education and household income were associated with higher and Black race was associated with lower working memory. The association between high parental education but not household income was less pronounced for Black than White children. This differential effect of parental education on working memory was explained by household income. *Conclusions.* For American children, parental education generates unequal working memory, depending on race. This means parental education loses some of its expected effects for Black families. It also suggests that while White children with highly educated parents have the highest working memory, Black children report lower working memory, regardless of their parental education. This inequality is mainly because of differential income in highly educated White and Black families. This finding has significant public policy and economic implications and suggests we need to do far more than equalizing education to eliminate racial inequalities in children's cognitive outcomes. While there is a need for multilevel policies that reduce the effect of racism and social stratification for middle-class Black families, equalizing income may have more returns than equalizing education.

Keywords: socioeconomic status; socioeconomic position; memory; working memory; social determinants of health; population groups

1. Background

Working memory is believed to be a core element of human cognition. Baddeley's original work on the multiple-component model [1] and executive function conceptualizes working memory as people's ability to bring information "online", which is core to thinking and thought. Working memory is our ability to hold information in short-term memory and maintain the required information "in mind" while processing them [2]. Over the past decades, working memory has received much scientific interest, which has resulted in a large body of empirical evidence. This research suggests that working memory is essential for cognitive tasks, math ability, and school performance. Working memory is closely associated with executive functioning [3] and is mainly performed in higher cortical areas, especially the prefrontal cortex (PFC) [4]. Because of the close correlation with cognitive tasks, working memory is believed to be the primary determinant of children's educational success [5–8].

With cognitive flexibility and inhibitory control, working memory is a part of the executive function, also called cognitive control [9,10]. Executive function refers to the top-down neurocognitive processes involved in the conscious, goal-directed control of thought, action, and emotions. Effective executive function and functional working memory are both reliant upon the integrity of neural networks involving the prefrontal cortex (PFC), the anterior cingulate cortex, and other regions [11–13], and they are required for keeping the information in mind, attending selectively, ignoring distractions, and solving problems flexibly [14].

High socioeconomic status (SES) is associated with better school performance [15] and working memory [16–18]. These are in line with the overall positive effects of high SES on childhood cognition, emotions, and behaviors [19]. For example, children from higher SES families are less likely to show school drop-out [20] and emotional [21–23] and behavioral problems [24,25]. These SES effects are non-specific and are attributed to the protective effects of resources and lower stress in childhood.

The SES–memory/health scarcity hypothesis can be seen through SES effects on healthy children's brain development. According to the scarcity hypothesis, low SES is a proxy of early adversity, stress, economic insecurity, and lack of resources, increasing the risk of low child development. In this view, stress, adversity, and scarce resources explain the SES–brain development link [26]. Low parental education and household income are proxies of living in stressful environments, food insecurity, environmental toxins, and parental risk behaviors that can jeopardize healthy brain development in children [27–29]. As a result of inadequate brain development, children from low SES are at an increased risk of poor memory, emotion regulation, learning disorders, and psychopathology [30–32]. In contrast, children from high SES backgrounds experience less stress and have more access to stimulating environments and better parenting [33–35].

According to the Minorities' Diminished Returns (MDRs) [36,37], Black and White families differ in the protective effect of high SES on health outcomes. Compared to their White counterparts, Black children show lower parental education effects on a wide range of developmental outcomes [38], such as school performance [38], mental health [39], emotion regulation [40,41], aggression [42], and substance use [39,43]. While income may also generate differential effects for Black and White children [44], most research has shown that parental education generates fewer Blacks outcomes than Whites [45–49].

MDRs are not due to behaviors or personalities but societal barriers. For Black families, high SES increases vulnerability to the effect of discrimination, meaning that if discrimination occurs, it is more likely to result in depression [50]. High SES is also associated with high discrimination, which is partly due to the increased proximity of high SES Blacks to Whites [51,52]. High SES Black families experience higher discrimination because they are at higher proximity to White people [51–54]. The positive link between SES and discrimination [51,52,55–58] reduces high SES Black families' health. As a result, SES effects are weaker for Blacks than Whites.

Research has established racial/ethnic differences in each SES indicator's role in children's brain development [33,59–61]. In several studies, the magnitude of parental education's effects on a wide range of developmental and health outcomes is weaker for Blacks than Whites [49,55,58,62–66]. As a result of MDRs, middle-class ethnic minority children remain at risk for poor developmental and health outcomes [45,67–70]. For example, high SES Black children remain at risk of anxiety [71], depression [44], poor health [62], poor school performance [72,73], and high-risk behaviors [45] such as aggression [45] and tobacco use [74,75]. Differential effects of SES across racial and ethnic groups of children are robust [49,62,63,76,77]. Data from the Fragile Families and Child Wellbeing Study (FFCWS) shows that high parental education and family income is associated with better outcomes in impulsivity, school performance, school bonding, attention-deficit/hyperactivity disorder (ADHD), obesity, aggression, depression, and self-rated health for White children than Black American children [69,77–79]. Subjective SES and parental education each impact brain imaging findings in a certain way [33,59–61]. Various SES indicators may also be the underlying mechanisms by which racial and ethnic disparities emerge in children's development [49,62,80].

At least some of the effects of high SES on school performance [81] can be attributed to the role of family SES on structure and function of the brain [33] and SES effect on memory [82–84]. Many brain structures, such as the amygdala [33,60,85], hippocampus [86], and PFC, carry the effects of SES on cognitive and behavioral outcomes. The amygdala is more involved in emotion regulation [87–91], while the hippocampus [86] and PFC [92–94] are more involved in cognitive tasks, executive function, and memory.

Aims

To investigate the complexities of social determinants of children's brain development in the US, we explored racial variation in the effects of two family SES indicators, namely parental education and household income, on working memory among 9- and 10-year-old children. We expected racial differences in the magnitude of the association between parental education on working memory, in line with the observed MDRs [36,37,45]. More specifically, we expected the weaker effects of parental education on working memory for Black than White children. This expectation is in line with the other research on a wide range of phenotypes and behaviors [36,37,45].

2. Methods

2.1. Design and Settings

This secondary analysis was a cross-sectional analysis of the baseline data of the ABCD study [95–99]. ABCD is a national, state-of-the-art brain imaging study of childhood brain development [95,100].

2.2. Participants and Sampling

The ABCD study sample was recruited from 21 cities across states. ABCD sampling was primarily through school systems. For sampling in the ABCD study, school selection was informed by race, ethnicity, sex, SES, and urbanicity [101]. Inclusion criteria were having data on our variables. Participants could be included regardless of race or ethnicity (*n* = 10,418). As this is a general population study of children, participants have been enrolled regardless of their psychopathologies. That means participants were not included or excluded from the sample based on the presence of psychopathology.

2.3. Study Variables

2.3.1. Primary Outcome

The primary outcome was working memory, measured by NIH Toolbox, the Dimensional Change Card Sort [102]. This measure [103] has shown high reliability and validity [9,104]. The NIH Toolbox card-sorting test is a part of the NIH Toolbox Cognition Battery (NIHTB-CB). This measure evaluates the executive function. The NIHTB-CB is designed for use in epidemiologic studies and clinical trials for ages 3 to 85. Some studies have documented very acceptable psychometric properties of the NIHTB-CB and card sort test. These are computer-based instruments assessing executive function: the Dimensional Change Card Sort, which measures cognitive flexibility, and a flanker task, which measures inhibitory control and selective attention. These measures show convergent and discriminant validity and correlate with SES. These measures also show excellent sensitivity to age-related changes during adulthood, excellent test-retest reliability. As a result, the Dimensional Change Card Sort can be used effectively in epidemiologic and clinical studies. Our outcome was a continuous variable in this study, with a higher score indicating higher cognitive flexibility [103,105].

2.3.2. Independent Variable

Parental Educational Attainment. Participants reported their years of schooling. This variable was operationalized as a five-level nominal variable: less than a high school diploma, high school diploma, some college, bachelor degree, graduate studies.

Household Income. Parents reported their overall annual income. This was a three-level nominal variable: <$50,000, $50,000–$100,000, and $100,000+.

2.3.3. Moderator

Race. Race was reported by parents, and operationalized as a nominal variable: Black, Asian, Other/Mixed, and White (reference group).

2.3.4. Confounders

Ethnicity. Parents were asked if they were of Latino ethnic background. This variable was coded as Latino = 1 and non-Latino = 0.

Age. Age was a dichotomous variable coded 1 or 0 for 10 years and 9 years of age. Parents reported the age of the children.

Sex. Sex was 1 for males and 0 for females.

Parental marital status. Parental marital status was 1 for married and 0 for any other condition (reference).

2.4. Data Analysis

We used SPSS for data analysis. Frequencies (n and %) and mean [standard deviations (SDs)] were reported for descriptive purposes. To estimate bivariate associations between the study variables, we used the Chi-square and Analysis of Variance (ANOVA) test in the pooled sample. To perform our multivariable analyses, we performed mixed-effects regressions. First, we tested the assumptions. We excluded collinearity between the study variables. We also tested the distribution of our outcome and error terms and quantiles (Figure 1). We ran six models. All models were performed in the pooled sample. *Model 1* to *Model 3* did not have interaction effects. *Model 1* had education but not income. *Model 2* had income but not education. *Model 3* had both education and income. *Model 4* had interactive effects of education and race but not income. *Model 5* had interactive effects of income and race. *Model 6* had interactive effects of race and education and also controlled for income. Box 1 lists our model formulas. Unstandardized regression coefficient (b), standard error (SE), and *p*-values were reported for each model. A *p*-value of equal or less than 0.05 was significant.

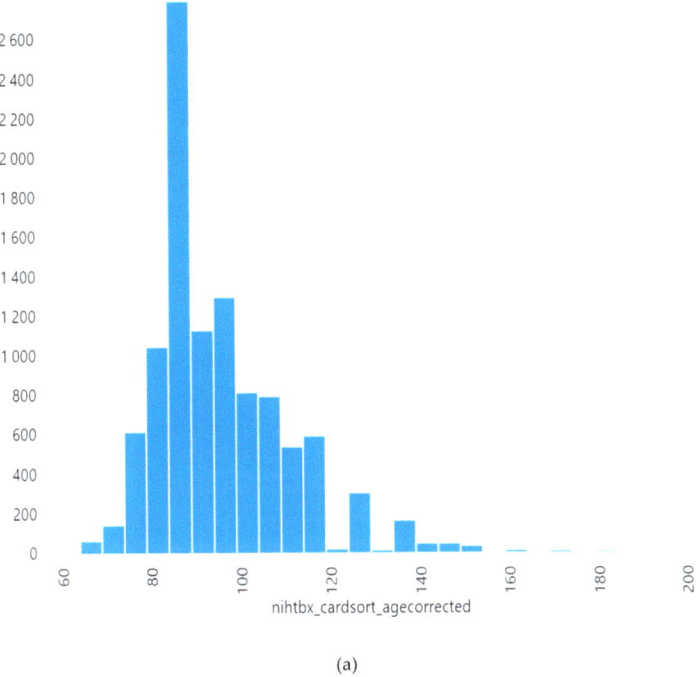

(a)

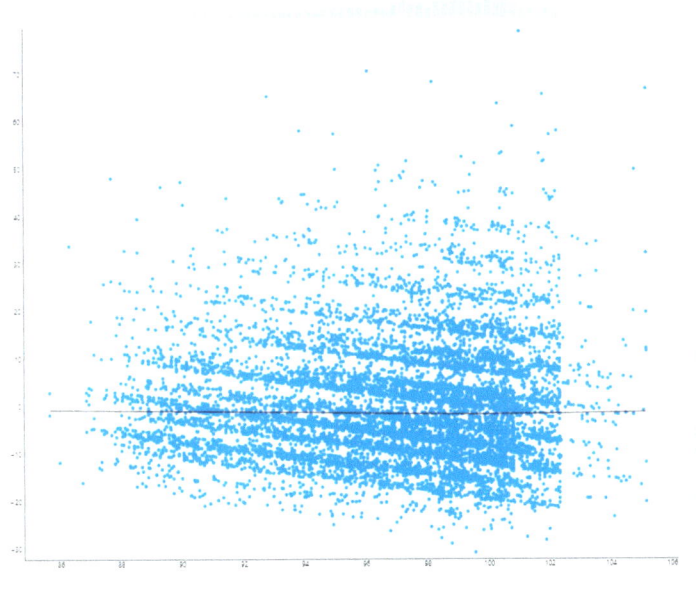

(b)

Figure 1. *Cont.*

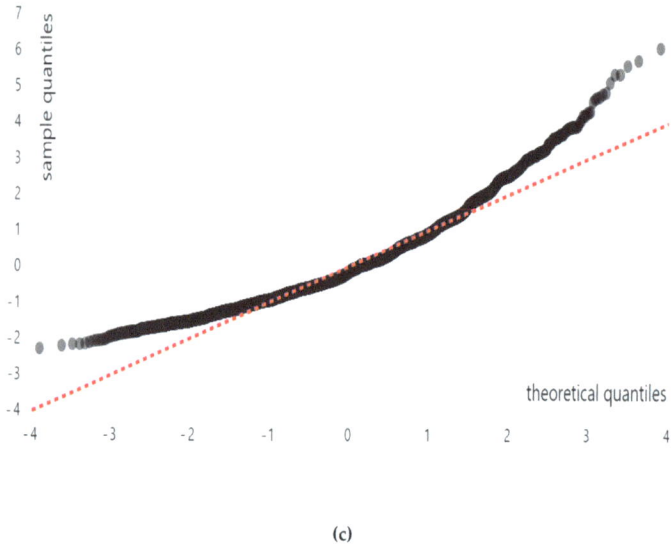

(c)

Figure 1. Testing our model's assumptions: (**a**) distribution of our outcome, (**b**) residuals, and (**c**) quantiles.

Box 1. Model Formula.

Model 1
nihtbx_cardsort_agecorrected ~ race.4level + sex + age + married.bl + hisp + high.educ.bl
Model 2
nihtbx_cardsort_agecorrected ~ + race.4level + sex + age + married.bl + hisp + household.income.bl
Model 3
nihtbx_cardsort_agecorrected ~ + race.4level + sex + age + married.bl + hisp + high.educ.bl + household.income.bl
Model 4
nihtbx_cardsort_agecorrected ~ + race.4level + sex + age + married.bl + hisp + high.educ.bl + high.educ.bl × race.4level
Model 5
nihtbx_cardsort_agecorrected ~ + race.4level + sex + age + married.bl + hisp + high.educ.bl + high.educ.bl × race.4level + household.income.bl
Model 6
nihtbx_cardsort_agecorrected~ race.4level + sex + age + married.bl + hisp + high.educ.bl + household.income.bl + high.educ.bl × race.4level
Random: ~(1|abcd_site/rel_family_id)

2.5. Ethical Aspect

Our analysis was exempt from a full review. However, the ABCD study protocol was approved by the University of California, San Diego (UCSD) Institutional Review Board (IRB) [100].

3. Results

3.1. Descriptives

The sample included 10,418 9- and 10-year-old children. Our participants were White (n = 6897; 66.2%), Black (n = 1515; 14.5%), Asian (n = 234; 2.2%), or other/mixed race (n = 1768; 17.0%). Card sorting was significantly different across racial groups. While Asian and White children had the highest card sorting scores, Black children scored worst in card sorting (Table 1).

Table 1. Presents the descriptive statistics of the pooled sample and by race.

Level	All	White	Black	Asian	Other/Mixed	p
	n = 10,414 Mean (SD)	n = 6897 Mean (SD)	n = 1515 Mean (SD)	n = 234 Mean (SD)	n = 1768 Mean (SD)	
Age (Months)	118.96 (7.46)	119.03 (7.49)	118.89 (7.23)	119.40 (7.77)	118.65 (7.51)	0.187
Card Sorting Score	97.10 (15.26)	98.29 (15.07)	91.31 (13.98)	102.36 (17.94)	96.73 (15.46)	<0.001
	n (%)	n (%)	n (%)	n (%)	n (%)	
Parental education						<0.001
<HS Diploma	385 (3.7)	145 (2.1)	123 (8.1)	6 (2.6)	111 (6.3)	
HS Diploma/GED	862 (8.3)	327 (4.7)	340 (22.4)	3 (1.3)	192 (10.9)	
Some College	2674 (25.7)	1462 (21.2)	600 (39.6)	18 (7.7)	594 (33.6)	
Bachelor	2766 (26.6)	2057 (29.8)	230 (15.2)	65 (27.8)	414 (23.4)	
Post Graduate Degree	3727 (35.8)	2906 (42.1)	222 (14.7)	142 (60.7)	457 (25.8)	
Household Income						<0.001
<50 K	2997 (28.8)	1259 (18.3)	999 (65.9)	36 (15.4)	703 (39.8)	
>= 50 K & <100 K	2974 (28.6)	2104 (30.5)	335 (22.1)	54 (23.1)	481 (27.2)	
>= 100 K	4443 (42.7)	3534 (51.2)	181 (11.9)	144 (61.5)	584 (33.0)	
Latino						<0.001
No	8451 (81.2)	5737 (83.2)	1439 (95.0)	215 (91.9)	1060 (60.0)	
Yes	1963 (18.8)	1160 (16.8)	76 (5.0)	19 (8.1)	708 (40.0)	
Sex						0.128
Female	4996 (48.0)	3254 (47.2)	760 (50.2)	117 (50.0)	865 (48.9)	
Male	5418 (52.0)	3643 (52.8)	755 (49.8)	117 (50.0)	903 (51.1)	
Married Family						<0.001
No	3165 (30.4)	1415 (20.5)	1058 (69.8)	33 (14.1)	659 (37.3)	
Yes	7249 (69.6)	5482 (79.5)	457 (30.2)	201 (85.9)	1109 (62.7)	

3.2. Regression Results

Tables 2 and 3 report the results of six pooled sample mixed-effects regression models. All models are significant. Effect sizes as shown in Table 2. *Model 1*, which only included the main effect of race and parental education and covariates, showed that high parental education is associated with higher working memory. *Model 2* showed that high income is associated with higher working memory. *Model 3* showed that parental education and household income have both associations with working memory. *Model 4* showed that parental education and race interact, meaning that parental education's boosting effect on working memory was less pronounced for Black than White children. *Model 5* did not show an interaction between race and household income. *Model 6* showed that household income explains why parental education and race interact with our outcome. (Figures 2–5).

Table 2. Effect sizes and % variance explained.

	Model 1	Model 2	Model 3	Model 4	Model 5	Model 6
n	11,315	10,418	10,414	10,418	11,315	10,414
R-squared	0.0454	0.03947	0.04545	0.03963	0.04696	0.04681
ΔR-squared	0.01244	0.00804	0.0062	0.02256	0.02922	0.01717
% Variance	1.24%	0.8%	0.62%	2.26%	2.92%	1.72%

Table 3. Mixed-effects regressions in the pooled sample ($n = 10418$).

Characteristics	b	SE	p	Sig
Model 1				
Parental Education (HS Diploma)	1.58	0.83	0.056	#
Parental Education (Some College)	2.86	0.75	<0.001	***
Parental Education (Bachelor)	4.84	0.78	<0.001	***
Parental Education (Graduate Degree)	6.69	0.77	<0.001	***
Model 2				
Household Income (50–100 K)	3.02	0.44	<0.001	***
Household Income (100 + K)	4.20	0.46	<0.001	***
Model 3				
Parental Education (HS Diploma)	0.95	0.94	0.311	
Parental Education (Some College)	2.04	0.85	0.017	*
Parental Education (Bachelor)	3.46	0.91	<0.001	***
Parental Education (Graduate Degree)	5.18	0.92	<0.001	***
Household Income (50–100 K)	2.21	0.52	<0.001	***
Household Income (100 + K)	1.88	0.47	<0.001	***
Model 4				
Household Income (50–100 K)	3.92	0.56	<0.001	***
Household Income (100 + K)	2.82	0.57	<0.001	***
Race (Black)	−4.96	0.69	<0.001	***
Race (Asian)	3.76	2.55	0.140	
Race (Other/Mixed)	−0.77	0.72	0.284	
Household Income (50–100 K) × Black	0.26	1.11	0.818	
Household Income (100 + K) × Black	0.66	1.34	0.624	
Household Income (50–100 K) × Asian	−2.18	3.27	0.505	
Household Income (100 + K) × Asian	−0.08	2.84	0.977	
Household Income (50–100 K) × Other/Mix	0.66	1.05	0.527	
Household Income (100 + K) × Other/Mix	0.86	0.99	0.385	
Model 5				
Parental Education (HS Diploma)	3.49	1.31	0.008	**
Parental Education (Some College)	3.87	1.14	0.001	***
Parental Education (Bachelor)	6.30	1.15	<0.001	***
Parental Education (Graduate Degree)	7.55	1.14	<0.001	***
Race (Black)	−1.77	1.66	0.286	
Race (Asian)	1.86	5.64	0.742	
Race (Other/Mixed)	0.49	1.64	0.768	
Parental Education (HS Diploma) × Black	−4.45	1.94	0.022	*
Parental Education (Some College) × Black	−2.44	1.77	0.169	
Parental Education (Bachelor) × Black	−3.62	1.93	0.060	#
Parental Education (Graduate Degree) × Black	−2.92	1.94	0.132	
Parental Education (HS Diploma) × Asian	−11.19	9.30	0.229	
Parental Education (Some College) × Asian	0.62	6.63	0.926	
Parental Education (Bachelor) × Asian	−1.26	5.90	0.831	
Parental Education (Graduate Degree) × Asian	1.83	5.76	0.751	
Parental Education (HS Diploma) × Other/Mix	−1.34	2.07	0.517	
Parental Education (Some College) × Other/Mix	−0.81	1.79	0.650	
Parental Education (Bachelor) × Other/Mix	−2.32	1.82	0.203	
Parental Education (Graduate Degree) × Other/Mix	0.80	1.80	0.659	
Model 6				
Parental Education (HS Diploma)	2.58	1.51	0.089	#
Parental Education (Some College)	2.80	1.35	0.038	*
Parental Education (Bachelor)	4.71	1.37	0.001	***
Parental Education (Graduate Degree)	5.86	1.37	<0.001	***
Household Income (50–100 K)	1.85	0.47	<0.001	***
Household Income (100 + K)	2.14	0.52	<0.001	***
Race (Black)	−2.34	1.89	0.216	
Race (Asian)	2.09	6.16	0.735	
Race (Other/Mixed)	0.80	1.89	0.673	

Table 3. Cont.

Characteristics	b	SE	p	Sig
Parental Education (HS Diploma) × Black	−3.60	2.20	0.101	
Parental Education (Some College) × Black	−1.23	2.01	0.542	
Parental Education (Bachelor) × Black	−2.74	2.16	0.203	
Parental Education (Graduate Degree) × Black	−1.86	2.16	0.389	
Parental Education (HS Diploma) × Asian	−10.60	10.58	0.316	
Parental Education (Some College) × Asian	0.27	7.09	0.969	
Parental Education (Bachelor) × Asian	−1.36	6.44	0.833	
Parental Education (Graduate Degree) × Asian	2.11	6.29	0.738	
Parental Education (HS Diploma) × Other/Mix	−1.16	2.33	0.620	
Parental Education (Some College) × Other/Mix	−1.00	2.03	0.621	
Parental Education (Bachelor) × Other/Mix	−2.36	2.06	0.252	
Parental Education (Graduate Degree) × Other/Mix	0.52	2.04	0.800	

\# $p < 0.1$, * $p < 0.05$, ** $p < 0.01$, *** $p < 0.001$.

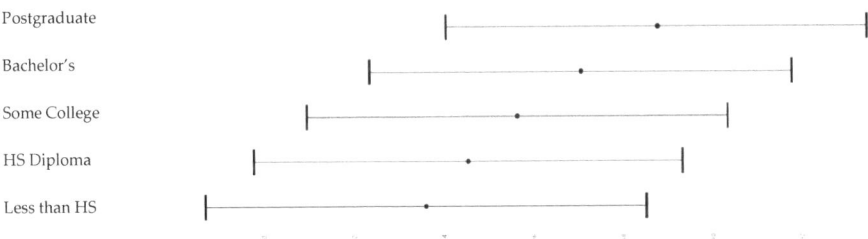

Figure 2. Parental education effects overall.

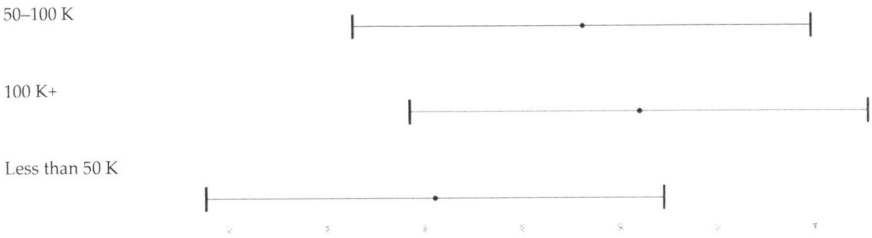

Figure 3. Income effects overall.

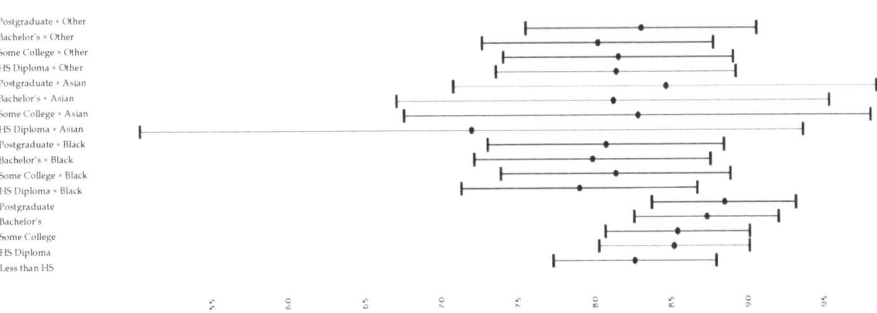

Figure 4. Parental education across groups.

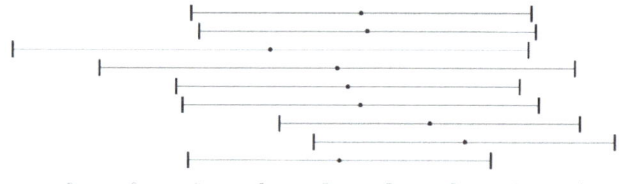

Figure 5. Income effects across groups.

4. Discussion

This study had three primary findings. Although higher parental education and household income predicted higher working memory (1st finding), parental education and household income showed weaker effects on Black children than White children's working memory (2nd finding). Third, income differentials (lower income levels of Black families with the same parental education and family structure) explain why parental education shows a weaker effect on working memory for Black than White children (3rd finding).

Our first results can be compared with the literature on the protective effects of high SES on children's cognitive outcomes [106]. A large body of literature has also documented poor educational outcomes in low SES than high SES children [107–110]. High SES is associated with better school performance [15] and working memory [16–18]. Literature has shown the effects of family SES indicators such as poverty and household income on the brain [111] and behavior [33,59–61,112]. The SES–health link may be because SES is a proxy of stress, adversities, trauma. Thus, many brain structures such as PFC, hippocampus, and amygdala [85,113–122] correlate with SES. The prefrontal cortex [33], hippocampus [86], and amygdala [123] have been shown to be under the influence of trauma. SES impacts reduced connectivity in neural networks involved in memory and emotion regulation [124]. In a recent study by Brody et al., data of 119 African American youths living in the rural South were used. The study measured poverty status and supportive parenting at ages 11–13 and 16–18. The study conducted brain imaging at age 25. This study applied resting-state fMRI to study two brain networks' functional connectivity: (1) central-executive and (2) emotion-regulation. The authors found that more years spent in poverty was associated with lower levels of connectivity in both neural networks; however, this was more robust among young adults who received low levels of supportive parenting. The study did not show an effect of income on connectivity in the presence of high levels of positive and supportive parenting [124]. In a study that analyzed data from a prospective longitudinal study of emotion development showed that lower income-to-needs ratio at preschool age was associated with reduced connectivity between hippocampus and amygdala and several regions at school age, including the cortex, lingual gyrus, posterior cingulate, and putamen. This study included preschoolers 3–5 years of age selected from the St. Louis area. Participants were followed for up to 12 years. Individuals underwent annual behavioral assessments. Participants also underwent neuroimaging at school age to measure brain resting-state functional connectivity with the left and right hippocampus and amygdala. This study showed that a lower income-to-needs ratio predicted a greater connectivity between the left hippocampus and the right superior frontal cortex and between the right amygdala and the right lingual gyrus. As this study showed, brain functional connectivity mediated the relationship between SES and depression [125]. Thus, low SES predicts reduced connectivity between the amygdala and hippocampus with brain regions, including the lingual gyrus, superior frontal cortex, posterior cingulate, as well as putamen [125]. Social adversities have cumulative (additive) effects on brain structures and functions that govern emotion regulation [85] and memory [126]; however, these effects may differ across demographic groups [60]. In part, these are due to parents' health [127] and behaviors [128].

While our first finding documented a link between SES and working memory, our second suggested that this effect differed across demographic groups. Most of the literature on the effects of race, parental education, and income on memory have focused on additive rather than multiplicative effects of SES indicators and race. Our second finding can also be seen as a reflection of the MDRs. Many studies have shown more significant effects of SES on outcomes for White than Black American children [49,62,129]. For example, family SES has shown larger effects on ADHD [79], anxiety [71], aggression [45], tobacco dependence [45], school bonding [130], school performance [73,131], obesity [69], and health [68] for White than Black American children.

As a result of our second finding, parental education shows a more salient role in shaping White's impulsivity than Black American children [67]. As a result of this pattern, higher than expected risk of poor self-rated health, obesity, poor mental health, chronic disease, impulsivity, aggression, smoking, and low school performance are observed in high SES Black American children [69,77,79]. These patterns are also called MDRs and seem robust as they hold across SES indicators, outcomes, population groups, birth cohorts, age groups, and settings [36,37]. The findings observed in this analysis, however, did not support MDRs.

As shown by this study and previous works [36], family SES differently influences Black and White children's outcomes [76,132], children [54], adults [133], and older adults [134,135]. A society is equal only if parental education [45], educational attainment [74,78,136], employment [137], marital status [63], and coping [138,139] generate equal outcomes for Blacks and Whites. Parental education seems to generate unequal effects for Blacks and Whites, a pattern that indicates inequality due to social stratification, segregation, and racism [140–149].

MDRs, differential effects of parental education across racial groups, maybe due to racial discrimination in high SES Black families. Racial and ethnic discrimination affect the amygdala's structure and function [150–155]. In a study in the US, 74 adults (43% women; 72% African American; 23% Hispanic; 32% homosexual/bisexual) reported their discrimination experience. The study also measured spontaneous amygdala activity and functional connectivity between the amygdala and other brain regions during resting-state functional magnetic resonance imaging (fMRI). In this study, greater experience of discrimination was associated with an increased level of spontaneous amygdala activity. Similarly, an increase in discrimination was associated with stronger functional connectivity between the amygdala and several neural regions such as the anterior insula, putamen, caudate, anterior cingulate, medial frontal gyrus. The most robust effect of discrimination was seen for the connectivity between the amygdala and thalamus [156]. As high SES, particularly high subjective SES, is a proxy of high not low discrimination [50–53,55–58,137], high SES Black American children still report lower than expected brain and behavior outcomes because of the effect of discrimination.

Differential effects of family SES indicators for Black and White families contribute to the transgenerational transmission of inequalities [45,67–70]. Differential effects of SES mean the same level of SES may generate unequal outcomes for the next generation, which results in the reproduction of inequalities across generations. However, most of the previous studies on MDRs have relied on self-reported outcomes. Thus, the evidence lacked biological studies that test the differential effects of SES on children's brain imaging. This paper documented complex, non-linear, multiplicative effects of SES, and race on working memory.

The observed MDRs suggest that Black American children suffer from three jeopardies. The first risk is that they live in low-SES families. The second risk is that they have worse outcomes (working memory in this study). The third jeopardy is their SES shows a weaker impact on their brain development. The weakened effect of SES for Black children suggests that it is very difficult to improve the health outcomes and close the Black-White gaps. Policymakers should not expect drastic effects as a result of their interventions. These diminishing returns are likely to be due to unique stressors in Black people's lives across all SES levels.

It should be emphasized that we see race as a social factor (as a proxy of social status, treatment by society, access to the opportunity structure, interpersonal discrimination, environmental injustices, societal obstacles, and historical injustice) on how people are treated by society. As our results suggested, race alters the implications of family SES for working memory not because Blacks are inferior or different than Whites, but because society has historically oppressed them and continues to discriminate against them. All these injustices take a toll in terms of health and development.

Our paper was on complex and multiplicative effects of social determinants on 9- and 10-year-old American children. Working memory is closely associated with executive functioning and is mainly performed in higher cortical areas, especially the prefrontal cortex (PFC) [157–159]. It is recognized that the PFC is one of the last regions of the brain to mature [157]. During preadolescence, the increase in gray matter volume is observed, especially in the PFC, among other frontal lobe regions [157]. Furthermore, it is recognized that females' brains develop about, on average two years earlier than male brains, so they are more likely to have a late developing male brain than females [157].

Limitations

All studies have some methodological and conceptual limitations. This study, which was a secondary analysis of existing data, is not an exception to this rule. Our first limitation was a cross-sectional analysis. As a result, we can only conclude associations, not causal effects. Our second limitation was a lack of inclusion of many confounders such as psychopathologies, learning disabilities, or physical health. Third, all our SES measures were reported by parents. Some measurement bias should be expected in the measurement of SES in this study. Also, the sample was not balanced regarding race and SES. Racial groups were also not comparable in their SES. Finally, brain development is behind in male than female children. This study, however, did not explore race by sex differences in social determinants of working memory. Built on intersectionality, future research may explore how groups based on the intersection of race, sex, SES, and place differ in the effects of SDoH on memory function.

5. Conclusions

Among American children, high parental education and household income correlate with better working memory. However, the effect of parental education is unequal across racial groups, with the marginal return of parental education being smaller for Black families than White people. Income, however, generates a similar outcome for Black and White families. Finally, parental education generates less outcome than the differential income of highly educated Black and White families. These findings have policy solutions for achieving equality. First, the solution to racial gaps lies beyond closing the SES inequalities. We should address barriers that interfere with the SES from generating equal outcomes for Blacks. Equalizing income may be a more effective way of equalizing outcomes than equalizing education, because more processes can interfere with the return of education than income. More research is needed on how we can equalize Black and White families for the effect of SES on brain development. Social determinants' influence on children's brain development is complicated and multiplicative rather than simple and additive. Moderated mediation and mediated moderation models are more realistic than simple additive models.

Author Contributions: G.A.: Conceptual design, first draft, and revision. S.A.: Conceptual design, data analysis, supervision, and revision. Both authors have read and agreed to the published version of the manuscript.

Funding: Author Funding: Assari received support from the following NIH grants: 2U54MD007598, U54 TR001627; CA201415-02, 5S21MD000103, R25 MD007610, 4P60MD006923, and 54MD008149. ABCD Funding: The ABCD Study is supported by the National Institutes of Health and additional federal partners under award numbers U01DA041022, U01DA041028, U01DA041048, U01DA041089, U01DA041106, U01DA041117, U01DA041120, U01DA041134, U01DA041148, U01DA041156, U01DA041174, U24DA041123, U24DA041147, U01DA041093, and U01DA041025. A full list of supporters is available at https://abcdstudy.org/federal-partners.html. A listing of participating sites and a complete listing of the study investigators can be found at https://abcdstudy.org/Consortium_Members.pdf. ABCD consortium investigators designed and implemented the study and/or provided data but did not necessarily participate in analysis or writing of this report. This manuscript reflects the views of the authors and may not reflect the opinions or views of the NIH or ABCD consortium investigators. The ABCD data repository grows and changes over time. The current paper used the Curated Annual Release 2.0, also defined in NDA Study 634 (doi:10.15154/1503209).

Conflicts of Interest: The authors declare no conflict of interest.

References

1. Baddeley, A.D.; Logie, R.H. *Working Memory: The Multiple-Component Model*; Cambridge University Press: Cambridge, UK, 1999.
2. Baddeley, A.D.; Hitch, G. Working memory. In *Psychology of Learning and Motivation*; Elsevier: Amsterdam, The Netherlands, 1974; Volume 8, pp. 47–89.
3. Gathercole, S.E.; Baddeley, A.D. *Working Memory and Language*; Psychology Press: New York, NY, USA, 2014.
4. Braver, T.S.; Cohen, J.D.; Nystrom, L.E.; Jonides, J.; Smith, E.E.; Noll, D.C. A parametric study of prefrontal cortex involvement in human working memory. *Neuroimage* **1997**, *5*, 49–62. [CrossRef] [PubMed]
5. Vandenbroucke, L.; Verschueren, K.; Desoete, A.; Aunio, P.; Ghesquière, P.; Baeyens, D. Crossing the bridge to elementary school: The development of children's working memory components in relation to teacher-student relationships and academic achievement. *Early Child. Res. Q.* **2018**, *42*, 1–10. [CrossRef]
6. Owens, M.; Stevenson, J.; Hadwin, J.A.; Norgate, R. Anxiety and depression in academic performance: An exploration of the mediating factors of worry and working memory. *Sch. Psychol. Int.* **2012**, *33*, 433–449. [CrossRef]
7. Dehn, M.J. *Working Memory and Academic Learning: Assessment and Intervention*; John Wiley & Sons: Hoboken, NJ, USA, 2011.
8. Lara, A.H.; Wallis, J.D. The role of prefrontal cortex in working memory: A mini review. *Front. Syst. Neurosci.* **2015**, *9*, 173. [CrossRef] [PubMed]
9. Zelazo, P.D.; Anderson, J.E.; Richler, J.; Wallner-Allen, K.; Beaumont, J.L.; Conway, K.P.; Gershon, R.; Weintraub, S. NIH toolbox cognition battery (CB): Validation of executive function measures in adults. *J. Int. Neuropsychol. Soc. JINS* **2014**, *20*, 620. [CrossRef]
10. Zelazo, P.D. The dimensional change card sort (DCCS): A method of assessing executive function in children. *Nat. Protoc.* **2006**, *1*, 297–301. [CrossRef]
11. Miller, E.K.; Cohen, J.D. An integrative theory of prefrontal cortex function. *Annu. Rev. Neurosci.* **2001**, *24*, 167–202. [CrossRef]
12. Zelazo, P.; Muller, U.; Goswami, U. *Handbook of Childhood Cognitive Development*; Blackwell: Oxford, UK, 2002.
13. Rosas, R.; Espinoza, V.; Porflitt, F.; Ceric, F. Executive functions can be improved in preschoolers through systematic playing in educational settings: Evidence from a longitudinal study. *Front. Psychol.* **2019**, *10*, 2024. [CrossRef]
14. Cowan, N. Evolving conceptions of memory storage, selective attention, and their mutual constraints within the human information-processing system. *Psychol. Bull.* **1988**, *104*, 163. [CrossRef]
15. Alexander, K.L.; Entwisle, D.R.; Bedinger, S.D. When expectations work: Race and socioeconomic differences in school performance. *Soc. Psychol. Q.* **1994**, *57*, 283–299. [CrossRef]
16. Engel, P.M.J.; Santos, F.H.; Gathercole, S.E. Are working memory measures free of socioeconomic influence? *J. Speech Lang. Hear. Res.* **2008**, *51*, 1580–1587. [CrossRef]
17. Sturge-Apple, M.L.; Suor, J.H.; Skibo, M.A. Maternal child-centered attributions and harsh discipline: The moderating role of maternal working memory across socioeconomic contexts. *J. Fam. Psychol.* **2014**, *28*, 645. [CrossRef] [PubMed]
18. Hackman, D.A.; Betancourt, L.M.; Gallop, R.; Romer, D.; Brodsky, N.L.; Hurt, H.; Farah, M.J. Mapping the trajectory of socioeconomic disparity in working memory: Parental and neighborhood factors. *Child Dev.* **2014**, *85*, 1433–1445. [CrossRef] [PubMed]
19. Oshri, A.; Hallowell, E.; Liu, S.; MacKillop, J.; Galvan, A.; Kogan, S.M.; Sweet, L.H. Socioeconomic hardship and delayed reward discounting: Associations with working memory and emotional reactivity. *Dev. Cogn. Neurosci.* **2019**, *37*, 100642. [CrossRef] [PubMed]
20. Sirin, S.R. Socioeconomic status and academic achievement: A meta-analytic review of research. *Rev. Educ. Res.* **2005**, *75*, 417–453. [CrossRef]
21. Mendelson, T.; Kubzansky, L.D.; Datta, G.D.; Buka, S.L. Relation of female gender and low socioeconomic status to internalizing symptoms among adolescents: A case of double jeopardy? *Soc. Sci. Med.* **2008**, *66*, 1284–1296. [CrossRef]

22. Yildiz, M.; Demirhan, E.; Gurbuz, S. Contextual socioeconomic disadvantage and adolescent suicide attempts: A multilevel investigation. *J. Youth Adolesc.* **2019**, *48*, 802–814. [CrossRef]
23. Eisenberg, D.; Gollust, S.E.; Golberstein, E.; Hefner, J.L. Prevalence and correlates of depression, anxiety, and suicidality among university students. *Am. J. Orthopsychiatry* **2007**, *77*, 534–542. [CrossRef]
24. Kaleta, D.; Usidame, B.; Dziankowska-Zaborszczyk, E.; Makowiec-Dabrowska, T. Socioeconomic disparities in age of initiation and ever tobacco smoking: Findings from Romania. *Cent. Eur. J. Public Health* **2015**, *23*, 299–305. [CrossRef] [PubMed]
25. Barreto, S.M.; de Figueiredo, R.C.; Giatti, L. Socioeconomic inequalities in youth smoking in Brazil. *BMJ Open* **2013**, *3*, e003538. [CrossRef]
26. Yaple, Z.A.; Yu, R. Functional and structural brain correlates of socioeconomic status. *Cereb. Cortex* **2019**. [CrossRef]
27. Assari, S.; Bazargan, M. Unequal associations between educational attainment and occupational stress across racial and ethnic groups. *Int. J. Environ. Res. Public Health* **2019**, *16*, 3539. [CrossRef] [PubMed]
28. Assari, S.; Bazargan, M. Second-hand exposure home second-hand smoke exposure at home in the united states; Minorities' diminished returns. *Int. J. Travel Med. Glob. Health* **2019**, *7*, 135. [CrossRef] [PubMed]
29. Assari, S.; Bazargan, M. Unequal effects of educational attainment on workplace exposure to second-hand smoke by race and ethnicity; Minorities' diminished returns in the national health interview survey (NHIS). *J. Med. Res. Innov.* **2019**, *3*. [CrossRef]
30. Chassin, L.; Presson, C.C.; Sherman, S.J.; Edwards, D.A. Parent educational attainment and adolescent cigarette smoking. *J. Subst. Abus.* **1992**, *4*, 219–234. [CrossRef]
31. Kocaoglu, B.; Moschonis, G.; Dimitriou, M.; Kolotourou, M.; Keskin, Y.; Sur, H.; Hayran, O.; Manios, Y. Parental educational level and cardiovascular disease risk factors in schoolchildren in large urban areas of Turkey: Directions for public health policy. *BMC Public Health* **2005**, *5*, 13. [CrossRef] [PubMed]
32. Padilla-Moledo, C.; Ruiz, J.R.; Castro-Pinero, J. Parental educational level and psychological positive health and health complaints in Spanish children and adolescents. *Child. Care Health Dev.* **2016**, *42*, 534–543. [CrossRef]
33. Javanbakht, A.; King, A.P.; Evans, G.W.; Swain, J.E.; Angstadt, M.; Phan, K.L.; Liberzon, I. Childhood poverty predicts adult amygdala and frontal activity and connectivity in response to emotional faces. *Front. Behav. Neurosci.* **2015**, *9*, 154. [CrossRef]
34. Masten, C.L.; Telzer, E.H.; Eisenberger, N.I. An FMRI investigation of attributing negative social treatment to racial discrimination. *J. Cogn. Neurosci.* **2011**, *23*, 1042–1051. [CrossRef]
35. Wu, X.; Zou, Q.; Hu, J.; Tang, W.; Mao, Y.; Gao, L.; Zhu, J.; Jin, Y.; Wu, X.; Lu, L.; et al. Intrinsic functional connectivity patterns predict consciousness level and recovery outcome in acquired brain injury. *J. Neurosci.* **2015**, *35*, 12932–12946. [CrossRef]
36. Assari, S. Unequal gain of equal resources across racial groups. *Int. J. Health Policy Manag.* **2017**, *7*, 1–9. [CrossRef] [PubMed]
37. Assari, S. Health disparities due to diminished return among black Americans: Public policy solutions. *Soc. Issues Policy Rev.* **2018**, *12*, 112–145. [CrossRef]
38. Spera, C.; Wentzel, K.R.; Matto, H.C. Parental aspirations for their children's educational attainment: Relations to ethnicity, parental education, children's academic performance, and parental perceptions of school climate. *J. Youth Adolesc.* **2009**, *38*, 1140–1152. [CrossRef] [PubMed]
39. Goodman, E.; Slap, G.B.; Huang, B. The public health impact of socioeconomic status on adolescent depression and obesity. *Am. J. Public Health* **2003**, *93*, 1844–1850. [CrossRef] [PubMed]
40. Morris, A.S.; Silk, J.S.; Steinberg, L.; Myers, S.S.; Robinson, L.R. The role of the family context in the development of emotion regulation. *Soc. Dev.* **2007**, *16*, 361–388. [CrossRef] [PubMed]
41. Park, S.; Holloway, S.D. No parent left behind: Predicting parental involvement in adolescents' education within a sociodemographically diverse population. *J. Educ. Res.* **2013**, *106*, 105–119. [CrossRef]
42. Pabayo, R.; Molnar, B.E.; Kawachi, I. The role of neighborhood income inequality in adolescent aggression and violence. *J. Adolesc. Health* **2014**, *55*, 571–579. [CrossRef]
43. Wills, T.A.; McNamara, G.; Vaccaro, D. Parental education related to adolescent stress-coping and substance use: Development of a mediational model. *Health Psychol.* **1995**, *14*, 464. [CrossRef]
44. Assari, S.; Caldwell, C.H. High risk of depression in high-income African American boys. *J. Racial Ethn. Health Dispar.* **2018**, *5*, 808–819. [CrossRef]

45. Assari, S.; Caldwell, C.H.; Bazargan, M. Association between parental educational attainment and youth outcomes and role of race/ethnicity. *JAMA Netw. Open* **2019**, *2*, e1916018. [CrossRef]
46. Assari, S.; Boyce, S.; Bazargan, M.; Caldwell, C.H. Diminished Returns of Parental Education in Terms of Youth School Performance: Ruling out Regression toward the Mean. *Children* **2020**, *7*, 74. [CrossRef] [PubMed]
47. Assari, S. Parental education and spanking of American children: Blacks' diminished returns. *World J. Educ. Res.* **2020**, *7*, 19–44. [CrossRef] [PubMed]
48. Assari, S. American Children's Screen Time: Diminished Returns of Household Income in Black Families. *Information* **2020**, *11*, 538. [CrossRef]
49. Assari, S. Parental education attainment and educational upward mobility; Role of race and gender. *Behav. Sci.* **2018**, *8*, 107. [CrossRef]
50. Assari, S.; Preiser, B.; Lankarani, M.M.; Caldwell, C.H. Subjective socioeconomic status moderates the association between discrimination and depression in African American youth. *Brain Sci.* **2018**, *8*, 71. [CrossRef] [PubMed]
51. Assari, S. Does School racial composition explain why high income black youth perceive more discrimination? A gender analysis. *Brain Sci.* **2018**, *8*, 140. [CrossRef]
52. Assari, S.; Moghani Lankarani, M. Workplace racial composition explains high perceived discrimination of high socioeconomic status African American men. *Brain Sci.* **2018**, *8*, 139. [CrossRef]
53. Assari, S.; Gibbons, F.X.; Simons, R.L. Perceived discrimination among black youth: An 18-year longitudinal study. *Behav. Sci.* **2018**, *8*, 44. [CrossRef]
54. Assari, S.; Gibbons, F.X.; Simons, R. Depression among black youth; Interaction of class and place. *Brain Sci.* **2018**, *8*, 108. [CrossRef]
55. Hudson, D.L.; Bullard, K.M.; Neighbors, H.W.; Geronimus, A.T.; Yang, J.; Jackson, J.S. Are benefits conferred with greater socioeconomic position undermined by racial discrimination among African American men? *J. Mens. Health* **2012**, *9*, 127–136. [CrossRef]
56. Hudson, D.L.; Puterman, E.; Bibbins-Domingo, K.; Matthews, K.A.; Adler, N.E. Race, life course socioeconomic position, racial discrimination, depressive symptoms and self-rated health. *Soc. Sci. Med.* **2013**, *97*, 7–14. [CrossRef] [PubMed]
57. Hudson, D.L.; Neighbors, H.W.; Geronimus, A.T.; Jackson, J.S. Racial discrimination, John Henryism, and depression among African Americans. *J. Black Psychol.* **2016**, *42*, 221–243. [CrossRef] [PubMed]
58. Assari, S.; Lankarani, M.M.; Caldwell, C.H. Does discrimination explain high risk of depression among high-income African American men? *Behav. Sci.* **2018**, *8*, 40. [CrossRef]
59. D'Angiulli, A.; Lipina, S.J.; Olesinska, A. Explicit and implicit issues in the developmental cognitive neuroscience of social inequality. *Front. Hum. Neurosci.* **2012**, *6*, 254. [CrossRef] [PubMed]
60. Javanbakht, A.; Kim, P.; Swain, J.E.; Evans, G.W.; Phan, K.L.; Liberzon, I. Sex-specific effects of childhood poverty on neurocircuitry of processing of emotional cues: A neuroimaging study. *Behav. Sci.* **2016**, *6*, 28. [CrossRef] [PubMed]
61. Kim, P.; Evans, G.W.; Angstadt, M.; Ho, S.S.; Sripada, C.S.; Swain, J.E.; Liberzon, I.; Phan, K.L. Effects of childhood poverty and chronic stress on emotion regulatory brain function in adulthood. *Proc. Natl. Acad. Sci. USA* **2013**, *110*, 18442–18447. [CrossRef] [PubMed]
62. Assari, S. Parental educational attainment and mental well-being of college students; Diminished returns of blacks. *Brain Sci.* **2018**, *8*, 193. [CrossRef] [PubMed]
63. Assari, S. Race, intergenerational social mobility and stressful life events. *Behav. Sci.* **2018**, *8*, 86. [CrossRef]
64. Fuller-Rowell, T.E.; Doan, S.N. The social costs of academic success across ethnic groups. *Child. Dev.* **2010**, *81*, 1696–1713. [CrossRef]
65. Fuller-Rowell, T.E.; Curtis, D.S.; Doan, S.N.; Coe, C.L. Racial disparities in the health benefits of educational attainment: A study of inflammatory trajectories among African American and white adults. *Psychosom. Med.* **2015**, *77*, 33–40. [CrossRef]
66. Hudson, D.L.; Neighbors, H.W.; Geronimus, A.T.; Jackson, J.S. The relationship between socioeconomic position and depression among a US nationally representative sample of African Americans. *Soc. Psychiatry Psychiatr. Epidemiol.* **2012**, *47*, 373–381. [CrossRef]
67. Assari, S.; Caldwell, C.H.; Mincy, R. Family socioeconomic status at birth and youth impulsivity at age 15; Blacks' diminished return. *Child* **2018**, *5*, 58. [CrossRef]

68. Assari, S.; Caldwell, C.H.; Mincy, R.B. Maternal educational attainment at birth promotes future self-rated health of white but not black youth: A 15-year cohort of a national sample. *J. Clin. Med.* **2018**, *7*, 93. [CrossRef] [PubMed]
69. Assari, S.; Thomas, A.; Caldwell, C.H.; Mincy, R.B. Blacks' diminished health return of family structure and socioeconomic status; 15 years of follow-up of a national urban sample of youth. *J. Urban Health* **2018**, *95*, 21–35. [CrossRef] [PubMed]
70. Assari, S.; Boyce, S.; Bazargan, M.; Mincy, R.; Caldwell, C.H. Unequal protective effects of parental educational attainment on the body mass index of black and white youth. *Int. J. Environ. Res. Public Health* **2019**, *16*, 3641. [CrossRef] [PubMed]
71. Assari, S.; Caldwell, C.H.; Zimmerman, M.A. Family structure and subsequent anxiety symptoms; Minorities' diminished return. *Brain Sci.* **2018**, *8*, 97. [CrossRef]
72. Assari, S. Mental Rotation in American Children: Diminished Returns of Parental Education in Black Families. *Pediatr. Rep.* **2020**, *12*, 130–141. [CrossRef]
73. Assari, S.; Caldwell, C.H. Parental educational attainment differentially boosts school performance of American adolescents: Minorities' diminished returns. *J. Fam. Reprod. Health* **2019**, *13*, 7–13. [CrossRef]
74. Assari, S.; Mistry, R. Educational attainment and smoking status in a national sample of American adults; Evidence for the blacks' diminished return. *Int. J. Env. Res. Public Health* **2018**, *15*, 763. [CrossRef]
75. Assari, S.; Mistry, R.; Bazargan, M. Race, educational attainment, and e-cigarette use. *J. Med. Res. Innov.* **2020**, *4*, e000185. [CrossRef]
76. Assari, S.; Moghani Lankarani, M. Poverty status and childhood asthma in white and black families: National survey of children's health. *Healthcare* **2018**, *6*, 62. [CrossRef] [PubMed]
77. Assari, S. Multiplicative effects of social and psychological risk factors on college students' suicidal behaviors. *Brain Sci.* **2018**, *8*, 91. [CrossRef] [PubMed]
78. Assari, S. Socioeconomic status and self-rated oral health; Diminished return among Hispanic whites. *Dent. J.* **2018**, *6*, 11. [CrossRef] [PubMed]
79. Assari, S.; Caldwell, C.H. Family income at birth and risk of attention deficit hyperactivity disorder at age 15: Racial differences. *Children* **2019**, *6*, 10. [CrossRef] [PubMed]
80. Assari, S. Parental education better helps white than black families escape poverty: National survey of children's health. *Economies* **2018**, *6*, 30. [CrossRef]
81. Sackett, P.R.; Kuncel, N.R.; Arneson, J.J.; Cooper, S.R.; Waters, S.D. Does socioeconomic status explain the relationship between admissions tests and post-secondary academic performance? *Psychol. Bull.* **2009**, *135*, 1. [CrossRef]
82. Brito, N.H.; Fifer, W.P.; Myers, M.M.; Elliott, A.J.; Noble, K.G. Associations among family socioeconomic status, EEG power at birth, and cognitive skills during infancy. *Dev. Cogn. Neurosci.* **2016**, *19*, 144–151. [CrossRef]
83. Last, B.S.; Lawson, G.M.; Breiner, K.; Steinberg, L.; Farah, M.J. Childhood socioeconomic status and executive function in childhood and beyond. *PLoS ONE* **2018**, *13*, e0202964. [CrossRef]
84. Moorman, S.M.; Carr, K.; Greenfield, E.A. Childhood socioeconomic status and genetic risk for poorer cognition in later life. *Soc. Sci. Med.* **2018**, *212*, 219–226. [CrossRef]
85. Evans, G.W.; Swain, J.E.; King, A.P.; Wang, X.; Javanbakht, A.; Ho, S.S.; Angstadt, M.; Phan, K.L.; Xie, H.; Liberzon, I. Childhood cumulative risk exposure and adult amygdala volume and function. *J. Neurosci. Res.* **2016**, *94*, 535–543. [CrossRef]
86. Assari, S.; Boyce, S.; Bazargan, M.; Caldwell, C.H. Family income mediates the effect of parental education on adolescents' hippocampus activation during an n-back memory task. *Brain Sci.* **2020**, *10*, 520. [CrossRef] [PubMed]
87. Dotterer, H.L.; Hyde, L.W.; Swartz, J.R.; Hariri, A.R.; Williamson, D.E. Amygdala reactivity predicts adolescent antisocial behavior but not callous-unemotional traits. *Dev. Cogn. Neurosci.* **2017**, *24*, 84–92. [CrossRef] [PubMed]
88. Gard, A.M.; Waller, R.; Swartz, J.R.; Shaw, D.S.; Forbes, E.E.; Hyde, L.W. Amygdala functional connectivity during socioemotional processing prospectively predicts increases in internalizing symptoms in a sample of low-income, urban, young men. *Neuroimage* **2018**, *178*, 562–573. [CrossRef] [PubMed]

89. Morawetz, C.; Bode, S.; Baudewig, J.; Heekeren, H.R. Effective amygdala-prefrontal connectivity predicts individual differences in successful emotion regulation. *Soc. Cogn. Affect. Neurosci.* **2017**, *12*, 569–585. [CrossRef] [PubMed]
90. Szczepanik, J.; Nugent, A.C.; Drevets, W.C.; Khanna, A.; Zarate, C.A., Jr.; Furey, M.L. Amygdala response to explicit sad face stimuli at baseline predicts antidepressant treatment response to scopolamine in major depressive disorder. *Psychiatry Res. Neuroimaging* **2016**, *254*, 67–73. [CrossRef]
91. Venta, A.; Sharp, C.; Patriquin, M.; Salas, R.; Newlin, E.; Curtis, K.; Baldwin, P.; Fowler, C.; Frueh, B.C. Amygdala-frontal connectivity predicts internalizing symptom recovery among inpatient adolescents. *J. Affect. Disord.* **2018**, *225*, 453–459. [CrossRef]
92. Lei, Y.; Su, J.; Jiang, H.; Guo, Q.; Ni, W.; Yang, H.; Gu, Y.; Mao, Y. Aberrant regional homogeneity of resting-state executive control, default mode, and salience networks in adult patients with moyamoya disease. *Brain Imaging. Behav.* **2017**, *11*, 176–184. [CrossRef]
93. Rougemont-Bucking, A.; Linnman, C.; Zeffiro, T.A.; Zeidan, M.A.; Lebron-Milad, K.; Rodriguez-Romaguera, J.; Rauch, S.L.; Pitman, R.K.; Milad, M.R. Altered processing of contextual information during fear extinction in PTSD: An fMRI study. *CNS Neurosci.* **2011**, *17*, 227–236. [CrossRef]
94. Reijmer, Y.D.; Schultz, A.P.; Leemans, A.; O'Sullivan, M.J.; Gurol, M.E.; Sperling, R.; Greenberg, S.M.; Viswanathan, A.; Hedden, T. Decoupling of structural and functional brain connectivity in older adults with white matter hyperintensities. *Neuroimage* **2015**, *117*, 222–229. [CrossRef]
95. Alcohol Research: Current Reviews Editorial Staff. NIH's adolescent brain cognitive development (ABCD) study. *Alcohol Res.* **2018**, *39*, 97.
96. Casey, B.J.; Cannonier, T.; Conley, M.I.; Cohen, A.O.; Barch, D.M.; Heitzeg, M.M.; Soules, M.E.; Teslovich, T.; Dellarco, D.V.; Garavan, H.; et al. The adolescent brain cognitive development (ABCD) study: Imaging acquisition across 21 sites. *Dev. Cogn. Neurosci.* **2018**, *32*, 43–54. [CrossRef] [PubMed]
97. Karcher, N.R.; O'Brien, K.J.; Kandala, S.; Barch, D.M. Resting-state functional connectivity and psychotic-like experiences in childhood: Results from the adolescent brain cognitive development study. *Biol. Psychiatry* **2019**, *86*, 7–15. [CrossRef]
98. Lisdahl, K.M.; Sher, K.J.; Conway, K.P.; Gonzalez, R.; Feldstein Ewing, S.W.; Nixon, S.J.; Tapert, S.; Bartsch, H.; Goldstein, R.Z.; Heitzeg, M. Adolescent brain cognitive development (ABCD) study: Overview of substance use assessment methods. *Dev. Cogn. Neurosci.* **2018**, *32*, 80–96. [CrossRef] [PubMed]
99. Luciana, M.; Bjork, J.M.; Nagel, B.J.; Barch, D.M.; Gonzalez, R.; Nixon, S.J.; Banich, M.T. Adolescent neurocognitive development and impacts of substance use: Overview of the adolescent brain cognitive development (ABCD) baseline neurocognition battery. *Dev. Cogn. Neurosci.* **2018**, *32*, 67–79. [CrossRef]
100. Auchter, A.M.; Hernandez Mejia, M.; Heyser, C.J.; Shilling, P.D.; Jernigan, T.L.; Brown, S.A.; Tapert, S.F.; Dowling, G.J. A description of the ABCD organizational structure and communication framework. *Dev. Cogn. Neurosci.* **2018**, *32*, 8–15. [CrossRef]
101. Garavan, H.; Bartsch, H.; Conway, K.; Decastro, A.; Goldstein, R.Z.; Heeringa, S.; Jernigan, T.; Potter, A.; Thompson, W.; Zahs, D. Recruiting the ABCD sample: Design considerations and procedures. *Dev. Cogn. Neurosci.* **2018**, *32*, 16–22. [CrossRef] [PubMed]
102. Tulsky, D.S.; Carlozzi, N.; Chiaravalloti, N.D.; Beaumont, J.L.; Kisala, P.A.; Mungas, D.; Conway, K.; Gershon, R. NIH toolbox cognition battery (NIHTB-CB): The list sorting test to measure working memory. *J. Int. Neuropsychol. Soc. JINS* **2014**, *20*, 599. [CrossRef]
103. Heaton, R.K.; Akshoomoff, N.; Tulsky, D.; Mungas, D.; Weintraub, S.; Dikmen, S.; Beaumont, J.; Casaletto, K.B.; Conway, K.; Slotkin, J. Reliability and validity of composite scores from the NIH toolbox cognition battery in adults. *J. Int. Neuropsychol. Soc. JINS* **2014**, *20*, 588. [CrossRef]
104. Hessl, D.; Sansone, S.M.; Berry-Kravis, E.; Riley, K.; Widaman, K.F.; Abbeduto, L.; Schneider, A.; Coleman, J.; Oaklander, D.; Rhodes, K.C. The NIH toolbox cognitive battery for intellectual disabilities: Three preliminary studies and future directions. *J. Neurodev. Disord.* **2016**, *8*, 35. [CrossRef]
105. Weintraub, S.; Dikmen, S.S.; Heaton, R.K.; Tulsky, D.S.; Zelazo, P.D.; Bauer, P.J.; Carlozzi, N.E.; Slotkin, J.; Blitz, D.; Wallner-Allen, K. Cognition assessment using the NIH toolbox. *Neurology* **2013**, *80*, S54–S64. [CrossRef]
106. Roberts, E.; Bornstein, M.H.; Slater, A.M.; Barrett, J. Early cognitive development and parental education. *Infant Child Dev. Int. J. Res. Pract.* **1999**, *8*, 49–62. [CrossRef]

107. Grant, M.D.; Kremen, W.S.; Jacobson, K.C.; Franz, C.; Xian, H.; Eisen, S.A.; Toomey, R.; Murray, R.E.; Lyons, M.J. Does parental education have a moderating effect on the genetic and environmental influences of general cognitive ability in early adulthood? *Behav. Genet.* **2010**, *40*, 438–446. [CrossRef] [PubMed]
108. Parisi, P.; Verrotti, A.; Paolino, M.C.; Miano, S.; Urbano, A.; Bernabucci, M.; Villa, M.P. Cognitive profile, parental education and BMI in children: Reflections on common neuroendrocrinobiological roots. *J. Pediatric Endocrinol. Metab.* **2010**, *23*, 1133–1141. [CrossRef] [PubMed]
109. Barnett, W.S. Long-term cognitive and academic effects of early childhood education on children in poverty. *Prev. Med.* **1998**, *27*, 204–207. [CrossRef] [PubMed]
110. Barajas, R.G.; Philipsen, N.; Brooks-Gunn, J. Cognitive and emotional outcomes for children in poverty. In *Handbook of Families and Poverty*; Sage: Thousand Oaks, CA, USA, 2007; pp. 311–333.
111. Finn, A.S.; Minas, J.E.; Leonard, J.A.; Mackey, A.P.; Salvatore, J.; Goetz, C.; West, M.R.; Gabrieli, C.F.O.; Gabrieli, J.D.E. Functional brain organization of working memory in adolescents varies in relation to family income and academic achievement. *Dev. Sci.* **2017**, *20*. [CrossRef] [PubMed]
112. Silverman, M.E.; Muennig, P.; Liu, X.; Rosen, Z.; Goldstein, M.A. The impact of socioeconomic status on the neural substrates associated with pleasure. *Open Neuroimag. J.* **2009**, *3*, 58–63. [CrossRef]
113. Calem, M.; Bromis, K.; McGuire, P.; Morgan, C.; Kempton, M.J. Meta-analysis of associations between childhood adversity and hippocampus and amygdala volume in non-clinical and general population samples. *Neuroimage. Clin.* **2017**, *14*, 471–479. [CrossRef]
114. Gianaros, P.J.; Sheu, L.K.; Matthews, K.A.; Jennings, J.R.; Manuck, S.B.; Hariri, A.R. Individual differences in stressor-evoked blood pressure reactivity vary with activation, volume, and functional connectivity of the amygdala. *J. Neurosci.* **2008**, *28*, 990–999. [CrossRef]
115. Gilliam, M.; Forbes, E.E.; Gianaros, P.J.; Erickson, K.I.; Brennan, L.M.; Shaw, D.S. Maternal depression in childhood and aggression in young adulthood: Evidence for mediation by offspring amygdala-hippocampal volume ratio. *J. Child Psychol. Psychiatry.* **2015**, *56*, 1083–1091. [CrossRef]
116. Merz, E.C.; Tottenham, N.; Noble, K.G. Socioeconomic status, amygdala volume, and internalizing symptoms in children and adolescents. *J. Clin. Child Adolesc. Psychol.* **2018**, *47*, 312–323. [CrossRef]
117. Morey, R.A.; Haswell, C.C.; Hooper, S.R.; De Bellis, M.D. Amygdala, hippocampus, and ventral medial prefrontal cortex volumes differ in maltreated youth with and without chronic posttraumatic stress disorder. *Neuropsychopharmacology* **2016**, *41*, 791–801. [CrossRef] [PubMed]
118. Rojas, D.C.; Smith, J.A.; Benkers, T.L.; Camou, S.L.; Reite, M.L.; Rogers, S.J. Hippocampus and amygdala volumes in parents of children with autistic disorder. *Am. J. Psychiatry* **2004**, *161*, 2038–2044. [CrossRef] [PubMed]
119. Taren, A.A.; Creswell, J.D.; Gianaros, P.J. Dispositional mindfulness co-varies with smaller amygdala and caudate volumes in community adults. *PLoS ONE* **2013**, *8*, e64574. [CrossRef]
120. Assari, S.; Boyce, S.; Bazargan, M. Subjective Socioeconomic Status and Children's Amygdala Volume: Minorities' Diminish Returns. *NeuroSci* **2020**, *1*, 59–74. [CrossRef] [PubMed]
121. Trotman, G.P.; Gianaros, P.J.; Veldhuijzen van Zanten, J.; Williams, S.E.; Ginty, A.T. Increased stressor-evoked cardiovascular reactivity is associated with reduced amygdala and hippocampus volume. *Psychophysiology* **2019**, *56*, e13277. [CrossRef]
122. Walton, E.; Cecil, C.A.M.; Suderman, M.; Liu, J.; Turner, J.A.; Calhoun, V.; Ehrlich, S.; Relton, C.L.; Barker, E.D. Longitudinal epigenetic predictors of amygdala:hippocampus volume ratio. *J. Child Psychol. Psychiatry* **2017**, *58*, 1341–1350. [CrossRef]
123. Tottenham, N.; Hare, T.A.; Quinn, B.T.; McCarry, T.W.; Nurse, M.; Gilhooly, T.; Millner, A.; Galvan, A.; Davidson, M.C.; Eigsti, I.M. Prolonged institutional rearing is associated with atypically large amygdala volume and difficulties in emotion regulation. *Dev. Sci.* **2010**, *13*, 46–61. [CrossRef]
124. Brody, G.H.; Yu, T.; Nusslock, R.; Barton, A.W.; Miller, G.E.; Chen, E.; Holmes, C.; McCormick, M.; Sweet, L.H. The protective effects of supportive parenting on the relationship between adolescent poverty and resting-state functional brain connectivity during adulthood. *Psychol. Sci.* **2019**. [CrossRef]
125. Barch, D.; Pagliaccio, D.; Belden, A.; Harms, M.P.; Gaffrey, M.; Sylvester, C.M.; Tillman, R.; Luby, J. Effect of hippocampal and amygdala connectivity on the relationship between preschool poverty and school-age depression. *Am. J. Psychiatry* **2016**, *173*, 625–634. [CrossRef]
126. Qian, W.; Schweizer, T.A.; Fischer, C.E. Impact of socioeconomic status on initial clinical presentation to a memory disorders clinic. *Int. Psychogeriatr.* **2014**, *26*, 597–603. [CrossRef]

127. Lupien, S.J.; Parent, S.; Evans, A.C.; Tremblay, R.E.; Zelazo, P.D.; Corbo, V.; Pruessner, J.C.; Séguin, J.R. Larger amygdala but no change in hippocampal volume in 10-year-old children exposed to maternal depressive symptomatology since birth. *Proc. Natl. Acad. Sci. USA* **2011**, *108*, 14324–14329. [CrossRef]
128. Moutsiana, C.; Johnstone, T.; Murray, L.; Fearon, P.; Cooper, P.J.; Pliatsikas, C.; Goodyer, I.; Halligan, S.L. Insecure attachment during infancy predicts greater amygdala volumes in early adulthood. *J. Child Psychol. Psychiatry* **2015**, *56*, 540–548. [CrossRef] [PubMed]
129. Assari, S. Educational attainment better protects African American women than African American men against depressive symptoms and psychological distress. *Brain Sci.* **2018**, *8*, 182. [CrossRef] [PubMed]
130. Assari, S. Family socioeconomic position at birth and school bonding at age 15; Blacks' diminished returns. *Behav. Sci.* **2019**, *9*, 26. [CrossRef]
131. Assari, S. Parental educational attainment and academic performance of American college students; Blacks' diminished returns. *J. Health Econ. Dev.* **2019**, *1*, 21–31. [PubMed]
132. Assari, S. Family income reduces risk of obesity for white but not black children. *Children* **2018**, *5*, 73. [CrossRef]
133. Assari, S. Blacks' diminished return of education attainment on subjective health; Mediating effect of income. *Brain Sci.* **2018**, *8*, 176. [CrossRef]
134. Assari, S.; Lankarani, M.M. Education and alcohol consumption among older Americans; Black-white differences. *Front. Public Health* **2016**, *4*, 67. [CrossRef]
135. Assari, S.; Moghani Lankarani, M.; Caldwell, C.H.; Zimmerman, M.A. Fear of neighborhood violence during adolescence predicts development of obesity a decade later: Gender differences among African Americans. *Arch. Trauma. Res.* **2016**, *5*, e31475. [CrossRef]
136. Assari, S. Education attainment and obesity differential returns based on sexual orientation. *Behav. Sci.* **2019**, *9*, 16. [CrossRef]
137. Assari, S.; Caldwell, C.H. Social determinants of perceived discrimination among black youth: Intersection of ethnicity and gender. *Children* **2018**, *5*, 24. [CrossRef] [PubMed]
138. Assari, S.; Lankarani, M.M. Reciprocal associations between depressive symptoms and mastery among older adults; Black-white differences. *Front. Aging Neurosci.* **2016**, *8*, 279. [CrossRef]
139. Assari, S. General self-efficacy and mortality in the USA.; Racial differences. *J. Racial Ethn. Health Dispar.* **2017**, *4*, 746–757. [CrossRef] [PubMed]
140. Krieger, N.; Williams, D.; Zierler, S. "Whiting out" white privilege will not advance the study of how racism harms health. *Am. J. Public Health* **1999**, *89*, 782–783. [CrossRef] [PubMed]
141. Krieger, N. Epidemiology, racism, and health: The case of low birth weight. *Epidemiology* **2000**, *11*, 237–239. [CrossRef] [PubMed]
142. Rich-Edwards, J.; Krieger, N.; Majzoub, J.; Zierler, S.; Lieberman, E.; Gillman, M. Maternal experiences of racism and violence as predictors of preterm birth: Rationale and study design. *Paediatr. Perinat. Epidemiol.* **2001**, *15* (Suppl. 2), 124–135. [CrossRef] [PubMed]
143. Krieger, N. Does racism harm health? Did child abuse exist before 1962? On explicit questions, critical science, and current controversies: An ecosocial perspective. *Am. J. Public Health* **2003**, *93*, 194–199. [CrossRef]
144. Parrott, R.L.; Silk, K.J.; Dillow, M.R.; Krieger, J.L.; Harris, T.M.; Condit, C.M. Development and validation of tools to assess genetic discrimination and genetically based racism. *J. Natl. Med. Assoc.* **2005**, *97*, 980–990.
145. Krieger, N.; Smith, K.; Naishadham, D.; Hartman, C.; Barbeau, E.M. Experiences of discrimination: Validity and reliability of a self-report measure for population health research on racism and health. *Soc. Sci. Med.* **2005**, *61*, 1576–1596. [CrossRef]
146. Assari, S. Age-Related Decline in Children's Reward Sensitivity: Blacks' Diminished Returns. *Res Health Sci.* **2020**, *5*, 112–128. [CrossRef]
147. Krieger, N. Living and dying at the crossroads: Racism, embodiment, and why theory is essential for a public health of consequence. *Am. J. Public Health* **2016**, *106*, 832–833. [CrossRef] [PubMed]
148. Bassett, M.T.; Krieger, N.; Bailey, Z. Charlottesville: Blatant racism, not grievances, on display. *Lancet* **2017**, *390*, 2243. [CrossRef]
149. Bailey, Z.D.; Krieger, N.; Agenor, M.; Graves, J.; Linos, N.; Bassett, M.T. Structural racism and health inequities in the USA: Evidence and interventions. *Lancet* **2017**, *389*, 1453–1463. [CrossRef]

150. Clark, U.S.; Miller, E.R.; Hegde, R.R. Experiences of discrimination are associated with greater resting amygdala activity and functional connectivity. *Biol. Psychiatry Cogn. Neurosci. Neuroimaging* **2018**, *3*, 367–378. [CrossRef] [PubMed]
151. Fourie, M.M.; Stein, D.J.; Solms, M.; Gobodo-Madikizela, P.; Decety, J. Effects of early adversity and social discrimination on empathy for complex mental states: An fMRI investigation. *Sci. Rep.* **2019**, *9*, 1–14. [CrossRef] [PubMed]
152. Han, S.D.; Lamar, M.; Fleischman, D.; Kim, N.; Bennett, D.A.; Lewis, T.T.; Arfanakis, K.; Barnes, L.L. Self-reported experiences of discrimination in older black adults are associated with insula functional connectivity. *Brain Imaging Behav.* **2020**, 1–10. [CrossRef] [PubMed]
153. Phelps, E.A.; O'Connor, K.J.; Cunningham, W.A.; Funayama, E.S.; Gatenby, J.C.; Gore, J.C.; Banaji, M.R. Performance on indirect measures of race evaluation predicts amygdala activation. *J. Cogn. Neurosci.* **2000**, *12*, 729–738. [CrossRef]
154. Wheeler, M.E.; Fiske, S.T. Controlling racial prejudice: Social-cognitive goals affect amygdala and stereotype activation. *Psychol. Sci.* **2005**, *16*, 56–63. [CrossRef]
155. Chekroud, A.M.; Everett, J.A.; Bridge, H.; Hewstone, M. A review of neuroimaging studies of race-related prejudice: Does amygdala response reflect threat? *Front. Hum. Neurosci.* **2014**, *8*, 179. [CrossRef]
156. Assari, S. Socioeconomic Status Inequalities Partially Mediate Racial and Ethnic Differences in Children's Amygdala Volume. *Stud. Soc. Sci. Res.* **2020**, *1*, 62–79. [CrossRef]
157. Uytun, M.C. Development period of prefrontal cortex. In *Prefrontal Cortex*; IntechOpen: London, UK, 2018.
158. Pennington, B.F.; Bennetto, L.; McAleer, O.; Roberts, R.J., Jr. Executive functions and working memory: Theoretical and measurement issues. In *Attention, Memory, and Executive Function*; Lyon, G.R., Krasnegor, N.A., Eds.; Paul H Brookes Publishing Co.: Baltimore, MD, USA, 1996.
159. Kesner, R.P.; Churchwell, J.C. An analysis of rat prefrontal cortex in mediating executive function. *Neurobiol. Learn. Mem.* **2011**, *96*, 417–431. [CrossRef] [PubMed]

Publisher's Note: MDPI stays neutral with regard to jurisdictional claims in published maps and institutional affiliations.

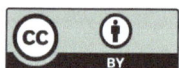

© 2020 by the authors. Licensee MDPI, Basel, Switzerland. This article is an open access article distributed under the terms and conditions of the Creative Commons Attribution (CC BY) license (http://creativecommons.org/licenses/by/4.0/).

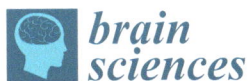

Article

Emotional Availability and Play in Mother–Child Dyads with ASD: Changes during a Parental Based Intervention

Silvia Perzolli [1,*], Giulio Bertamini [1,2], Simona de Falco [1], Paola Venuti [1] and Arianna Bentenuto [1]

1. Laboratory of Observation, Department of Psychology and Cognitive Science, Diagnosis and Education (ODFLab), University of Trento, 38068 Rovereto, Italy; giulio.bertamini@unitn.it (G.B.); simona.defalco@unitn.it (S.d.F.); paola.venuti@unitn.it (P.V.); arianna.bentenuto@unitn.it (A.B.)
2. Center for Information Technology, Bruno Kessler Foundation (FBK), University of Trento, 38123 Trento, Italy
* Correspondence: silvia.perzolli@unitn.it

Received: 26 October 2020; Accepted: 18 November 2020; Published: 24 November 2020

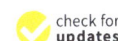

Abstract: (1) Background: Parental involvement during intervention with children with Autism Spectrum Disorder (ASD) has been demonstrated to be fundamental for children's developmental outcomes. However, most research focused on child gains especially considering cognitive functioning and symptoms severity, whereas parental and dyadic changes during intervention need further investigation. (2) Methods: 29 mothers in interaction with their preschool children with ASD were analyzed through two standardized behavioral and observational measures to evaluate the dyadic Emotional Availability (EA) and play skills before (T1) and after (T2) a parental-based intervention. (3) Results: Results revealed mothers increased affective quality and major awareness in understanding the signals produced by the child, that in turn was more responsive, involving also using more complex play strategies. Interestingly, the role of specific factors able to predict parental characteristics was investigated, pointing out the important contribution of mothers' perceptions of having a difficult child and child language communicative abilities. (4) Conclusions: the study enhances knowledge about child and caregiver variables that impact on dyadic outcomes, identifying important target areas to be addressed during intervention. Further, our results suggest that a parental-based intervention supports and facilitates improvements in both children's and caregivers' affective quality and cognitive abilities.

Keywords: Autism Spectrum Disorder (ASD); mother–child interaction; parental involvement; predictors of change

1. Introduction

Autism Spectrum Disorder (ASD) is a neurodevelopmental disorder characterized by qualitative impairments in social interaction and communication alongside a pattern of restricted and repetitive behaviors and interests [1]. The fundamental role of caregiver–child interactions on child cognitive, social and affective development is well established considering children with Typical Development (TD) [2,3], with other Developmental Disabilities (DD) such as Down Syndrome [4,5] and with Autism Spectrum Disorder (ASD) [6,7]. However, core symptoms of ASD dramatically impact on the child's ability to interact with significant others, especially with parents, inducing maladaptive caregiver–child interactive circuits that need to be restored in order to guarantee effective emotional exchanges [8,9]. Children with ASD tend to be socially less involving, less responsive and they have the tendency to decline, reject or ignore their caregivers' social initiatives [9]. Furthermore, children with ASD have difficulties in sharing attention on an object with an interactive partner [10] and they often appear to be wholly focused on objects [8,11]. Consequently, interventions teaching parents strategies designed to increase time in joint engagement might be crucial [12]. Interestingly, recent at-risk studies pointed out a developmental picture revealing that children with eventual autism and their primary caregiver interact with each other in some ways that depart from a typical trajectory early in the child's first years of life [13]. In addition to this, ASD symptomatology impacts significantly also on children's play abilities, in fact children with ASD often engage with objects in repetitive ways and fail to develop creative and symbolic engagement with objects [14]. Also, play provides a platform for social engagement with others [15], and indeed, socially connected play and social behavior with others are particularly impaired in children with autism [8,14,16]. Taken together, these difficulties constitute a daily challenge for parents to engage children in joyful syntonic activities, influencing stress levels perceived by parents as well as the general emotional climate to which the child is exposed [17].

1.1. Affective Quality in Mother–Child Dyads with ASD

First interactions with parents have a unique and fundamental function for the overall development of children with typical development and of children with autism. Several research works investigated the role of parent–infant interaction focusing on mothers as primary caregiver. However, the recent socio-cultural changes implicate an increasing involvement of fathers in child rearing. In line with this, scientific literature highlights the relevance of fathering for child psychological development in children with and without developmental disabilities [18–22]. These results pointed out both similarities and differences in the interactive modalities that may support specific aspects of child development. In the context of ASD, some research highlighted that mothers tend to be more directive [23,24], displaying more intrusive and controlling behaviors and physical attempts to catch the child's attention [4,25]. Mothers of children with ASD were also found to be as sensitive as mothers of children with typical development [26] or other developmental disabilities [27]. These findings result as particularly important, given the impact of parent scaffolding and sensitivity, for the emotional development of children with ASD [17]. However, recent studies showed that mothers in the group of children with ASD demonstrated lower sensitivity, assessed through the scheme of Karreman, highlighting their difficulties with timing and quality of play intervention [28]. This scale contains seven dimensions of maternal parenting rated on a 7-point Likert scale including warmth, sensitivity, provision of structure and limit-setting and it is applied on video-recorded observations during home-visit mother–child interactions using different play materials. This instrument was found to be particularly sensitive in capturing mothers' characteristics, but it does not capture how children respond to their mother's interactive strategies.

In the last few years, research focused on the dyadic nature of the mother–child relationship, in which the child clearly plays an active role [29,30]. In line with this, the construct of the Emotional Availability (EA) refers to a solid empirical basis (attachment theory, theory of emotions, maternal sensitivity) but focuses on the quality of emotional exchanges between parent and child, on their reciprocal accessibility, as well as their ability to understand and respond to each other communicative signals [31]. The construct was later operationalized by Biringen and colleagues in the Emotional Availability Scales (EAS, [32] see measures for details). Research on EA Scales has been conducted in a variety of contexts and validated in over twenty countries (Europe, Asia, subcultures of the United States etc.) [33–36] and because of this the EA Scales are one of the most widely used instruments for assessing the interaction within the parent–child dyad. However, to our knowledge only few studies have analyzed EA in mother–child with ASD dyads [21,27,37–39] and no studies investigated EA in a longitudinal design in these dyads. Furthermore, EA is found to be predictive of various positive developmental outcomes such as attachment security [39,40], emotion expressions and regulation [41] and school readiness [40]. EA parental levels seem also to modulate the functionality of neural circuits involved in executive functioning, especially in response inhibition [42]. These results suggest that intervention aiming to increase maternal EA should begin early in the child's life [43].

1.2. Cognitive Elements in Mother–Child Dyads with ASD: The Role of Play

Another important context for the child's early social and cognitive development is play. It provides a motivating opportunity for child learning and advanced levels of play are associated with greater cognitive and language development [16]. At first, children are generally more focused on physical properties of toys and their exploration, but later they engage more in symbolic activities that need higher representational abilities and cognitive skills. Despite deviations in play behaviors in children with ASD, more skills in symbolic play are reported when play is scaffolded by an adult [44] and more systemic instructions are required to support the play with peers [45]. Recent findings revealed also that mothers of children with ASD adapted their activities to their child's sophistication level [46]. These mothers seem to use fewer symbolic solicitations than mothers of children with typical development but a positive correlation between maternal verbal solicitations of symbolic play and children's actual symbolic play was found only in children with ASD, highlighting a fundamental role of the caregivers in cognitive aspects in dyads with children with ASD. Considering this, [47] operationalized a scale for play behavior that follows the progression from simple manipulation of toys, to recognition of conceptual relationships between objects (i.e., functional play and combinatory play), to increasingly decontextualized play (i.e., symbolic or pretend play). This code allows individual scoring of caregiver and child levels of play to see how parents adapt their level to child functioning, and also to investigate how the child responds to a caregiver's behavioral characteristics.

In general, mother–child interactions may be influenced by the fact that mothers of children with ASD tend to have higher levels of stress compared to mothers of children with typical development [28,48]. Consequently, stress levels may lead parents to feel more negative emotions and to be more irritable and upset [49], directly influencing child behavioral problems [28,50]. In line with this, maternal stress and negative feelings over the child were negatively associated with the emotional availability and particularly on structuring skills using verbal and non-verbal techniques [38]. All together these findings strengthen the importance of finding shared strategies for parents in dealing with their children, given their positive impact on stress reduction [51].

1.3. Parental Involvement during Intervention with Children with ASD

Given the influence of parent's qualities and dyadic characteristics on child developmental outcomes, recent findings strengthened the importance of involving caregivers during the intervention in order to increase dyadic levels of syntonization and to extend the acquisition of competencies also in naturalistic contexts (e.g., home) [52–54]. Further, parental involvement during intervention seemed to be extremely important in order to guarantee the adaptation to child's difficulties and impairments, allowing the child to respond with enhanced communicative and social development [55], long-term symptom reduction [56], and to generalize these outcomes across settings [57]. Further, recent literature documented that marked difficulties in social communication and responsiveness in parents of children with ASD [58] might create a potential barrier to care for their children. In line with this, recent findings suggested that an enhanced version of parental involvement was able to guarantee more prominent results considering caregivers. Interestingly, the authors found a significant relationship between the degree of change in parental interaction and the rate of child's improvement [59], underlying the importance of the dyadic relational aspects in child developmental outcomes. Moreover, some research showed that without involving caregivers these variables tend to remain more stable over time [55–57]. Because parents are so important in ensuring success and good prognosis, it is critical to include them throughout the intervention process. As a matter of fact, these findings shed new light on the idea that if parents are adequately informed during intervention and if they constantly deliver intervention strategies in naturalistic contexts, the intensity of the intervention dwindles on intervention outcomes. Caregivers, in fact, may carry on teaching competencies to their children in the home context, improving parent–child interactions and actually increasing the amount of treatment they receive. Recently, Naturalistic Developmental Behavioral Interventions (NDBI) are underlying the role of interactive aspects. Different works on efficacy showed significant gains in developmental outcomes and in symptoms severity [60–65]. However, in general the evaluation of treatment response is mainly focused on child outcomes demonstrating the improvements in both child' social engagement and their cognitive development [66], often without deepening dyadic and caregivers' variables associated with the response. Child gains are, in fact, predominantly assessed through developmental outcome measures using standardized instruments such as Autism Diagnostic Observation Schedule (ADOS-2, [67]) and Griffiths Scales (GMDS-ER, [68]). However, these instruments in the assessment of treatment's outcomes might suffer from the issue of sensitivity [69]. Standardized diagnostic and cognitive test items are, in fact, neither proximal to the treatment nor necessarily sensitive to small changes in social communication and interactive skills that may be occurring as treatment progresses. For this, the detection of change may be enhanced by using observational measures of social responsiveness [70]. In line with this, the analysis of the dyad's interactive component through observational and behavioral measures might represent a very sensitive-to-change instrument to assess caregiver and child improvements in the relational context.

To conclude, at this point it is also important to identify caregivers' characteristics that impact on intervention outcomes given the paucity of empirical research. For example, some research pointed out that higher parental age may be linked to more successful interactions and this could be due to their greater experience in parenting [71]. Further, higher educational level [71] and lower stress levels in parents [72] seemed to be associated with greater developmental outcomes. Also, different caregiving styles, such as higher levels of parental sensitivity, were also found to be related with better child communications abilities [27,29] and joint engagement [73]. Further, the increase of maternal age is associated with the increase of structuring abilities in interaction with the child with typical development [74–76]. In fact, as pointed out in three longitudinal studies that monitor mothers' interactive skills at different time points, it seems that the increase of maternal age may be associated with increased structuring abilities. Moreover, mothers' stress and depressive symptoms predicted the warmth and criticism toward their child, and the general well-being of the primary caregiver seemed to restrict or promote the involvement of the other caregiver in the ASD context [77]. More empirical evidence and more exploration is needed considering caregivers characteristics and dyadic factors.

1.4. Aims and Hypotheses

In accordance with the above, the aim of the present work is to assess an Early Intensive Intervention with Parent Involvement focusing on caregivers and dyadic outcomes through two observational standardized instrument that allow the evaluation of the affective quality (measured through the Emotional Availability Scales, EAS, [32]) within the dyad and the play skills abilities (assessed through the play code, [47]). First of all, in the present study we want to examine how the implementation of a parental-based intervention, that provides active participation of the caregiver into the therapeutic setting, impacts on interactive characteristics within the dyad and how this relationship evolves over time, given that the majority of empirical work is conducted on child outcomes only. Then, we want to examine the impact of child and caregiver factors on the emotional availability and on the play skills abilities given the persistent need to examine in details some factors that might predict, moderate and mediate intervention effectiveness for children and their parents. On this basis, we hypothesize as follows. First of all, we want to investigate if mothers and their children will improve specific interactive modalities during intervention.

1. In line with previous findings that include caregivers into the therapeutic setting [55–57], and in line with the theoretical framework of the implemented intervention that focuses on the syntonization between adult and child's needs, we expect that mothers will increase their awareness of timing during the interaction with the child, catching child's signals and respecting his/her time given the possibility for parents to experiment themselves in functional interaction with their children.
2. Further, considering that during intervention therapists provide caregivers appropriate hints and suggestions to interact and play with their children in a functional way, we also predict

that mothers will increase their general levels of Emotional Availability, especially considering structuring and non-intrusiveness scales.

3. With respect to the child, in line with previous findings that depicted positive change in child socio-communicative behaviors [78–81] we expect to find improvements in the child's level of responsiveness and in the use of different communicative strategies (e.g., eye-contact looking, body positioning, verbal involvement) to involve the caregiver during an interactive exchange.

Second, we want to examine the evolution of child cognitive play abilities during intervention.

1. In particular, we expect that during the intervention children will increase their level of symbolic play, consequently decreasing their level of exploratory play during the interaction with the caregiver, given that the intervention focuses also on a specific work on cognitive abilities necessary to be able to play with more advanced skills.
2. We further expect that mother and child scores will be more related after intervention, indicating an increased adaptation by the adult to the child's level of play.

Finally, we want to investigate the impact of child and caregivers' factors on the affective quality during their interaction measured through the Emotional Availability Scales. In particular,

1. Considering the child, we expect that the communicative aspects of the child in interaction with the caregiver may impact on the child's scales of Emotional Availability, given the impact of verbal and non-verbal communicative aspects on dyadic functional relationships.
2. Further, on the basis of previous literature that reported that higher levels of parental stress may impact on adult interactive modalities considering children with typical development [82] and children with ASD [83], we want to investigate the parental stress with respect to the adult Emotional Availability, and the specific stress dimensions that may impact on parent's modalities during the interplay with the child.

2. Materials and Methods

2.1. Participants

This study involved 29 Italian preschool children (27 males and 2 females) with Autism Spectrum Disorder (ASD) (M chronological age = 46.65 months, SD = 11.1; M mental age = 33.76 months, SD = 9.15) and their mothers, exposed to an early intensive treatment with parent involvement (M chronological age = 38.31 years, SD = 4.89) (see Table 1). All participants were recruited at the Laboratory of Observation, Diagnosis and Education (ODFLab), a clinical and research center of the Department of Psychology and Cognitive Science (University of Trento, Italy) specialized in functional diagnosis of neurodevelopmental disorders, in particular ASD, where families voluntarily go to in order to receive an assessment of their child functional profile. Moreover, the laboratory currently implements a parental based early intensive intervention in line with Naturalistic Developmental Behavioral Interventions (NDBI) [66].

Table 1. Demographic Statistics of the sample.

	Mean (SD)	
	T1	T2
Child Chronological Age (months)	37.793 (9.108) range (22–55)	55.500 (13.063) range (32–81)
Child Mental Age (months)	26.750 (7.006) range (15–43)	40.760 (11.296) range (23–63)
Parental Age (years)	38.071 (4.799) range (27–45)	39.996 (5.071) range (27–46)
Socio Economic Status	35.214 (13.600) range (14.5–59.5)	35.600 (14.361) range (14.5–66.0)

The diagnosis of ASD of the children in the present work was confirmed through clinical judgment by an independent clinician based on the DSM-5 criteria for Autism Spectrum Disorder, as well as through the administration of the Autism Diagnostic Observation Schedule (ADOS-2; [67]). Recruitment of participants was done on a voluntary basis through advertisements in the waiting room of the Laboratory. Then, a dedicated meeting will be scheduled with a referent not involved in the clinical process in order to explain the objectives of the research. Finally, participants had to sign a written consent.

2.2. Procedure

All procedures of this study were in accordance with the ethical standards of the Italian Association of Psychology (AIP), with the ethical standards of the Ethics Committee of the University of Trento (Italy) and the last version of the Declaration of Helsinki [84]. In order to determine children's developmental level, the Griffith Mental Development Scale-Edition Revised [68] was administered to all children. Further, Autism Diagnostic Observation Schedule (ADOS-2; [67]) was administered in order to certify the presence of Autism Spectrum Disorder and to specify the severity level. On the basis of the level of language development and the chronological age of children, ADOS Toddler, Module 1 and Module 2, were applied. Further, in order to assess the affective quality within the dyad the Emotional Availability Scales (EAS, [32]; see measures for details) were applied to ten minutes of video-recorded interactions between the child and the caregiver in which mothers were asked to spontaneously play with their child with a standard set of toys as if they were at home. In the same interaction sequence, the Play code ([47] see measures for details) was also applied in order to assess the levels of both child and caregiver's exploratory and symbolic play. The coding is randomly assigned to two independent observers that codify the interactions after receiving a specific training considering both the application of the Emotional Availability Scales (EAS) and the Play Code, and after having reached a significant level of interrater reliability. Two-way mixed effects ICC with absolute agreement has been used [85]. Two independent observers codified four target videos with a total duration of about 120 min as indicated in the EAS training [32]. The coefficient ranged from 0.84 to 0.92.

Considering play the average kappa's between coders for the play levels ranged from 0.79 to 0.88 for training videos. The above-mentioned measures are applied before intervention (T1), during the first diagnostic and functional assessment and after an average of 11.03 (SD = 3.00) months of intervention (T2) to both children and caregivers, in order to investigate the evolution of dyadic factors during intervention and the impact of affective characteristics on cognitive play skills.

2.3. ODFLab Parental Based Intensive Intervention

ODFLab implements an "Italian Model of Intervention" which combines empirically validated scientific principles together with guidelines in accordance with the Italian sanitary system [52,86,87]. This intervention integrates behavioral, developmental and relationship-based principles, according to the key elements of the American Early Start Denver Model [81,88]. Further, in order to restore caregiver–child maladaptive interactive circuits and to strengthen the generalization of child competencies, the intervention involves caregivers into the therapeutic setting together with the child. The ground idea is that if caregivers have the possibility to learn adequate strategies to deal with their children, they may effectively make use of them in more naturalistic contexts (e.g., home). With this in mind, the intervention includes specific activities for the child (speech therapy, music therapy, cognitive activities and emotional and social play for 4–6 h per week) and parent involvement into the therapy room (at least 2 h per week). Differently from parent-mediated intervention and parent training, the parental involvement does not require home assignments nor fidelity schedules and the intervention is entirely delivered by the therapist. In fact, during these weekly sessions the therapist remains the key figure that structures activities but he/she also creates opportunities for the caregivers and the child to interact and play together. Consequently, the caregivers have the possibility to experience more functional interactions with the child characterized by more adequate proposals and major awareness of the child's individual timing. In turn, such changes may increase dyadic shared pleasure, parents' self-efficacy and motivation to interact with their child, while reducing stress and frustration levels.

Importantly, these interactions between adult and child are discussed together with a psychotherapist every two weeks through the video-feedback procedure. Thanks to this, the intervention works on functional dyadic characteristics and consequently on parental representation of both the child and the caregivers in their role. In fact, during these meetings the parents have the possibility to analyze specific child's avoidant, non-respondent or other problematic behaviors, understanding child's signals together with the therapist. Therefore, they have the possibility to build a more truthful image of the child and of himself/herself as a parent. In addition to this, meetings with parents of all children are organized in order to create a moment of sharing feelings, emotions, experiences, fears and uncertainties and experiencing the sensation of not being alone in dealing with children with ASD. The intervention is delivered by trained psychologists after receiving specific licenses on developmental models of intervention for children with ASD. Finally, the team is constantly supervised at least once every month by an expert psychotherapist.

2.4. Measures

2.4.1. Griffiths Mental Development Scales

Child cognitive development before and after intervention is assessed through the Griffiths Mental Development Scales (GMDS-ER; [68], see Table 2). The GMDS-ER are developmental scales normalized also in an Italian sample and are administered to the child in a laboratory setting through semi-structured activities designed to evaluate different aspects of mental development in infants and children. They provide Z-scores relative to 6 subscales in the main developmental areas: Locomotion; Personal–Social; Communication and Listening; Eye–Hand Coordination; Performance; and Practical Reasoning. These scales provide a Global Quotient and a developmental age-equivalent—allowing to detect developmental delays—as well as specific quotients and developmental age-equivalents for each of the 6 subscales. All scores are standardized (M = 100; SD = 15).

Table 2. Developmental child's outcomes before and after intervention.

	T1 M(SD)	T2 M(SD)	p-Value-r^2	BF
Ados Social Affect	12.931 (2.939)	11.357 (2.599)	$T(27) = 3.827$, $p = 0.0007$; $r^2 = 0.352$	BF = 46.309
ADOS Restrictive and Repetitive Behabiors	3.552 (1.824)	3.500 (1.876)	$T(27) = 0$; p-value = 1; $r^2 = 0$	BF = 0.200
Ados Total Score	16.700 (3.809)	14.893 (3.370)	$T(27) = 2.718$; $p = 0.011$; $r^2 = 0.215$	BF = 4.146
ADOS Comparison Score	6.407 (1.394)	5.786 (1.101)	$T(25) = 2.476$; $p = 0.020$; $r^2 = 0.197$	BF = 2.606
GMDS-General Quotient	71.964(13.675)	75.037(21.636)	$T(26) = -1.311$, $p = 0.201$, $r^2 = 0.062$	BF = 0.439
GMDS–Language and Communication Scale	54 (23.764)	69.84 (37.121)	$W = 77.5$, $p = 0.023$; $r^2 = 0.458$	BF = 6.671

2.4.2. Autism Diagnostic Observation Schedule-2

Child severity of symptoms is assessed before and after intervention through the Autism Diagnostic Observation Schedule (ADOS-2; [67], see Table 2), golden standard instrument for the diagnosis of ASD. The administration of this tool is carried out by trained psychologists after an official ADOS course. The instrument provides different modules according to child chronological age and expressive level of language. Each module gives a total score used for the ADOS diagnostic classification (Autism–Autism Spectrum–Non Spectrum). This score is transformed in the comparison score in order to perform comparisons among different modules and classify the severity of symptoms in three categories (mild, moderate or severe).

2.4.3. Emotional Availability Scales

Mother–child Emotional Availability (EA) is assessed before and after the early intensive intervention with parent involvement through the Emotional Availability Scales (EAS; [32]). EA is a relational construct that refers to the quality of emotional exchanges between parent and child. It focuses on their reciprocal accessibility and their ability to understand and respond appropriately to each other's communicative signals (31). The EA Scales are created to observationally measure and operationalize the construct of Emotional Availability and consist of four scales for adults that include sensitivity, structuring, non-intrusiveness and non-hostility, as well as two scales for children, responsiveness and involvement, with 7 subscales that measures specific dimensions of the main scale (see Table 3). The main scales are scored from 1 (lowest EA) to 7 (highest EA) on a Likert scale; the first two subscales are scored from 1 to 7, however the other 5 subscales are scored from 1 (lowest EA) to 3 (highest EA). Midpoints were also used in the present study as they are highly recommended especially for children with disabilities [89,90]. Adult Sensitivity refers to the ability to capture and respond adequately to the child's communicative signals and to the caregiver's ability to be emotionally connected to the child [91]. Adult Structuring refers to the parent's ability to promote and organize the child's activities by furnishing appropriate prompts and suggestions during interaction, without limiting the child's autonomy. Non-intrusiveness refers to the ability of the parent to be aware of the best time to fit in the interaction without being too demanding nor directive. Finally, Non-hostility refers to the ability to interact with the child without showing over nor covert signs of hostility. The child's scales comprise Responsiveness and Involvement. Responsiveness refers to the child's manifestation of clear signs of pleasure during the interaction with the caregiver and measures how often the child responds to parents' suggestions. Finally, Involvement refers to the child's ability to actively engage and involve the parent into interaction through different modalities (eye-contact looking, verbal involvement, body positioning). In general, optimal levels of EA (7) are characterized by the presence of an ideal quality of affect and support, as well as child's optimal levels of responsiveness and involvement. Moderate levels (5–6) refers to good modalities of parents in interaction with the child that shows appropriate but not ideal strategies for involving caregivers. Apparent/inconsistent levels of EA (4) are characterized by the adult's inconsistency in their ability to lead the child, that, in turn, shows both positive and negative approaches to draw the adult's attention. Low levels (3/2.5) or very low levels (2–1) of EA are typical of caregivers that show insensitive and unavailable affect and children are characterized by worry, anxiety and distress in their responsiveness and their involving strategies might be inappropriate or nonexistent.

Table 3. Scales and subscales of the Emotional Availability Scales.

Adult Sensitivity	Adult Structuring	Adult Non-Intrusiveness	Adult Non-Hostility
Affect	Provides appropriate guidance and suggestions	Follows child's lead	Adult lacks negativity in face or voice
Clarity of perceptions and appropriate responsiveness	Success of attempts	Non-interruptive ports of entry into interaction	Lack of mocking, ridiculing, or other disrespectful statement and/or behavior and general demeanor
Awareness of timing	Amount of structure	Commands, directives	Lack of threats of separation
Flexibility, variety, and creativity in modes of play or interaction	Limit setting proactively	Adult talking	Does not lose cool during low and high challenge/stress times
Acceptance	Remaining firm in the face of pressure	Didactic teaching	Frightening behavior/tendencies
Amount of interaction	Verbal vs. non-verbal structuring	Physical vs. verbal interferences	Silence

Table 3. *Cont.*

Adult Sensitivity	Adult Structuring	Adult Non-Intrusiveness	Adult Non-Hostility
Conflicts situations	Peer vs. adult role	The adult is made to "feel" or "seem" intrusive	Themes or plat themes hostile
Child Responsiveness	**Child Involvement**		
Affect/emotion regulation, organization of behavior	Simple initiative		
Responsiveness	Elaborative initiative		
Age-appropriate autonomy seeking and exploration	Use of adult		
Positive physical positioning	Lack of over-involvement		
Lack of role reversal/over-responsiveness	Eye contact, looking		
Lack of avoidance	Body positioning		
Task oriented/concentrate	Verbal involvement		

2.5. Play

Mother–child Play skills are assessed before and after intervention through the Play code [47], an operationalized scale that follows the sequence of play from simple exploration of toys, to identification of relationships between objects (i.e., functional play and combinatory play), to increasingly decontextualized play (i.e., symbolic or pretend play). The code allows to score caregiver and child levels of play individually, but also to investigate whether parents appropriately adapt to the child's intentionality and level of functioning, as well as how he/she responds to parent's interactive proposals. The play levels considered in this code are described briefly as follows:

Level 1. Unitary functional activity: considers effects that are unique to a single object (e.g., dialing a telephone).

Level 2. Inappropriate combinatorial activity: refers to the inappropriate juxtaposition of two or more objects (e.g., putting the cup on the telephone).

Level 3. Appropriate combinatorial activity: concerns the appropriate juxtaposition of two or more objects (e.g., putting the handset on the telephone).

Level 4. Transitional play: refers to the approximation of pretend play but the action is not concluded (e.g., putting the telephone handset to ear without vocalization).

Level 5. Self-directed pretense: relates to the pretense activity that is directed toward self (e.g., drinking from an empty cup).

Level 6. Other-directed pretense: pertains to the pretense activity that is now directed towards someone or something else (e.g., putting a doll to sleep).

Level 7. Sequential pretense: concerns child's ability to connect two or more pretense actions (e.g., pouring into an empty cup from the teapot and then drinking).

Level 8. Substitution pretense: refers to the child's ability to include one or more object substitutions (e.g., pretending a cup is a telephone and talking into it).

Level 9. When no action is taken within the dyad (e.g., child is running around the room in an afinalistic way and no object is touched).

Play levels from 1 to 4 are considered an index of the child's exploratory play, whereas levels from 5 to 8 reflect the quantity of symbolic play displayed during the interaction. The trained observers used BORIS (Behavioral Observation Research Interactive Software, [92], an open-source event logging software for video/audio coding and live observations. It allows to code continuously by noting play level as well as start and end times (accurate to 1 s). Minimum play time is fixed at 1 s, after that a specific level of play is coded until there is a break longer than 10 s during which neither the child nor the caregiver touches an object. For each level of play four measures are extracted: the absolute frequency, the proportional frequency, the absolute duration, and the proportional duration. These scores are later normalized through the proportion of maximum scaling ("POMS"), a min-max normalization method [93,94] that transforms each index to a metric from 0 to 1 through the following formula: POMS = [(observed − minimum)/(maximum − minimum)]. This method is therefore useful to have a monotonic metric and to avoid problems concerning "classical" standardization in longitudinal design [89]. A general index for each play level is then computed averaging the standardized scores of the four measures (i.e., absolute frequencies, proportional frequencies, absolute durations and proportional durations). POMS indexes are then grouped in two main indexes: exploratory play, computed as the average of levels from 1 to 4, and symbolic play, computed as the average of levels from 5 to 8. These indexes represent quantitative measures of both the amount and duration of the different types of play, accounting both for absolute and proportional measures of the interplay.

2.6. Parental Stress Index-Short Form

The Parental Stress Index-Short Form (PSI/SF, [95]) is a standardized instrument widely used in the clinical context for the early identification of stress in the parent–child relationship. It contains 36 items on a five-point Likert scale and it yields a Total Stress score from three scales: Parental Distress, Parent–Child Dysfunctional Interaction, and Difficult Child. In particular, the Parental Distress (PD) defines stress levels of the caregiver in his/her role as a parent but considering only personal factors, independently from the child. Parent–Child Dysfunctional Interaction (P–CDI) analyses the interaction with the child perceived by the parent as difficult and problematic (e.g., when parents consider themselves rejected by the child). Difficult Child (DC) examines some characteristics of the child's behaviors and the perception the parent has to have a child with a difficult temperament.

2.7. Statistical Analysis

Data has been checked for normality (i.e., Shapiro test) and homogeneity of variances (i.e., Levene test). When assumptions for parametric tests were met, Welch T test for dependent samples has been used for longitudinal analysis, as it is recommended in psychological research with relatively small samples to reduce the probability of Type I Error [96]. Otherwise, paired Wilcoxon signed rank with continuity correction has been used to verify differences between T1 and T2. Effect sizes have been calculated using R-squared.

A Bayes Factor analysis has been performed to investigate evidence supporting the null vs. alternative hypothesis given the observed data as a way to improve inferential statistics.

Data has been analyzed using R [97]. The Bayes Factor (BF) analysis has been performed using the package 'Bayes Factor' and will be interpreted following the proposal of Harold Jeffreys revised by Lee and Wagenmakers [98].

Linear mixed-models have been fitted to investigate longitudinal relationships between child's play abilities on developmental outcomes and, in turn, child's cognitive skills on caregiver Emotional Availability Scales together with parental stress levels. Models have been fitted using the 'lme4' package, with the 'lmerTest' and the 'car' packages to compute *p*-values, Bayesian Information Criteria (BIC), marginal R-squared and the ANOVA with Wald F test to check for model significance. Futher, the models have been checked for significance against baseline (χ^2).

Linear correlation analysis has been performed using Pearson product-moment correlation coefficient and tested for significance.

3. Results

3.1. Longitudinal Changes: Emotional Availability Scales

3.1.1. Adult's Scales

Wilcoxon signed rank test with continuity correction revealed a significant (V(28) = 13; p = 0.002; r^2 = 0.596; BF = 25.097) change in adult's Sensitivity scale during intervention, indicating a medium effect. Bayes Factor (BF) analysis suggests strong evidence for the alternative hypothesis.

Considering Sensitivity subscales, results revealed that "the awareness of timing" showed significant increase (V(28) = 0; $p = 0.026$; $r^2 = 0.454$; BF = 2.952). Further, the subscale "amount of interaction" revealed a significant (V(28) = 0; $p < 0.001$; $r^2 = 0.669$; BF > 100) change before and after the intervention, indicating a strong effect. BF analysis suggests extreme evidence for the alternative hypothesis. Considering adult Structuring scale, results exhibit a significant (V(28) = 0; $p < 0.0001$; $r^2 = 0.892$; BF > 100) change between T1 and T2, indicating a strong effect and extreme evidence for the alternative hypothesis through the BF analysis. The investigation of the subscales revealed that the "appropriate guidance and suggestions" increased significantly (V(28) = 24; $p < 0.0001$; $r^2 = 0.795$; BF > 100) during time, indicating a strong effect and extreme evidence for the alternative hypothesis. Also, the rate of "success of attempts" emerged to be significant (V(28) = 16; $p = 0.003$; $r^2 = 0.559$; BF = 23.428) and the "amount of structure" also increased significantly (V(28) = 0; $p < 0.001$; $r^2 = 0.641$; BF > 100) during play with the child, indicating a strong effect and suggesting extreme evidence for the alternative hypothesis. The subscales "remaining firm in the face of pressure" and "verbal vs. non-verbal structuring" are both significant, respectively (V(28) = 5; $p = 0.023$; $r^2 = 0.433$; BF = 2.952) (V(28) = 0; $p = 0.010$; $r^2 = 0.523$; BF = 2.108). With respect to the adult Non-Intrusiveness scale, results showed a significant (V(28) = 0; $p < 0.0001$; $r^2 = 0.886$; BF > 100) change during intervention, indicating a strong effect and supporting extreme evidence for the alternative hypothesis. The subscales, and particularly results considering the ability of "following child's lead" showed significant (V(28) = 38.5; $p = 0.019$; $r^2 = 0.504$; BF = 5.069) increase during intervention, together with the ability to "not interrupt the child into interaction" (V(28) = 31; $p = 0.014$; $r^2 = 0.549$; BF = 7.699) and the reduction of "physical vs. verbal interferences" (V(28) = 0; $p = 0.019$; $r^2 = 0.454$; BF = 4.031). Finally, also the subscale "the adult is made to feel or seem intrusive" showed a significant change during intervention, revealing that the adult is less intrusive in the interplay (V(28) = 0; $p = 0.003$; $r^2 = 0.586$; BF = 30.755), indicating a strong effect and a very strong evidence supporting the alternative hypothesis. Adult Non-Hostility scale revealed no differences in the main domain nor in the subscales (see Table 4).

Table 4. Descriptive and Inferential Statistics of Adult Emotional Availability Scales-Main Scales and Subscales.

	Mean (SD)		p-Value–R^2	Bayes Factor
	T1	T2	T1–T2	T1–T2
Total Sensitivity	4.552 (0.588)	4.914 (0.669)	$p = 0.002$ ** $r^2 = 0.596$	BF = 25.097
Sensitivity 3: Awareness of timing	1.966 (0.421)	2.207 (0.412)	$p = 0.0262$ * $r^2 = 0.454$	BF = 2.952
Sensitivity 6: Amount of interaction	1.0690 (0.604)	2.138 (0.516)	$p < 0.001$ *** $r^2 = 0.669$	BF > 100
Total Structuring	4.276 (0.560)	5.121 (0.529)	$p < 0.0001$ *** $r^2 = 0.892$	BF > 100
Structuring 1: Appropriate guidance	4.103 (0.724)	5.034 (0.731)	$p < 0.0001$ *** $r^2 = 0.795$	BF > 100
Structuring 2: Success of attempts	4.103 (0.724)	4.552 (0.985)	$p = 0.003$ ** $r^2 = 0.559$	BF = 23.42
Structuring 3: Amount of structure	1.690 (0.541)	2.138 (0.516)	$p < 0.001$ *** $r^2 = 0.641$	BF > 100
Structuring 5: Remaining firm during pressure	2.310 (0.471)	2.552 (0.506)	$p = 0.023$ * $r^2 = 0.433$	BF = 2.952
Total Non–Intrusiveness	4.466 (0.654)	5.345 (0.769)	$p < 0.0001$ *** $r_2 = 0.886$	BF > 100
Non–Intrusiveness 1: Follows child's lead	4.379 (0.775)	4.931 (0.961)	$p = 0.019$ * $r^2 = 0.504$	BF = 5.069

Table 4. Cont.

	Mean (SD)		p-Value–R^2	Bayes Factor
	T1	T2	T1-T2	T1–T2
Non-Intrusiveness 2: Non-interruptive entry in interaction	4.552 (0.783)	5.103 (1.113)	$p = 0.014$ * $r^2 = 0.549$	BF = 7.699
Non-Intrusiveness 6: Physical vs. verbal interferences	2.103 (0.409)	2.310 (0.471)	$p = 0.019$ * $r^2 = 0.454$	BF = 4.031
Non-Intrusiveness 7: The adult is made to feel intrusive	2.172 (0.602)	2.552 (0.506)	$p = 0.003$ ** $r^2 = 0.586$	BF = 30.755
Total Non–Hostility	5.431 (0.578)	5.379 (0.883)	p = ns	BF = 0.210

* $p < 0.05$; ** $p < 0.01$; *** $p < 0.001$.

3.1.2. Child's Scales

With regards to child Responsiveness scale, results showed a significant (V(28) = 21.5; $p < 0.001$; $r^2 = 0.716$; BF > 100) improvement during intervention, indicating a strong effect. BF supports extreme evidence for the alternative hypothesis. The analysis of the subscales pointed out that "the emotional regulation of affect and behavior" resulted to be significantly (V(28) = 1; $p = 0.022$; $r^2 = 0.432$; BF = 2.880) greater during the intervention, together with the increased "positive physical positioning" of the child towards adult (V(28) = 11; $p = 0.036$; $r^2 = 0.479$; BF = 1.836). Moreover, the subscale that considers the degree of "quantitative responsiveness" of the child results to be highly significant (V(28) = 19; $p = 0.001$; $r^2 = 0.675$; BF = 21.431) indicating a strong effect and strong evidence supporting the alternative hypothesis through the BF analysis. Moreover, the degree of "task orientation and concentration" without excluding the adult during the interaction is significant (V(28) = 7; $p = 0.003$; $r^2 = 0.566$; BF = 30. 755) indicating a strong effect, with the BF analysis indicating very strong evidence for the alternative hypothesis.

To conclude, considering the child Involvement scale, the analysis revealed a significant increase (V (28) = 0; $p = 0.002$; $r^2 = 0.613$; BF = 24.648), indicating a strong effect and a BF supporting strong evidence for the alternative hypothesis. With respect to the different subscales, results pointed out that the "simple initiative" toward the caregiver is significantly increased (V(28) = 0; $p = 0.003$; $r^2 = 0.557$; BF = 25.097) indicating strong effect and a BF supporting strong evidence for the alternative hypothesis. Further, the subscale of the "elaborative initiative" is significantly changed as well (V(28) = 2; $p = 0.036$; $r^2 = 0.425$; BF = 2.313). The subscale that considers the "use of adults" results significant (V(28) = 0; $p = 0.010$; $r^2 = 0.491$; BF = 7.206) and BF analysis indicates moderate evidence for the alternative hypothesis. This indicates an increase in the degree to which the child goes to the adult for both the emotional and playful exchange. Finally, results revealed that during intervention children seemed to increase also their involving strategies to interact with the caregiver through different channels of communication such as "eye-contact looking" (V(28) = 4.5; $p = 0.024$; $r^2 = 0.435$; BF = 2.776), "body positioning" (V(28) = 5; $p = 0.009$; $r^2 = 0.471$; BF = 4.598) and "verbal involvement" (V(28) = 0; $p < 0.0001$; $r^2 = 0.742$; BF > 100), the latter one indicating a strong effect. BF analysis indicates extreme evidence supporting the alternative hypothesis with respect to "verbal involvement" (see Table 5).

3.2. Longitudinal Changes: Play Skills

Paired sample T-tests revealed a significant decrease (t(27) = 2.922; $p = 0.007$; $r^2 = 0.234$; BF = 6.319) in the index of child exploratory play that includes the first four levels of the Play Code during intervention. Further, the Wilcoxon signed rank test with continuity correction revealed that the index of child symbolic play, that contains more advanced levels of play skills, resulted to be significantly increased (V(27) = 79; $p = 0.0255$; $r^2 = 0.392$; BF = 3.449) during intervention. Interestingly, we found out that the amount of exploratory play exhibited by caregivers and child is not correlated at T1 ($r = 0.063$; t(27) = −0.326; p = ns) but the correlation between adult and child indexes is significant at T2 ($r = 0.591$; t(27) = 3.022; $p = 0.005$) (see Table 6). Finally, we found out a moderate correlation

($r = 0.424$; $t(27) = 2.436$; $p = 0.022$) between the amount of symbolic play displayed by the caregiver and by the child at T1, but the correlation resulted to be particularly increased after intervention ($r = 0.669$; $t(27) = 4.673$; $p < 0.001$) falling into the strong range. The level of non-play, that refers to level 9 of the code, resulted to be non-significant both before and after intervention.

Table 5. Descriptive and Inferential Statistics of the Child Emotional Availability Scales–Main Scales and Subscales.

	Mean (SD)		p-Value–R^2	Bayes Factor
	T1	T2	T1–T2	T1–T2
Total Responsiveness	3.552 (0.817)	4.034 (0.844)	$p < 0.001$ ** $r^2 = 0.716$	BF > 100
Responsiveness 1: Emotional regulation of affect and behavior	3.241 (0.872)	3.552 (1.088)	$p = 0.022$ * $r^2 = 0.432$	BF = 2.880
Responsiveness 2: quantity of responsiveness	3.069 (1.163)	3.655 (1.143)	$p = 0.001$ ** $r^2 = 0.675$	BF = 21.431
Responsiveness 4: Positive physical positioning	1.724 (0.649)	2.000 (0.535)	$p = 0.036$ $r^2 = 0.479$	BF = 1.836
Responsiveness 7: Task orientation-concentration	1.448 (0.686)	1.828 (0.539)	$p = 0.003$ ** $r^2 = 0.566$	BF = 30.755
Total Involvement	3.138 (0.823)	3.379 (0.690)	$p = 0.02$ * $r^2 = 0.613$	BF = 24.648
Involvement 2: Elaborative initiative	1.655 (0.974)	1.828 (1.071)	$p = 0.036$ * $r^2 = 0.425$	BF = 2.313
Involvement 3: Use of adult	1.448 (0.632)	1.690 (0.660)	$p = 0.010$ * $r^2 = 0.491$	BF = 7.206
Involvement 5: Eye–contact looking	1.310 (0.604)	1.586 (0.733)	$p = 0.024$ * $r^2 = 0.435$	BF = 2.776
Involvement 6: Body positioning	1.759 (0.689)	2.069 (0.593)	$p = 0.009$ ** $r^2 = 0.471$	BF = 4.698
Involvement 7: Verbal involvement	1.517 (0.688)	2.069 (0.651)	$p < 0.0001$ *** $r^2 = 0.742$	BF > 100

* $p < 0.05$; ** $p < 0.01$; *** $p < 0.001$.

Table 6. Descriptive and Inferential Statistics for Play skills.

	Mean (SD)		p-Value-R^2	Bayes Factor
	T1	T2	T1–T2	T1–T2
Child Exploratory Play	0.194 (0.0715)	0.133 (0.095)	$p = 0.007$ ** $r^2 = 0.234$	BF = 6.319
Child Symbolic Play	0.0721 (0.0833)	0.125 (0.115)	$p = 0.014$ * $r^2 = 0.197$	BF = 3.449
Adult Exploratory Play	0.1666 (0.090)	0.0126 (0.087)	p = ns	BF = 0.837
Adult Symbolic Play	0.160 (0.102)	0.148 (0.124)	p = ns	BF = 0.231

* $p < 0.05$; ** $p < 0.01$.

3.3. Linear Mixed Models

3.3.1. Parents' Structuring Ability is Linked to Chronological Age and Their Perception of Having a Difficult Child

The linear mixed-effect model (Model 1, see Table 7) has been fitted considering the Structuring Total Score of the Emotional Availability Scales (EAS) as dependent variable, with time, the Difficult Child Score of the Parent Stress Index (PSI) and the caregiver chronological age as fixed effects and a random effect of participants to account for repeated measures.

Table 7. Results of Mixed Linear Models.

	Beta	T	p-Value (T)	Wald F	p-Value (W)	Chi² (Baseline Model)	Marginal R²	BIC
Model 1: Structuring						X² (6) = 9.364, p = 0.009	0.485	55.365
Intercept	1.900	t(25.474) = 2.340	p = 0.027	F (27.315) = 5.344	p = 0.029			
Predictor 1: time	0.718	t(12.196) = 9.954	p < 0.0001	F (14.543) = 96.451	p < 0.0001			
Predictor 2: Psi–Difficult Child	0.016	t(24.079) = 2.255	p = 0.034	F (26.096) = 4.531	p = 0.043			
Age caregiver	0.050	t(21.529) = 2.510	p = 0.0.020	F (23.798) = 6.226	p = 0.020			
Model 2: Non Intrusiveness						X² (5) = 26.709, p < 0.0001	0.400	101.400
Intercept	4.090	t(46.979) = 21.277	p < 0.0001	F (47.394) = 429.756	p < 0.0001			
Predictor 1: Time	0.771	t(26.111) = 7.045	p < 0.0001	F (28.052) = 48.834	p < 0.0001			
Predictor 2: GMDS-Language and Communication	0.008	t(50.000) = 2.677	p = 0.010	F (50.000) = 6.610	p = 0.013			
Model 3: language and communications scale						X²(5) = 16.218, p = 0.0003	0.164	508.120
Intercept	47.218	t(41.660) = 8.046	p < 0.0001	F (41.157) = 63.895,	p < 0.0001			
Predictor 1: Time	8.186	t(29.848) = 1.526	p = 0.138					
Predictor 2: Child symbolic play	104.376	t(46.240) = 2.810	p = 0.008	F (45.987) = 7.321,	p = 0.010			
Model 4: child Responsiveness						X² (5) = 10.086, p = 0.001	0.260	118.020
Intercept	2.947	t(46.702) = 13.129	p < 0.0001	F (47.260) = 163.592	p < 0.0001			
Predictor 1: Time	3.22	t(25.642) = 2.504	p = 0.019	F (28.093) = 28.093	p = 0.019			
Predictor 3: GMDS-Language and communication scale	0.011	t(49.983) = 3.389	p = 0.001	F (49.986) = 10.590	p = 0.002			

The model showed a significant intercept (b = 1.900; t(25.474) = 2.340; $p = 0.027$). All the predictors were significant: time (b = 0.718; t(12.196) = 9.954; $p < 0.0001$); the Difficult Child Score of the PSI (b = 0.016; t(24.079) = 2.255; $p = 0.034$) and the chronological age of the caregiver (b = 0.050; t(21.529) = 2.510; $p = 0.020$).

Anova with Wald F test confirmed significance of the intercept (F(27.315) = 5.344; $p = 0.029$) and all the predictors: time (F(14.543) = 96.451; $p < 0.0001$); the Difficult Child Score (F(26.096) = 4.5313; $p = 0.0429$) and the chronological age of the caregiver (F(23.798) = 6.226; $p = 0.020$).

The model has been compared against a baseline model (BIC = 57.402) considering only the time, and resulted to be significant (χ^2 (6) = 9.364; $p = 0.009$; BIC = 55.365) showing an increase in the goodness of fit, with a marginal R-squared of 0.485.

3.3.2. Parents' Non-Intrusiveness is Linked to Child's Language Ability

Model 2 (see Table 6) has been fitted considering the Non-intrusiveness Total Score of the Emotional Availability Scales (EAS) as dependent variable, with time and the child's Language Quotient of the Griffiths Mental Development Scale (GMDS) as fixed effects, and a random effect of participants to account for repeated measures.

The model showed a significant intercept (b = 4.090; t(46.979) =2 1.277; $p < 0.0001$). All the predictors are significant: time (b = 0.771; t(26.111) = 7.045; $p < 0.0001$) and the child's Language Quotient (b = 0.008; t(50.000) = 2.677; $p = 0.010$).

Anova with Wald F test confirmed significance of the intercept (F (47.394) = 429.756; $p < 0.0001$), time (F(28.052) = 48.834; $p < 0.0001$) and the Language Quotient (F(50.000) = 6.610; $p = 0.013$).

The model has been compared against a baseline model (BIC = 123.140) considering only the time, and resulted to be significant (χ^2 (5) = 26.709; $p < 0.0001$; BIC = 101.400) showing an increase in the goodness of fit, with a marginal R-squared of 0.400.

3.3.3. Child's Symbolic Play Level is Predictive of Child's Language Ability

Model 3 (see Table 6) has been fitted considering the child's Language Quotient as dependent variable, with time and the child's symbolic play index as fixed effects, and a random effect of participants to account for repeated measures.

The model showed a significant intercept (b = 47.218; t(41.660) = 8.046; $p < 0.0001$). Time resulted to be non-significant (b = 8.186; t(29.848) = 1.526; $p = 0.138$). The symbolic play index was significant (b = 104.376; t(46.240) = 2.810; $p = 0.008$).

Anova with Wald F test confirmed the significance of the intercept (F(41.157) = 63.895; $p < 0.0001$) and the symbolic play index (F(45.987) = 7.321; $p = 0.010$).

The model has been compared against a baseline model (BIC = 516.400) considering only the intercept, and resulted to be significant (χ^2 (5) = 16.218; $p = 0.0003$; BIC = 508.12) showing an increase in the goodness of fit, with a marginal R-squared of 0.164.

3.3.4. Child's Responsivity is Linked to Child's Language Ability

Model 4 (see Table 6) has been fitted considering the Responsivity Total Score of the Emotional Availability Scales (EAS) as dependent variable, with time and the child's Language Quotient of the Griffiths Mental Development Scale (GMDS) as fixed effects and a random effect of participants to account for repeated measures.

The model showed a significant intercept (b = 2.947; t(46.702) = 13.129; $p < 0.0001$). All the predictors were significant: time (b = 0.322; t(25.642) = 2.504; $p = 0.019$) and the child's Language Quotient (b = 0.011; t(49.983) = 3.389; $p = 0.001$).

Anova with Wald F test confirmed significance of the intercept (F(47.260) = 163.592; $p < 0.0001$), time (F(28.093) = 6.171; $p = 0.019$) and the Language Quotient (F(49.986) = 10.590; $p = 0.002$).

The model has been compared against a baseline model (BIC = 124.140) considering only the time, and resulted to be significant (χ^2 (5) = 10.086; p = 0.001; BIC = 118.020) showing an increase in the goodness of fit, with a marginal R-squared of 0.260.

4. Discussion

Given the importance of parental involvement into the therapeutic setting [53,55–57,79,99,100] and the paucity of studies highlighting parental and dyadic changes during intervention, the main purpose of the present study was to investigate mother–child dyads with ASD through two standardized behavioral instruments that allow to assess both the affective quality and play skills abilities of these dyads.

With respect to our first aim, we wanted to analyze the dyadic aspects of mother–child interaction and the bidirectional influence during the exchange. These elements were assessed through the Emotional Availability Scales (EAS) before and after intervention and revealed a significant improvement in the mother's general level of Sensitivity, especially in the subscale of awareness of timing during the interaction, waiting for the appropriate moment to propose or interrupt the child. In line with this, other studies, using different instruments than the EAS in the evaluation of treatment, reported major parent's acceptance of the child and positive dyadic pattern [53,99]. Further, our results are also in line with findings suggesting that parents seem to show changes in their interactive strategies pre and post intervention [78,79]. In fact, we found a significant increase in mothers' general Structuring abilities from inconsistent to moderate–good levels. Interestingly, the analysis of the subscales revealed that the improvement concerned an enhanced quality of proactive guidance and varied suggestions that lead the child in an appropriate way. Also, parents seem to adequately structure just the right amount according to the child's need, using both verbal but also non-verbal strategies. This result could be even more important in the context of ASD. In fact, communicative abilities are often impaired, and thus verbal indications are generally not enough to effectively scaffold an appropriate interaction, making the use of nonverbal strategies play a crucial role. Consequently, interaction attempts are more appropriate and, therefore, more successful during the interaction with the child. Because EA is a dyadic construct which describes both the sending and receiving emotional signs, the structure is considered adequate when parent's attempts are successful, in the sense that these are appreciated and welcomed by the child.

While Structuring is about guidance and mentoring, Non-Intrusiveness is about the actual over-direction, over stimulation and interference into child's behaviors and, in the literature, these scales resulted to be particularly correlated one to the other [101]. Our results suggested that non-intrusive behaviors increased from "inconsistent" to "moderate–good" over time. In particular, mothers seemed to be more able to follow the child's needs without interfering too much with his/her activity. In fact, fewer interruptions were observed, in favor of waiting for the perfect timing to interrupt or to propose another activity to the child. Further, the verbal and or physical interferences decreased significantly, indicating more appropriateness in the way of dealing with the child, that in turn showed fewer signs indicating that the adult is intrusive in his/her activity. This result appears to be particularly relevant considering that literature about parenting in the context of neurodevelopmental disorders consistently underlined the tendency of caregivers to be more intrusive during the interpersonal interchange [4,25]. In this framework, a significant improvement of this parental behavior, together with better scaffolding strategies and skills, represent two important elements that may actually impact on the dyadic quality of the interplay. Furthermore, in line with previous literature that depicted the Non-Hostility scale as particularly stable and difficult to detect compared to the other scales [90,102] we did not find changes over time. In fact, an expert observer may also have some difficulties in noting subtle and covert signs of hostility (e.g., boredom, discomfort) in an adult's tone of voice or in face, and more time for an appropriate and accurate evaluation is needed [102]. Also, even if parents are particularly uncomfortable during the interaction, they are aware of the fact that they are video-recorded, and for this they unlikely will show clear signs of hostility and/or aggression toward the child. However, our results highlighted the substantial absence of hostile behaviors and signs, with scores being in the range "moderate–good" both pre- and post-intervention [38,102].

The child's increases in the responsiveness domains might be influenced by parental involvement, which gives them the possibility to experience positive exchanges, first of all mediated by the therapist and then gradually alone with the child. In this sense, the therapist somehow acts as a promoter of the exchange, supporting both the partners in establishing effective and adaptive social routines in which they can experiment themselves in a functional and pleasant manner. Therefore, the therapist gradually leaves space to the dyad, supporting them only when necessary to facilitate reciprocal attunement. Experimenting with these positive changes, parents might be more motivated and facilitated to reproduce specific social routines also in the domestic context.

Concerning the child's scales, in general we expected that a specific work on adult abilities would impact also on child's abilities to respond positively to the more adequate and functional proposals. On the basis of our hypothesis and considering the dyadic nature of the relationship in which both the partners play an active role, we also expected a subsequent increase in the child's Responsiveness scale. In fact, the significant increases found in parents may indicate having acquired better abilities to understand, interpret and respond to their communicative signals, often impaired or atypical in ASD.

In line with this, results in literature showed how children exhibit better play skills when the activities were scaffolded by an adult [44,103]. Within a more supported environment, children are provided more opportunities to request and comment on objects than they would have if they played alone. Coherently, our results revealed an increase in child's general affective regulation, even if scores are still in the inconsistent range of the Responsiveness scale. In fact, it may be still present a quality of inappropriateness and the child may get dysregulated in front of particularly challenging situations. Nevertheless, the general amount of the child's responsiveness to parents' initiative significantly increased over time, and this was also confirmed by the significant increase in the subscale that assesses the amount of physical contact sought by the child. The framework of the intervention focuses on two main aspects: establishing virtuous circles in the dyad and promoting intentionality and reciprocity. The results discussed so far seem to support the first one. With respect to the second, results seemed to depict a more intentional child. In fact, even if general levels of the Involvement scale generally fall into the "inconsistent–low" range both before and after intervention, it is interesting to notice that children significantly enhanced their involving strategies towards their caregivers. Child's involving strategies comprise: the use of non-verbal channels such as eye-contact or verbal involvement, using both talking and babbling, and also through the physical positioning of their body in a way that does not exclude the other. These results suggest an enhancement in child's functional strategies to involve the social partner, effectively expressing communicative intentionality.

As we expected, the child responds to more effective caregiver strategies progressively increasing his/her degree of motivation to begin socio-communicative routines in the first place, therefore actively engaging the social partner in the interchange.

As highlighted by literature, more functional and effective interactions also have an impact on cognitive abilities and, in general, on child development [2,3] also in the context of ASD [8,14,16]. Further, it is well established that play skills are related to cognitive skills and play is considered as a primary opportunity of learning, especially when shared in the context of child–adult interactions [102]. On this basis, in the context of intervention, shared play represents a key mediator of the whole process [10]. In line with this, children did not show significant changes in the quantity of play, demonstrated by the fact that "non-play levels" seem to be stable before and after the intervention. Nonetheless, as we expected, child's play exhibited significant changes in quality over time. In fact, we found out a significant increase in children's symbolic play together with the reduction in the levels of the exploratory play. Hence, results suggest a significant evolution in the quality of play in the direction of the typical milestones of play development. Interestingly, mothers' and children's play levels are related to each other. In fact, child's exploratory play was moderately correlated with that of the mother after intervention, but not before, suggesting the presence of a greater ability of dyadic synchronization. Further, mothers' and children's symbolic play levels resulted to be significantly correlated both before and after intervention. Even more importantly, correlation increases from moderate to strong over time with respect to symbolic play. This change goes in the direction of the reinforcement of higher levels of reciprocal syntonization, supporting the importance of directly intervening on the dyad to promote bidirectional exchange.

So far, we pointed out significant changes in affective and cognitive aspects of the relationship in the context of intervention. In line with previous literature, we investigated both child and caregivers' factors that might be relevant for the intervention. Particularly, we expected that parental stress levels could have an influence on adult Emotional Availability. We found out that the general stress levels seemed not predictive of parents' abilities. Interestingly, among the different subdimensions of parental stress, a significant negative relationship emerged between the perception of having a difficult child and the ability of the caregiver to adequately structure the interaction. From a clinical standpoint, this result might emphasize the relevance of caregivers' perception of the child, as well as the need of taking into account parents' mental representation during the implementation of the parental based early intensive intervention.

Further, we also explored the impact of child's variables on caregivers' behaviors. From our analysis, it emerged that the child's language communicative abilities seemed to be positively associated with parents' ability to not be intrusive, interfering with the child's activity. In addition to this, linguistic and communicative elements seemed to impact also on the child's relational aspects, in particular in his/her modalities to respond to the mother. More specifically, language abilities seemed to be in turn linked to play abilities. In particular, greater symbolic play skills appear to be predictive of better language. From this analysis, it emerges that linguistic aspects showed a general influence on both parent and child interactive behaviors. In particular, when a child has the possibility to directly communicate in a more effective way, the parent, in turn, gives the impression to show a lower necessity to directly interfere with his/her activity. It is also worth noting that, in line with literature on developmental psychology, our results seemed to support the role of play competencies in cognitive development, which in turn entirely happens in the context of the interpersonal relationship mediated by affective exchanges.

Limitations

This study presents some limitations. A main limit of the present work is represented by the small sample size, consequently, further studies should be conducted with larger samples size in order to achieve more generalizable results. Our study also focused only on mothers, while fathers may show different characteristics and changes. Moreover, our sample is unbalanced with respect to gender and therefore, this limits the generalization of the results to females, that may have different characteristics. Another main limitation consists in the absence of a comparison group subjected to an intervention with a different theoretical framework (e.g., treatment "as-usual") or another clinical group that was not exposed to any intervention. However, given the importance of guaranteeing an early intervention as soon as possible especially for preschool children with neurodevelopmental disorders, waiting lists were not a possibility. Another limitation of this study concerns the presence of only two time points for the evaluation of the dyadic changes, in fact more assessments will be able to better describe the process of change in both affective quality and play during interventions.

In this sense, we aim to conduct next studies including a bigger sample comprising fathers and more balanced with respect to gender. We will also work on building a comparison group made by children that are regularly monitored by ODFLab, but that receive the intervention in their local community services since they come from other regions. Since such interventions usually do not provide parental involvement, this can be considered as a treatment "as usual" and therefore constitutes a suitable comparison group. Further research should also include more longitudinal time points in order to better understand trajectories' trend. Finally, next works will include different subgroups of patients with different characteristics in cognitive functioning and symptoms severity, as well as intervention outcomes variables.

5. Conclusions

Investigating the longitudinal changes in parent–child affective quality and play skills during a parental based early intervention may have important implications. From a theoretical perspective, it enhances knowledge about child's and caregiver's variables that impact on dyadic outcomes. In particular, our findings are in line with a reciprocal interdependence between the social partners, in which play skills are linked to child's language development that, in turn, have an impact on parent's interactive skills. Further, these abilities seem also to be influenced by the caregiver's perceptions and representations of their children. From a clinical standpoint, our results suggest that parental-based intervention supports and facilitates improvements in both children's and caregivers' affective quality and cognitive abilities. In particular, parents and children exhibit greater levels of syntonization during play, as well as a trajectory that follows the milestones of typical development towards progressively more evolved interactive modalities. Further, studying dyadic aspects allows to identify important target areas to be addressed during intervention. Through this, it may be possible to identify peculiar outcome trajectories associated with different profiles and this, in turn, might help planning individualized intervention programs that directly influence parent–child interaction. To conclude, our results support the importance of actively involving caregivers during the intervention.

Author Contributions: Conceptualization and Methodology: A.B., S.P., G.B., P.V. Formal Analysis: G.B., S.P. Patient recruitment: A.B., S.P. Data Curation: G.B., S.P. Writing—Original Draft Preparation: S.P., G.B., A.B. Writing—Review and Editing: P.V., S.P., G.B., A.B. Supervision: A.B., P.V., S.d.F. All authors have read and agreed to the published version of the manuscript.

Funding: This research received no external funding.

Acknowledgments: We gratefully acknowledge the families participating in our research and all the clinical psychologists and psychotherapists of the Laboratory of Observation, Diagnosis and Education (ODFLab).

Conflicts of Interest: The authors declare no conflict of interest.

References

1. American Psychiatric Association. *Diagnostic and Statistical Manual of Mental Disorders*, 5th ed.; American Psychiatric Publishing: Washington, DC, USA, 2014.
2. Gartstein, M.A.; Crawford, J.; Robertson, C.D. Early Markers of Language and Attention: Mutual Contributions and the Impact of Parent–Infant Interactions. *Child Psychiatry Hum. Dev.* **2008**, *39*, 9–26. [CrossRef] [PubMed]
3. Cyr, C.; Dubois-Comtois, K.; Moss, E. Mother-child conversations and the attachment of children in the pre-school period. *Can. J. Behav. Sci.* **2008**, *40*, 140–152. [CrossRef]
4. Blacher, J.; Baker, B.L.; Kaladjian, A. Syndrome Specificity and Mother–Child Interactions: Examining Positive and Negative Parenting across Contexts and Time. *J. Autism Dev. Disord.* **2013**, *43*, 761–774. [CrossRef] [PubMed]
5. Slonims, V.; McConachie, H. Analysis of Mother–Infant Interaction in Infants with Down Syndrome and Typically Developing Infants. *Am. J. Ment. Retard.* **2006**, *111*, 273. [CrossRef]
6. Leclère, C.; Viaux, S.; Avril, M.; Achard, C.; Chetouani, M.; Missonnier, S.; Cohen, D. Why Synchrony Matters during Mother-Child Interactions: A Systematic Review. *PLoS ONE* **2014**, *9*, e113571. [CrossRef] [PubMed]
7. Karst, J.S.; Van Hecke, A.V. Parent and Family Impact of Autism Spectrum Disorders: A Review and Proposed Model for Intervention Evaluation. *Clin. Child Fam. Psychol. Rev.* **2012**, *15*, 247–277. [CrossRef]
8. Kasari, C.; Gulsrud, A.C.; Wong, C.; Kwon, S.; Locke, J. Randomized controlled caregiver mediated joint engagement intervention for toddlers with autism. *J. Autism Dev. Disord.* **2010**, *40*, 1045–1056. [CrossRef]
9. Adamson, L.B.; Deckner, D.F.; Bakeman, R. Early Interests and Joint Engagement in Typical Development, Autism, and Down Syndrome. *J. Autism Dev. Disord.* **2010**, *40*, 665–676. [CrossRef]
10. Wong, C.; Kasari, C. Play and Joint Attention of Children with Autism in the Preschool Special Education Classroom. *J. Autism Dev. Disord.* **2012**, *42*, 2152–2161. [CrossRef]

11. Dawson, G.; Toth, K.; Abbott, R.; Osterling, J.; Munson, J.; Estes, A.; Liaw, J. Early Social Attention Impairments in Autism: Social Orienting, Joint Attention, and Attention to Distress. *Dev. Psychol.* **2004**, *40*, 271–283. [CrossRef]
12. Kaale, A.; Smith, L.; Nordahl-Hansen, A.; Fagerland, M.W.; Kasari, C. Early Interaction in Autism Spectrum Disorder: Mothers' and Children's Behaviours during Joint Engagement. *Child Care Health Dev.* **2018**, *44*, 312–318. [CrossRef] [PubMed]
13. Wan, M.W.; Green, J.; Scott, J. A Systematic Review of Parent–Infant Interaction in Infants at Risk of Autism. *Autism* **2019**, *23*, 811–820. [CrossRef] [PubMed]
14. Zlomke, K.R.; Bauman, S.; Edwards, G.S. An Exploratory Study of the Utility of the Dyadic Parent-Child Interaction Coding System for Children with Autism Spectrum Disorder. *J. Dev. Phys. Disabil.* **2019**, *31*, 501–518. [CrossRef]
15. Bornstein, M.H.; Venuti, P.; Hahn, C.-S. Mother-Child Play in Italy: Regional Variation, Individual Stability, and Mutual Dyadic Influence. *Parenting* **2002**, *2*, 273–301. [CrossRef]
16. Pierucci, J.M. Mothers' Scaffolding Techniques Used During Play in Toddlers with Autism Spectrum Disorder. *J. Dev. Phys. Disabil.* **2016**, *28*, 217–235. [CrossRef]
17. Ting, V.; Weiss, J.A. Emotion Regulation and Parent Co-Regulation in Children with Autism Spectrum Disorder. *J. Autism Dev. Disord.* **2017**, *47*, 680–689. [CrossRef] [PubMed]
18. Cabrera, N.J.; Fitzgerald, H.E.; Bradley, R.H.; Roggman, L. The Ecology of Father-Child Relationships: An Expanded Model. *J. Fam. Theory Rev.* **2014**, *6*, 336–354. [CrossRef]
19. Volling, B.L.; Cabrera, N.J.; Feinberg, M.E.; Jones, D.E.; McDaniel, B.T.; Liu, S.; Almeida, D.; Lee, J.; Schoppe-Sullivan, S.J.; Feng, X.; et al. Advancing Research and Measurement on Fathering and Children's Development. *Monogr. Soc. Res. Child* **2019**, *84*, 7–160. [CrossRef] [PubMed]
20. Rankin, J.A.; Paisley, C.A.; Tomeny, T.S.; Eldred, S.W. Fathers of Youth with Autism Spectrum Disorder: A Systematic Review of the Impact of Fathers' Involvement on Youth, Families, and Intervention. *Clin. Child Fam. Psychol. Rev.* **2019**, *22*, 458–477. [CrossRef]
21. Bentenuto, A.; Perzolli, S.; de Falco, S.; Venuti, P. The Emotional Availability in Mother-Child and Father-Child Interactions in Families with Children with Autism Spectrum Disorder. *Res. Autism Spectr. Disord.* **2020**, *75*, 101569. [CrossRef]
22. Sethna, V.; Perry, E.; Domoney, J.; Iles, J.; Psychogiou, L.; Rowbotham, N.E.L.; Stein, A.; Murray, L.; Ramchandani, P.G. Father-child interactions at 3 months and 24 months: Contributions to children's cognitive development at 24 months: Fathers' and Children's Cognitive Development. *Infant Ment. Health J.* **2017**, *38*, 378–390. [CrossRef] [PubMed]
23. Spiker, D.; Boyce, G.C.; Boyce, L.K. Parent-Child Interactions When Young Children Have Disabilities. In *International Review of Research in Mental Retardation*; Elsevier: Amsterdam, The Netherlands, 2002; Volume 25, pp. 35–70. [CrossRef]
24. Meirsschaut, M.; Warreyn, P.; Roeyers, H. What Is the Impact of Autism on Mother-Child Interactions within Families with a Child with Autism Spectrum Disorder? *Autism Res.* **2011**, *4*, 358–367. [CrossRef]
25. Freeman, S.; Kasari, C. Parent–Child Interactions in Autism: Characteristics of Play. *Autism* **2013**, *17*, 147–161. [CrossRef] [PubMed]
26. Campbell, S.B.; Mahoney, A.S.; Northrup, J.; Moore, E.L.; Leezenbaum, N.B.; Brownell, C.A. Developmental Changes in Pretend Play from 22- to 34-Months in Younger Siblings of Children with Autism Spectrum Disorder. *J. Abnorm. Child Psychol.* **2018**, *46*, 639–654. [CrossRef] [PubMed]
27. Van IJzendoorn, M.H.; Rutgers, A.H.; Bakermans-Kranenburg, M.J.; Swinkels, S.H.N.; van Daalen, E.; Dietz, C.; Naber, F.B.A.; Buitelaar, J.K.; van Engeland, H. Parental Sensitivity and Attachment in Children With Autism Spectrum Disorder: Comparison with Children with Mental Retardation, with Language Delays, and With Typical Development. *Child Dev.* **2007**, *78*, 597–608. [CrossRef] [PubMed]
28. Madarevic, M.; van Esch, L.; Lambrechts, G.; Van Leeuwen, K.; Noens, I. Mothers of Pre-Schoolers with ASD: Parenting Behaviours, Parenting Stress, and Externalising Behaviour Problems. *PsyArXiv Prepr.* **2020**. [CrossRef]
29. Siller, M.; Sigman, M. Modeling Longitudinal Change in the Language Abilities of Children with Autism: Parent Behaviors and Child Characteristics as Predictors of Change. *Dev. Psychol.* **2008**, *44*, 1691–1704. [CrossRef] [PubMed]
30. Venuti, P. Percorsi Evolutivi, Roma, Carocci Editore. 2007. Available online: http://www.carocci.it/index.php?option=com_carocci&task=schedalibro&Itemid=72&isbn=9788843041602 (accessed on 23 November 2020).

31. Biringen, Z.; Easterbrooks, M.A. Emotional Availability: Concept, Research, and Window on Developmental Psychopathology. *Dev. Psychopathol.* **2012**, *24*, 1–8. [CrossRef]
32. Biringen, Z. The Emotional Availability (EA) Scales Manual: Part 1. Infancy/Early Childhood Version. 2008. Available online: https://www.google.com.hk/url?sa=t&rct=j&q=&esrc=s&source=web&cd=&ved=2ahUKEwj4otDHm5rtAhXRZt4KHWJcCdsQFjAAegQIARAC&url=http%3A%2F%2Fwww.emotionalavailability.com%2Fwp-content%2Fuploads%2F2009%2F08%2FEmotional-Availability-Trainings-Description.pdf&usg=AOvVaw3l9LfXhanv8pFe79hHYSo7 (accessed on 23 November 2020).
33. Bornstein, M.H.; Putnick, D.L.; Suwalsky, J.T.D.; Venuti, P.; de Falco, S.; de Galperín, C.Z.; Gini, M.; Tichovolsky, M.H. Emotional Relationships in Mothers and Infants: Culture-Common and Community-Specific Characteristics of Dyads From Rural and Metropolitan Settings in Argentina, Italy, and the United States. *J. Cross-Cult. Psychol.* **2012**, *43*, 171–197. [CrossRef]
34. Bornstein, M.H.; Suwalsky, J.T.D.; Putnick, D.L.; Gini, M.; Venuti, P.; de Falco, S.; Heslington, M.; Zingman de Galperín, C. Developmental Continuity and Stability of Emotional Availability in the Family: Two Ages and Two Genders in Child-Mother Dyads from Two Regions in Three Countries. *Int. J. Behav. Dev.* **2010**, *34*, 385–397. [CrossRef]
35. Easterbrooks, M.A.; Biringen, Z. Introduction to the Special Issue: Emotional Availability across Contexts. *Parenting* **2009**, *9*, 179–182. [CrossRef]
36. Bornstein, M.H.; Putnick, D.L.; Heslington, M.; Gini, M.; Suwalsky, J.T.D.; Venuti, P.; de Falco, S.; Giusti, Z.; Zingman de Galperín, C. Mother-Child Emotional Availability in Ecological Perspective: Three Countries, Two Regions, Two Genders. *Dev. Psychol.* **2008**, *44*, 666–680. [CrossRef] [PubMed]
37. Gul, H.; Erol, N.; Pamir Akin, D.; Ustun Gullu, B.; Akcakin, M.; Alpas, B.; Öner, Ö. Emotional availability in early mother-child interactions for children with autism spectrum disorders, other psychiatric disorders, and developmental delay: Emotional Availability in Early Interactions. *Infant Ment. Health J.* **2016**, *37*, 151–159. [CrossRef] [PubMed]
38. Dolev, S.; Oppenheim, D.; Koren-Karie, N.; Yirmiya, N. Emotional Availability in Mother-Child Interaction: The Case of Children with Autism Spectrum Disorders. *Parenting* **2009**, *9*, 183–197. [CrossRef]
39. Licata, M.; Zietlow, A.-L.; Träuble, B.; Sodian, B.; Reck, C. Maternal Emotional Availability and Its Association with Maternal Psychopathology, Attachment Style Insecurity and Theory of Mind. *Psychopathology* **2016**, *49*, 334–340. [CrossRef]
40. Saunders, H.; Kraus, A.; Barone, L.; Biringen, Z. Emotional Availability: Theory, Research, and Intervention. *Front. Psychol.* **2015**, *6*, 1069. [CrossRef]
41. Martins, E.C.; Soares, I.; Martins, C.; Tereno, S.; Osório, A. Can We Identify Emotion Over-Regulation in Infancy? Associations with Avoidant Attachment, Dyadic Emotional Interaction and Temperament: Emotion over-Regulation in Infancy. *Inf. Child Dev.* **2012**, *21*, 579–595. [CrossRef]
42. Schneider-Hassloff, H.; Zwönitzer, A.; Künster, A.K.; Mayer, C.; Ziegenhain, U.; Kiefer, M. Emotional Availability Modulates Electrophysiological Correlates of Executive Functions in Preschool Children. *Front. Hum. Neurosci.* **2016**, *10*. [CrossRef]
43. Célia, M.-G.; Stack, D.M.; Serbin, L.A. Developmental Patterns of Change in Mother and Child Emotional Availability from Infancy to the End of the Preschool Years: A Four-Wave Longitudinal Study. *Infant Behav. Dev.* **2018**, *52*, 76–88. [CrossRef]
44. Beurkens, N.M.; Hobson, J.A.; Hobson, R.P. Autism Severity and Qualities of Parent–Child Relations. *J. Autism Dev. Disord.* **2013**, *43*, 168–178. [CrossRef]
45. Lory, C.; Rispoli, M.; Gregori, E. Play Interventions Involving Children with Autism Spectrum Disorder and Typically Developing Peers: A Review of Research Quality. *Rev. J. Autism Dev. Disord.* **2018**, *5*, 78–89. [CrossRef]
46. Bentenuto, A.; De Falco, S.; Venuti, P. Mother-Child Play: A Comparison of Autism Spectrum Disorder, Down Syndrome, and Typical Development. *Front. Psychol.* **2016**, *7*, 1829. [CrossRef] [PubMed]
47. O'Reilly, A.W.; Bornstein, M.N. Caregiver-Child Interaction in Play. *New Dir. Child Adolesc. Dev.* **1993**, *1993*, 55–66. [CrossRef]
48. Hayes, S.A.; Watson, S.L. The Impact of Parenting Stress: A Meta-Analysis of Studies Comparing the Experience of Parenting Stress in Parents of Children With and Without Autism Spectrum Disorder. *J. Autism Dev. Disord.* **2013**, *43*, 629–642. [CrossRef] [PubMed]
49. Goetz, G.L.; Rodriguez, G.; Hartley, S.L. Actor-Partner Examination of Daily Parenting Stress and Couple Interactions in the Context of Child Autism. *J. Fam. Psychol.* **2019**, *33*, 554–564. [CrossRef]

50. Barroso, N.E.; Mendez, L.; Graziano, P.A.; Bagner, D.M. Parenting Stress through the Lens of Different Clinical Groups: A Systematic Review & Meta-Analysis. *J. Abnorm. Child Psychol.* **2018**, *46*, 449–461. [CrossRef]
51. Brown, M.; Whiting, J.; Kahumoku-Fessler, E.; Witting, A.B.; Jensen, J. A Dyadic Model of Stress, Coping, and Marital Satisfaction among Parents of Children with Autism. *Fam. Relat.* **2020**, *69*, 138–150. [CrossRef]
52. Venuti, P. *Intervento e Riabilitazione Nei Disturbi Dello Spettro Autistico*; Carocci Editore: Roma, Italy, 2012.
53. Oono, I.P.; Honey, E.J.; McConachie, H. Parent-Mediated Early Intervention for Young Children with Autism Spectrum Disorders (ASD): Parent-Mediated Early Intervention for Young Children with Autism Spectrum Disorders (ASD). *Evid.-Based Child Health* **2013**, *8*, 2380–2479. [CrossRef]
54. Parsons, L.; Cordier, R.; Munro, N.; Joosten, A.; Speyer, R. A Systematic Review of Pragmatic Language Interventions for Children with Autism Spectrum Disorder. *PLoS ONE* **2017**, *12*, e0172242. [CrossRef]
55. Green, J.; Charman, T.; McConachie, H.; Aldred, C.; Slonims, V.; Howlin, P.; Le Couteur, A.; Leadbitter, K.; Hudry, K.; Byford, S.; et al. Parent-Mediated Communication-Focused Treatment in Children with Autism (PACT): A Randomised Controlled Trial. *Lancet* **2010**, *375*, 2152–2160. [CrossRef]
56. Pickles, A.; Le Couteur, A.; Leadbitter, K.; Salomone, E.; Cole-Fletcher, R.; Tobin, H.; Gammer, I.; Lowry, J.; Vamvakas, G.; Byford, S.; et al. Parent-Mediated Social Communication Therapy for Young Children with Autism (PACT): Long-Term Follow-up of a Randomised Controlled Trial. *Lancet* **2016**, *388*, 2501–2509. [CrossRef]
57. Green, J.; Aldred, C.; Charman, T.; Le Couteur, A.; Emsley, R.A.; Grahame, V.; Howlin, P.; Humphrey, N.; Leadbitter, K.; McConachie, H.; et al. Paediatric Autism Communication Therapy-Generalised (PACT-G) against Treatment as Usual for Reducing Symptom Severity in Young Children with Autism Spectrum Disorder: Study Protocol for a Randomised Controlled Trial. *Trials* **2018**, *19*, 514. [CrossRef] [PubMed]
58. Page, J.; Constantino, J.N.; Zambrana, K.; Martin, E.; Tunc, I.; Zhang, Y.; Abbacchi, A.; Messinger, D. Quantitative Autistic Trait Measurements Index Background Genetic Risk for ASD in Hispanic Families. *Mol. Autism* **2016**, *7*, 39. [CrossRef] [PubMed]
59. Rogers, S.J.; Estes, A.; Lord, C.; Munson, J.; Rocha, M.; Winter, J.; Greenson, J.; Colombi, C.; Dawson, G.; Vismara, L.A.; et al. A Multisite Randomized Controlled Two-Phase Trial of the Early Start Denver Model Compared to Treatment as Usual. *J. Am. Acad. Child Adolesc. Psychiatry* **2019**, *58*, 853–865. [CrossRef]
60. Fuller, E.A.; Kaiser, A.P. The Effects of Early Intervention on Social Communication Outcomes for Children with Autism Spectrum Disorder: A Meta-Analysis. *J. Autism Dev. Disord.* **2020**, *50*, 1683–1700. [CrossRef]
61. Bentenuto, A.; Bertamini, G.; Perzolli, S.; Venuti, P. Changes in Developmental Trajectories of Preschool Children with Autism Spectrum Disorder during Parental Based Intensive Intervention. *Brain Sci.* **2020**, *10*, 289. [CrossRef]
62. Stringer, D.; Kent, R.; Briskman, J.; Lukito, S.; Charman, T.; Baird, G.; Lord, C.; Pickles, A.; Simonoff, E. Trajectories of Emotional and Behavioral Problems from Childhood to Early Adult Life. *Autism* **2020**, *24*, 1011–1024. [CrossRef]
63. Szatmari, P.; Georgiades, S.; Duku, E.; Bennett, T.A.; Bryson, S.; Fombonne, E.; Volden, J. Developmental trajectories of symptom severity and adaptive functioning in an inception cohort of preschool children with autism spectrum disorder. *JAMA Psychiatry* **2015**, *72*, 276–283. [CrossRef]
64. Klintwall, L.; Eldevik, S.; Eikeseth, S. Narrowing the gap: Effects of intervention on developmental trajectories in autism. *Autism* **2015**, *19*, 53–63. [CrossRef]
65. Venker, C.E.; Ray-Subramanian, C.E.; Bolt, D.M.; Weismer, S.E. Trajectories of autism severity in early childhood. *J. Autism Dev. Disord.* **2014**, *44*, 546–563. [CrossRef]
66. Tiede, G.; Walton, K.M. Meta-Analysis of Naturalistic Developmental Behavioral Interventions for Young Children with Autism Spectrum Disorder. *Autism* **2019**, *23*, 2080–2095. [CrossRef] [PubMed]
67. Lord, C.; Rutter, M.; DiLavore, P.C.; Risi, S.; Gotham, K.; Bishop, S. *Autism Diagnostic Observation Schedule–Second Edition (ADOS-2)*; Western Psychological Services: Los Angeles, CA, USA, 2012.
68. Luiz, D.; Barnard, A.; Knosen, N.; Kotras, N.; Horrocks, S.; McAlinden, P.; O'Connell, R. *GMDS-ER 2–8 Griffith Mental Developmental Scales-Extended Revised: 2 to 8 Years*; The Test Agency: Oxford, UK, 2006.
69. Anagnostou, E.; Jones, N.; Huerta, M.; Halladay, A.K.; Wang, P.; Scahill, L.; Horrigan, J.P.; Kasari, C.; Lord, C.; Choi, D.; et al. Measuring Social Communication Behaviors as a Treatment Endpoint in Individuals with Autism Spectrum Disorder. *Autism* **2015**, *19*, 622–636. [CrossRef] [PubMed]
70. MacDonald, R.; Parry-Cruwys, D.; Dupere, S.; Ahearn, W. Assessing Progress and Outcome of Early Intensive Behavioral Intervention for Toddlers with Autism. *Res. Dev. Disabil.* **2014**, *35*, 3632–3644. [CrossRef] [PubMed]

71. Ben Itzchak, E.; Zachor, D.A. Who Benefits from Early Intervention in Autism Spectrum Disorders? *Res. Autism Spectr. Disord.* **2011**, *5*, 345–350. [CrossRef]
72. Strauss, K.; Vicari, S.; Valeri, G.; D'Elia, L.; Arima, S.; Fava, L. Parent Inclusion in Early Intensive Behavioral Intervention: The Influence of Parental Stress, Parent Treatment Fidelity and Parent-Mediated Generalization of Behavior Targets on Child Outcomes. *Res. Dev. Disabil.* **2012**, *33*, 688–703. [CrossRef]
73. Patterson, S.Y.; Elder, L.; Gulsrud, A.; Kasari, C. The Association between Parental Interaction Style and Children's Joint Engagement in Families with Toddlers with Autism. *Autism* **2014**, *18*, 511–518. [CrossRef]
74. Bornstein, M.H.; Putnick, D.L.; Suwalsky, J.T.D. A Longitudinal Process Analysis of Mother-Child Emotional Relationships in a Rural Appalachian European American Community. *Am. J. Community Psychol.* **2012**, *50*, 89–100. [CrossRef]
75. Bornstein, M.H.; Putnick, D.L.; Suwalsky, J.T.D.; Gini, M. Maternal Chronological Age, Prenatal and Perinatal History, Social Support, and Parenting of Infants. *Child Dev.* **2006**, *77*, 875–892. [CrossRef]
76. Bornstein, M.H.; Gini, M.; Suwalsky, J.T.D.; Putnick, D.L.; Haynes, O.M. Emotional Availability in Mother-Child Dyads: Short-Term Stability and Continuity from Variable-Centered and Person-Centered Perspectives. *Merrill-Palmer Q.* **2006**, *52*, 547–571. [CrossRef]
77. Hickey, E.J.; Hartley, S.L.; Papp, L. Psychological Well-Being and Parent-Child Relationship Quality in Relation to Child Autism: An Actor-Partner Modeling Approach. *Fam. Proc.* **2020**, *59*, 636–650. [CrossRef]
78. Vismara, L.A.; McCormick, C.E.B.; Wagner, A.L.; Monlux, K.; Nadhan, A.; Young, G.S. Telehealth Parent Training in the Early Start Denver Model: Results From a Randomized Controlled Study. *Focus Autism Other Dev. Disabil.* **2018**, *33*, 67–79. [CrossRef]
79. Vismara, L.A.; Colombi, C.; Rogers, S.J. Can One Hour per Week of Therapy Lead to Lasting Changes in Young Children with Autism? *Autism* **2009**, *13*, 93–115. [CrossRef] [PubMed]
80. Dawson, G.; Jones, E.J.H.; Merkle, K.; Venema, K.; Lowy, R.; Faja, S.; Kamara, D.; Murias, M.; Greenson, J.; Winter, J.; et al. Early Behavioral Intervention Is Associated With Normalized Brain Activity in Young Children With Autism. *J. Am. Acad. Child Adolesc. Psychiatry* **2012**, *51*, 1150–1159. [CrossRef]
81. Dawson, G.; Rogers, S.; Munson, J.; Smith, M.; Winter, J.; Greenson, J.; Donaldson, A.; Varley, J. Randomized, Controlled Trial of an Intervention for Toddlers With Autism: The Early Start Denver Model. *Pediatrics* **2010**, *125*, e17–e23. [CrossRef]
82. Ward, K.P.; Lee, S.J. Mothers' and Fathers' Parenting Stress, Responsiveness, and Child Wellbeing among Low-Income Families. *Child. Youth Serv. Rev.* **2020**, *116*, 105218. [CrossRef] [PubMed]
83. Shawler, P.M.; Sullivan, M.A. Parental Stress, Discipline Strategies, and Child Behavior Problems in Families with Young Children with Autism Spectrum Disorders. *Focus Autism Other Dev. Disabil.* **2017**, *32*, 142–151. [CrossRef]
84. Mondiale, A.M. Dichiarazione di Helsinki. Principi etici per la ricerca medica che coinvolge soggetti umani. *Assist. Inferm. Ric.* **2014**, *33*, 36–41.
85. Koo, T.K.; Li, M.Y. A Guideline of Selecting and Reporting Intraclass Correlation Coefficients for Reliability Research. *J. Chiropr. Med.* **2016**, *15*, 155–163. [CrossRef] [PubMed]
86. Istituto Superiore di Sanità. *Il Trattamento dei Disturbi dello Spettro Autistico nei Bambini e Negli Adolescenti. Linea Guida 21, Sistema Nazionale per le Linee Guida*; Ministero della Salute: Roma, Italy, 2011.
87. Venuti, P.; Bentenuto, A. *Studi di caso—Disturbi Dello Spettro Autistico*; Erickson: Trento, Italy, 2017.
88. Rogers, S.J.; Vismara, L.A. Evidence-based comprehensive treatments for early autism. *J. Clin. Child Adolesc. Psychol.* **2008**, *37*, 8–38. [CrossRef] [PubMed]
89. Biringen, Z.; Damon, J.; Grigg, W.; Mone, J.; Pipp-Siegel, S.; Skillern, S.; Stratton, J. Emotional Availability: Differential Predictions to Infant Attachment and Kindergarten Adjustment Based on Observation Time and Context. *Infant Ment. Health J.* **2005**, *26*, 295–308. [CrossRef]
90. Easterbrooks, M.; Biringen, Z. Emotional availability: Extending the assessment of emotional availability to include gender, culture, and at-risk populations. *Infant Ment. Health J.* **2005**, *26*, 291–294. [CrossRef] [PubMed]
91. Biringen, Z. *Raising a Secure Child: Creating Emotional Availability between You and Your Child*; Perigee-Penguin Group: New York, NY, USA, 2004.
92. Friard, O.P.; Gamba, M. Behavioral Observation Research Interactive Software (BORIS). 2016. Available online: https://iris.unito.it/handle/2318/1589424#.X7x7grMRXIU (accessed on 23 November 2020).
93. Moeller, J. A Word on Standardization in Longitudinal Studies: Don't. *Front. Psychol.* **2015**, *6*, 1389. [CrossRef] [PubMed]
94. Little, T.D. *Longitudinal Structural Equation Modeling*; Guilford press: New York, NY, USA, 2013.

95. Abidin, R.; Flens, J.R.; Austin, W.G. The Parenting Stress Index. In *Forensic Uses of Clinical Assessment Instruments*; Archer, R.P., Ed.; Lawrence Erlbaum Associates Publishers: Mahwah, NJ, USA, 2006; pp. 297–328.
96. Delacre, M.; Lakens, D.; Leys, C. Why psychologists should by default use Welch's t-test instead of student's t-test. *Int. Rev. Soc. Psychol.* **2017**, *30*, 92–101. [CrossRef]
97. R Core Team. *A Language and Environment for Statistical Computing*; R Foundation for Statistical Computing: Vienna, Austria, 2015.
98. Lee, M.D.; Wagenmakers, E.-J. *Bayesian Cognitive Modeling: A Practical Course*; Cambridge University Press: Cambridge, UK, 2013. [CrossRef]
99. Schreibman, L.; Dawson, G.; Stahmer, A.C.; Landa, R.; Rogers, S.J.; McGee, G.G.; Kasari, C.; Ingersoll, B.; Kaiser, A.P.; Bruinsma, Y.; et al. Naturalistic Developmental Behavioral Interventions: Empirically Validated Treatments for Autism Spectrum Disorder. *J. Autism Dev. Disord.* **2015**, *45*, 2411–2428. [CrossRef]
100. Vismara, L.A.; McCormick, C.; Young, G.S.; Nadhan, A.; Monlux, K. Preliminary Findings of a Telehealth Approach to Parent Training in Autism. *J. Autism Dev. Disord.* **2013**, *43*, 2953–2969. [CrossRef]
101. Biringen, Z.; Derscheid, D.; Vliegen, N.; Closson, L.; Easterbrooks, M.A. Emotional Availability (EA): Theoretical Background, Empirical Research Using the EA Scales, and Clinical Applications. *Dev. Rev.* **2014**, *34*, 114–167. [CrossRef]
102. Bretherton, I. Emotional Availability: An Attachment Perspective. *Attach. Hum. Dev.* **2000**, *2*, 233–241. [CrossRef]
103. Bornstein, M.H. *Handbook of Parenting*, 3rd ed.; Routledge, Taylor and Francis Group: New York, NY, USA, 2019.

Publisher's Note: MDPI stays neutral with regard to jurisdictional claims in published maps and institutional affiliations.

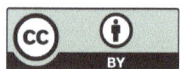

© 2020 by the authors. Licensee MDPI, Basel, Switzerland. This article is an open access article distributed under the terms and conditions of the Creative Commons Attribution (CC BY) license (http://creativecommons.org/licenses/by/4.0/).

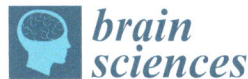

Article

Using Hybrid Telepractice for Supporting Parents of Children with ASD during the COVID-19 Lockdown: A Feasibility Study in Iran

Sayyed Ali Samadi [1,*], Shahnaz Bakhshalizadeh-Moradi [2], Fatemeh Khandani [3], Mehdi Foladgar [4], Maryam Poursaid-Mohammad [5] and Roy McConkey [1]

1. Institute of Nursing Research, University of Ulster, Newtownabbey BT37 0QB, UK; r.mcconkey@ulster.ac.uk
2. Raha Autism Education and Rehabilitation Center, Tabriz 51368, Iran; moradi.1151@yahoo.com
3. Fariha Autism Education and Rehabilitation Center, Tehran 25529, Iran; drkhandani@autismfariha.ir
4. Ordibehesht Autism Education and Rehabilitation Center, Isfahan 83714, Iran; Mehdi.fouladgar@yahoo.com
5. Director of the Daily Rehabilitation Centre Section, Iranian State Welfare Organization (ISWO), Tehran 25529, Iran; marypoury77@gmail.com
* Correspondence: s.samadi@ulster.ac.uk

Received: 22 October 2020; Accepted: 20 November 2020; Published: 22 November 2020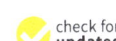

Abstract: During the three-month closure of clinics and day centers in Iran due to the coronavirus disease 2019 (COVID-19) lockdown, parents of children with Autism Spectrum Disorder (ASD) became solely responsible for their care and education. Although centers maintained telephone contact, it quickly became evident that parents needed more detailed advice and guidance. Staff from 30 daycare centers volunteered to take part in a two-month online support and training course for 336 caregivers of children with ASD of different ages. In addition to the provision of visual and written information, synchronous video sessions were used to coach parents on the learning goals devised for the children. Both qualitative and quantitative data were collected to understand the acceptability of using telepractice and the outcomes achieved. A low dropout rate and positive feedback from parents indicated that they perceived telepractice sessions to be useful. The factors contributing to parents' satisfaction were identified. Although the use of telepractice would be a good alternative for caregivers in any future lockdowns, it could also be used in conjunction with daycare center services to encourage greater parental participation, or with families living in areas with no day centers. Further studies are needed to compare telepractice to usual daycare face-to-face interventions, and to document its impact and cost-effectiveness for parents and children.

Keywords: telepractice; autism spectrum disorders; COVID-19; parental-mediated intervention; Coronavirus; daycare center

1. Introduction

Communication technology used by healthcare professionals is diverse [1]. Modern technologies offer a range of flexible modalities, ranging from simple daily applications (e.g., phone calls, email, and voice and video messaging) to complex technologies (e.g., interactive web-based software and interactive virtual classrooms). Smartphones, tablets, and laptops are more generally accessible to the general population at a reduced cost [2]. A recent review [3] explored the increasing usage of technology as a viable option in providing home health education and counseling to various populations in need of support. The uptake of these technologies has been lower in-person education, therapy, and social services—especially in services for children with special needs, who are mostly dependent on face-to-face interactions. Nevertheless, Camden et al. [4] concluded in their review that "available communication technology might be particularly well suited to implementing best practices for children with disabilities when the focus of the therapies is on supporting the children and their families, problem-solving with them to foster the child's development and functioning" [4].

Despite the dearth of applications in technologies for children with developmental disabilities, the available studies report promising results for children with Autism Spectrum Disorder (ASD) [5,6]. ASD is a neurodevelopmental disability that affects social communication and behavior development, and it typically manifests in the early stages of life [7]. Improved parental knowledge, parental intervention fidelity, and improved social behavior and communication skills for children with ASD were reported in a review of 15 studies on parent-mediated intervention training delivered remotely [8,9]. Moreover, parents appreciated being active agents in this approach; it gave them access to appropriate training and ongoing guidance so that they were able to deliver the intervention in a consistent manner [10]. Furthermore, evidence in using communication technology for individuals with ASD (at different age levels) is emerging, with preliminary findings suggesting that it has potential benefits in service delivery and cost savings, such as speedier set-up and coverage in rural areas [11,12].

1.1. Telepractice

The term telepractice is a general term that embraces other terms, such as telehealth and telemedicine, and has been defined as "the application of telecommunications technology to deliver professional services at a distance by linking service provider to a client, or supervisor to service providers for assessment, intervention, and/or consultation" [13]. Two approaches for delivering telepractice are defined as synchronous and asynchronous. When the telepractitioner and client are in a one-to-one or group setting, and are interacting in real-time via video and/or audio, this is referred to as a synchronous telepractice. Asynchronous telepractice occurs when information, such as videos, pictures, or audio files are recorded and exchanged via technology between the telepractitioner and client (and vice versa), with no live interaction between them. This approach is known as "store and forward". When both synchronous and asynchronous methods are used in combination, this is referred to as hybrid telepractice, which combines the benefits of both synchronous and asynchronous approaches.

1.2. Supporting Families in Iran

In Iran, there has been very limited use of telepractice with families of children with ASD. Rather, the focus has been on the preparation of written and visual materials, such as those produced by the first (SAS) and the last (RM) authors and their colleagues, which arose from a series of research studies into the needs of Iranian parents [14–16]. The tailored, parent-focused program that the mentioned authors devised [17,18] was based on the biopsychosocial model of disability. There were five booklets on different aspects of ASD, in lay language, plus a toolkit consisting of eight practical booklets to enhance parental reciprocity and interactive communication through everyday life activities and play. The booklets offer simple information and practical advice to enhance communication and its development in different stages. Simple, self-completed checklists were provided to parents, so they could have a better understanding of their child's level of functioning. Modifications to the home environment, to address the child's sensory preferences, along with strategies to manage unusual behaviors, were also covered in the booklets. It was also envisaged that the booklets would enable and empower parents to nurture their child's development at home, alongside the teaching and therapy the child would receive at school or a daycare center. Fortuitously, this resource was available when the COVID-19 lockdown commenced.

The Iranian Social Welfare Organization (ISWO) provides at least 110 daycare centers, across the 31 provinces in Iran, for children with autism spectrum disorder (ASD). The centers care for children aged 3 to 14 who usually attend, daily, under the supervision of these centers. The centers provide educational and rehabilitation services, and are open from 08.00 a.m. to 12.00 p.m. (4 h), to provide a wide range of daily services, which are mainly sponsored by the government. Most of the centers also provide afternoon extracurricular and rehabilitation services funded by parental fees. As the world became increasingly affected by the COVID-19 pandemic, Iran followed the advice of WHO [19] and UNESCO [20] in closing all of the educational and daycare centers (the closures started in March and lasted until May 2020). Telecommunication through mobile-based technology was the only possible approach to deliver professional services at a distance, by linking daycare centers to caregivers for assessment, intervention, and/or consultation.

1.3. Country Profile

The prevalence of ASD in Iranian children was reported to be 6.26 per 10,000, which is lower than that reported for some Western nations, but in line with rates from other countries [21]. ASD services in Iran fall under the Ministry of Health and Ministry of Social Welfare, with 90 percent of healthcare services provided through governmental services [22]. Improvements in recent decades have resulted in healthcare services covering the majority of the population [23]. The Iranian Social Welfare Organization (ISWO) provides clinical and daycare services to preschoolers with physical and intellectual disabilities, and older children with developmental disabilities, who were assessed by educational services as not suitable to attend mainstream schools. The government pays the attendance expenses for the majority of families, while other parents pay for a portion of the services they receive, based on their socioeconomic situation. Moreover, children with developmental disabilities who attend mainstream schools may also come to ISWO centers after school to receive therapy and specialist interventions from psychologists and therapists. Families contribute to these costs. The maximum capacity of daycare centers, based on the approved regulations in Iran, is fifty children. Iran ranks first in terms of the number of people in the Middle East with access to telecommunication services and satisfactory internet infrastructure, with an estimated 43 million users [24]. The widespread use of smartphones, social media [25], and computers throughout Iran enabled some daycare centers for adults (with mostly physical disabilities) to provide video-conferencing, to deliver rehabilitation services alongside consultations, advice, and guidance to their service-users [26].

1.4. Developing a Hybrid Telepractice for Families

The ISWO recognized the need for daycare centers for children with ASD to stay active, and to continue providing support for family caregivers who were in desperately need of assistance due to their around the clock caregiving because of the COVID lockdown. The only possible way was to use technology and available telecommunication services. Most daycare centers had already established mobile phone-based groups using Telegram or WhatsApp channels, in which they provided caregivers with one-way, non-interactive, and passive forms of daily center information, and news sharing. However, neither the daycare centers nor caregivers were ready for the newly imposed roles placed on them, but there was no other choice available to reduce the danger to children and families negatively impacted during the lockdown. ISWO quickly took the decision to pilot the use of telepractice services from their day centers by using mobile phone-based video technology. Caregivers during the lockdown would be observed in their homes while interacting with their children, with remote supervision and coaching provided by staff from the daycare center.

Previous studies on developing telepractice services have stressed the crucial preparatory role of organizational processes, in providing support and resources to prepare therapists and practitioners in implementing new models of practice [27]. However, the COVID-19 imposed closure of centers shortcut these preparations; thus, telepractice services had to be developed and implemented in a very short period using existing resources, such as the parent training resources as described above. More positively, family caregivers, who had previously been reluctant in engaging with their child's education and therapy, were asking the (then closed) daycare centers for practical advice and guidance for managing their child at home. This confirmed the assertion by Chorpita et al. [28] that parental advocacy and training is the most important element in the successful implementation of new models. ISWO invited the first author (SAS) to oversee the development of the telepractice materials and to supervise their staff in implementing them. SAS had previously acted as the senior consultant with the

ISWO on ASD research and training courses and was familiar with the staff and service users. The brief was to test the feasibility of using mobile phone-based telepractice services in a parent-implemented, home-based intervention program, under the supervision of the daycare center staff.

The feasibility study addressed three main questions.

- Is telepractice a feasible approach for providing services to family caregivers and children with ASD in a less affluent country such as Iran?
- What are the factors that contribute to caregivers' positive attitudes regarding the telepractice services provided to them and their children with ASD, in the absence of in-person daycare center services?
- Is it possible to increase the effectiveness of telepractice services for caregivers of children with ASD?

The present study was carried out over eight consecutive weeks—telepractice services in 30 daycare centers across the country with a maximum capacity of 50 individuals with ASD admission. This report can be considered a proof-of-concept study, in that it examines how telepractice was developed and implemented in a home setting through continuous support from a daycare center. It also provides a foundation in which further studies can be built regarding the effectiveness of telepractice.

2. Methods

2.1. Setting up the Telepractice Service

Three parties were engaged in the telepractice program: (i) the family caregivers; (ii) day center staff, and a course supervisor with extensive experience of ASD; and (iii) ISWO centers in Iran who provided support and supervision to the day centers. Following a literature review of existing telepractice studies involving families of children with ASD, the heads of 50 day centers (in Iran) for children with ASD were invited by the course supervisor to join an online discussion group, in which they were invited to share their perceptions on parental information and support needs during the closure of centers. The discussion, using online synchronous and asynchronous focus groups, continued for over one week, and resulted in a listing of priority issues required to implement a telepractice service, which included the following:

- Suitable resource materials from Iran—written and visual—were identified to act as a guide for center staff, as well as for sharing with caregivers as appropriate.
- Each participating center nominated a key person as the main coordinator of the center's telepractice. In most instances, this was a person with the required qualification to supervise the daycare center's daily services. During the lockdown, other center staff were involved with caregivers and children on a scheduled daily basis for routine contact, but the key person's responsibility was the coordination, supervision, and monitoring of the prepared online telepractice program.
- An online group was created for the course supervisor and daycare center staff for them to develop procedures relating to freeing up time from other clinical work; making different reading materials accessible for parents, the provision of high-quality supervision and training, establishing peer-learning working groups and planning periodic evaluation of the program.
- Identifying and creating video-based parental training materials for use alongside written materials. Videos are reported to be more effective [29].
- Caregivers needed to have smartphones or similar devices with home internet access and the freeware program, WhatsApp version 4.0.0 (Mountain View, CA, USA, 2009), with the free calling feature. This app was also used for documents and link sharing, online video calls, observing the home session, and coaching the parent.

The daycare centers provided online support in two forms, group and individual sessions, which were scheduled based on the center and parental preferences. Both individual and group sessions used the hybrid approach of support to provide both synchronous and asynchronous sessions.

2.1.1. The Main Aims of the Telepractice Service

The telepractice model for parent-implemented, home-based interventions was based around an online, daily, hybrid telepractice training session, for caregivers or parents, administered by the daycare center's key person. The aims and objectives were:

- To devise individual learning plans for a child with ASD in conjunction with caregivers to use at home.
- To boost the confidence of caregivers in managing their child with ASD at home.
- To answer caregivers' questions through the provision of accurate personalized information.
- To provide updated information relating to ASD.

The link below covered different areas of caregiving, with the main focus on communication and behavioral management in the natural home setting, through play, with a focus on daily living. For each part, there were separate tutorial videos, along with written and oral information, and self-rated scales, which was shared with caregivers. (http://www.behzisti.ir/news/12221). Parents were guided in the use of structured teaching, behavioral approaches, and environment modifications, which were adapted to the child's communication and sensory preferences, based on a parent-implemented intervention perspective.

2.1.2. Implementing the Telepractice Service

During the training sessions, daycare center staff aimed to encourage parent–child interaction in a modified natural home environment, using behavioral and structural strategies based around common pictures and objects. Training sessions for each child were developed and documented in a weekly training plan, focusing on communication, and sensory and cognitive domains. Caregivers were encouraged through video clips, pictures, and printed sources to replicate the program at home, and to make video recordings of interactions with their child. The daycare center's key person provided parents with feedback, cues, and coaching for the proper implementation of the intervention strategies. All of the home-based sessions were monitored by the center's key person, who in turn submitted fortnightly reports to the course supervisor (SAS). SAS also provided regular coaching and training to the key persons in each center.

In addition, there was also a virtual meeting place for key persons across the centers for social networking, exchanging information, and for contacting the therapists and clinicians to answer questions. All of these sessions were digitally video-recorded by each daycare center for later analysis.

2.1.3. Evaluating Telepractice

To allow for a more thorough understanding of the impact of telepractice on caregivers, a mixed-methods approach was used [30]. To date, concerning research on parent-mediated intervention, telepractice has generally adopted a quantitative approach, whereas parental and practitioner perceptions, as the main stakeholders of this service's delivery model, have yet to be examined as a primary outcome variable [31]. Therefore, caregivers who finished the course, as well as those who dropped out, were asked for their feedback regarding the course, and its shortcomings, via a WhatsApp questionnaire consisting of closed- and open-ended questions, which were possible for them to answer using voice messages or in written form. Caregivers who completed the online course were invited to answer six open-ended questions:

1. What is the most important advantage of the online training course?
2. What is the most obvious shortcoming of the online training course?

3. If you have to continue using online courses for a long time, what are your recommendations for improvement of the quality of the course?
4. Which part of the information was most useful for you?
5. Which part was less useful for you?
6. Do you have any further comments about the course?

Caregivers who dropped out were also asked about the reason for their leaving. In all, 15 (36%) voice recorded messages were transcribed along with 27 (64%) written comments, verbatim. A thematic content analysis approach was used to analyze the responses [32].

In addition, quantitative data were collected using pre- and post-course design. Assessment measures administered at pre- and post-course were as follows: a researcher-made questionnaire, regarding a main parental complaint about caregiving, online course, information provision, and the level of provided support. The video analyses were assessed based on a fidelity rubric, which considered the following 10 items—the most common and neglected items that might happen in a training or communicational session with children with ASD. The items were: (1) consistency with the environment (considered for a different type of training), (2) environment modification and stimulus control, (3) providing visual notification about the possible uncontrolled stimulus, (4) not forcing the child to do requests, (5) following the child's comfortable position, (6) understanding the child's reaction, (7) using visual icon for the start, (8) creativity in using toys and play, (9) parental temper control, using the visual icon to notify, and (10) finishing the task. Each item was rated on a five-point scale. After the course, caregivers were allowed to rate the course and the daycare center, to rate the parental level of engagement using a Likert scale, and to evaluate their experience as providers of intervention services to their child.

All procedures in the present study were in accordance with the ethical standards of the ISWO All caregivers signed an online consent form in which their rights to confidentiality, and to withdraw from the project at any stage of the study, were mentioned.

2.2. Participants

Parents and daycare center key persons were the key stakeholders in this feasibility study: namely 30 daycare coordinators from ASD centers and 336 caregivers of children with a confirmed diagnosis of ASD through the professionals of ISWO.

Key Persons

The 30 daycare centers were located in 19 (61%) of the 31 provinces across the country. The demographic information on the 30 key workers is presented in Table 1.

Table 1. The key persons' demographic data.

Variable	
Gender	Male 5 (17%)
	Female 25 (83%)
Age	Mean (37.10) SD (6.32)
	(Min 25 Max 55,)
Education	Undergraduate 5 (17%)
	Graduate 22 (73%)
	Postgraduate 3 (10%)
Profession	Psychologist 19 (63%)
	Occupational Therapist 5 (18%)
	Speech and Language Therapist 2 (7%)
	Educational Science 3 (10%)
	General Health 1 (3%)
Experience with ASD in years	Mean (8.26) SD (3.23)
	(Min 1, Max 15)

Twenty-one (70%) of the key persons had already participated in the Iranian Social Welfare Organization (ISWO) professional training courses for Autism Spectrum Disorder (ASD) [33], although 9 (30%) had not.

Concerning caregivers and children, Table 2 gives the demographic details of 417 (28%) out of 1500 caregivers (the maximum number of parents based on the registration volume permission granted by ISWO) who initially volunteered to be enrolled for the telepractice (an average of 11 caregivers participated from each center), and contrasts the 336 caregivers who completed two months of the online training course of the center, in which their child was registered, and the 81 caregivers (19%) who registered, but failed to complete the telepractice sessions. In Table 3, demographic information of children who both completed the online course and who dropped-out are presented.

Table 2. Demographic data of caregivers who completed the online course and the dropout groups.

Variable	Completed Course Group N = 336	Drop Out Group N = 81
Relationship with the child with ASD	Mother: 279 (83%) Father: 17 (5%) Sibling: 9 (3%) Grandparent: 1 (0.3%) Both Parents: 30 (9%)	Mother: 57 (70%) Father: 12 (15%) Sibling: 4 (5%) Grandparent: (–%) Both Parents: 8(10%)
Caregivers age	Mean (35.79) SD (6.51) (Max 70, Min 18)	Mean (37.88) SD (6.87) (Max 56, Min 22)
Caregivers education in years	Under-university education: 210 (62.5%) University Education: 126 (37.7%)	Under-university education: 57 (70%) University Education: 24 (30%)
Caregivers Profession	Housewife: 216 (64%) Public work: 60 (18%) Technician: 26 (8%) Education: 16 (5%) Medical and Health: 14 (4%) Unemployed: 4 (1%)	Housewife: 54 (67%) Public work: 14 (17%) Technician: 6 (7%) Education: 3 (4%) Medical and Health: 4 (5%) Unemployed: (–%)
Having assistance with caregiving from the family members	Yes: 192 (57%) No: 144 (43%)	Yes: 43 (53%) No: 38(47%)

Table 3. Demographic data of children who completed the online course and the dropout groups.

Variable	Completed Course Group N = 336	Drop Out Group N = 81
Children's Age	Mean (8.06) SD (2.78) (Max 14, Min 3)	Mean (10.81) SD (2.31) (Max 14, Min 3)
Children's Gender	Boys 261 (78%), Girls 75 (22%)	Boys 60 (74%), Girls 21 (26%)
Birth Order	First born: 203 (60%) Second born: 102 (30%) 3rd and above born: 31 (10%)	First born: 47 (58%) Second born: 29 (38%) 3rd and above born: 5 (4%)
Children's diagnosis	ASD: 158 (55.5%) Dual Diagnosis (diagnosis of ASD and other impairments such as Attention Deficit and Hyper Activity (ADHD), Cerebral Palsy (CP), or Intellectual Disability ID): 151 (45%)	ASD: 19 (23.5%) Dual Diagnosis: 62 (76.5%)

2.3. Activity Records

The number of days daycare centers offered individual services to family caregivers differed across centers (Mean = 5.60, days SD = 1.47 Max = 7, Min = 2) as did the number of daily hours the centers spent for each family and child (Mean = 1.20 h SD = 0.40 Max = 2 Min = 1). The number of days in which daycare centers were active each week over the eight weeks differed across centers (Mean = 5.36 days SD = 1.67 Max = 7 Min = 1). The number of hours spent on each call also varied (Mean = 1.70 h SD = 0.79 Max = 4 Min = 1). During the eight-week presentation of the course, the course supervisor was available for support in a WhatsApp group, in which all 30 daycare centers were members. An average of six contacts per centers in each week was recorded

3. Results

3.1. Qualitative Findings

At the end of the study period, all caregivers were invited to send their feedback on the effectiveness of the telepractice. Responses were received from 42 caregivers (12.5%) who finished the telepractice and 8 (9.9%) from caregivers who dropped out. In all, 30 responses came as written comments and 20 as voice messages.

All caregivers thought that the new mobile-based social media facilities were user-friendly and easy to use. A mother said (No.1): "Getting access to the course contents and contact with others through my mobile was not a challenge at all. This is turned to be a part of our daily life".

Caregivers generally said that the most important advantage of the course, for them, was to give caregivers a hand, when they were in the utmost need, with continuous caregiving. A father said: (No. 39) "Being engaged with my son and helping him to progress by my energy and at my pace while being directly engaged in the process and having more hope that I wanted for him in such a sudden unpredictable hard time. Thanks".

Almost all caregivers found no parts of the provided information useless and some mentioned special rehabilitation or educational information as being most applicable. They recommended different issues to improve the services, but mainly suggested hard copies and more video resources in the form of training packages. A mother said, "Internet package in the form of low price internet from Telecom system, and more hardcopy info before the course in CD and DVD format will be very helpful" (No. 3). Similar suggestions and recommendations were repeated in response to the final question. A mother said: "We have always been engaged with our children but not in a systematized way and with considering aims and objectives and under the guidance of professionals. Keep this good job continue. This was excellent" (No. 43).

Of the 41 caregivers who completed the telepractice, 38 (93%) caregivers thought that they would continue with the service, and would consider it as one of their choices, as well as recommend it to other caregivers as a very useful service. However, three caregivers (7%) were reluctant to continue the telepractice service because of the extra financial demands that it imposed on them, or technical problems, such as the internet speed. A father from the completed training course group said: "We had a serious problem with the internet and extra expenses we had to pay to top up the system on a weekly basis. This is important for us to be cautious about the extra expenses in this economically difficult time. I am unemployed because of the COVID-19 now" (No. 27).

The reasons given by caregivers who dropped out included the following. Some were not persuaded that online services were sufficient for children with ASD and their caregivers. Other issues were raised, such as extra pressure being placed on caregivers, or it being a beneficial service only for the daycare center, as they were still entitled to receive governmental financial assistance, while the pressure was mainly on caregivers instead of daycare provider centers. A mother from the dropout group said: "I do not approve of this online system. You are getting governmental financial help to work with our children not to force us to do it by ourselves" (No. 49).

Some undesired aspects of online services were mentioned, including the sharing of videos and pictures of the children, even if was assured that they would not be used or seen by the others.

A mother from the dropout group said: "Open the daycare centers. I do not want to take videos of my child and to share it online to be seen by the entire world!" (No.19).

Parents who dropped out were asked for their suggestions regarding the training courses for them or their children. They mostly requested for the reopening of the daycare centers, or requested private home services. A mother said, "Just try to make safe places at school and reopen the centers as before" (No. 50). A father from the same group said: "I think you should look at your services to cover a wide range of children with Autism. What was offered was not suitable for all. These children are unique. He was also critical of the amount of information caregivers were asked to provide. I think you wanted to test a new service for us. I am a scholar myself and familiar with these activities. You forgot about the service and paid more attention to the data you wanted to collect. You cannot test a service while you are providing it" (No. 30).

3.2. Quantitative Findings

Daycare centers asked caregivers about the main difficulties regarding caregiving during the lockdown. They also rated parental perception of the severity of ASD in caregivers through a self-rated scale. Key persons also rated the parental level of engagement, in the process, through their level of activity and their provision of requested records. Parental satisfaction with the support course, after the course, was evaluated, as was caregiver and daycare center staff attitudes to the online course.

Parental reaction to telepractice: caregivers were asked to rate their perception of online training courses by choosing between three choices: positive, negative, and having no ideas. These ratings were repeated at the end of the telepractice session. Before the course started, 7.4% of respondents rated it as positive; after the course, this had risen to 61.0%—a statistically significant change in attitude (chi-square (4) = 71.16, $p < 0.001$).

Parental reactions were further investigated in relation to the children's characteristics. Parents of the younger children were more satisfied with the course (86%) than those with older children (28%) (chi-square (2) = 1.17, $p < 0.001$. Moreover, caregivers whose child with ASD had another accompanying diagnosis were less positive about the course (52%) than those with a single diagnosis of ASD (68%) (chi-square (2) = 9.79, $p = 0.007$).

At the outset, younger aged parents were more positive (10%) than were older parents (2%) about the telepractice course (chi-square (2) = 21.15, $p < 0.000$), but afterwards, the percentages of positive ratings had reduced in younger parents (68%) and increased for older parents (51%) (chi-square 2) = 10.68, $p = 0.005$).

Likewise, caregivers who had assistance with caregiving were more positive regarding the online course at the outset (11%) compared to those without assistance (0.5%), but for both sets of caregivers, these percentages rose to 71% and 47%, respectively, although they were still statistically significant (chi-square (2) = 23.57, $p < 0.001$).

Comparing children's gender indicated that girls were more likely than boys to have dual diagnosis (48% of boys compared to 62.5% of girls (chi-square (1) = 6.51, $p = 0.007$). There was no statistical significance reported between the child's gender and the birth order.

Parents concerns: caregivers' specific concerns were grouped into behavioral, communication/talking, restlessness (including difficulty keeping their child inside), and a combination of all the areas. After the lockdown, and before the telepractice course started, the percentage of parents reported each type of concern was: Behavior (51%), Communication (14%), Restlessness (9%), and All areas (61%). After the course, the percentages had changed significantly: Behavior (12%), Communication (35%), Restlessness (17%), All areas (16%). Table 3 summarizes these findings. Concerns about behavior had reduced markedly (t = 10.67, df = 335 $p < 0.001$); while "has concerns in all areas" was (t = 18.35: df = 335 $p < 0.001$); whereas concerns about communication (t = 6.43, df = 335 $p < 0.001$, had increased and, to a lesser extent, so had restlessness (t = 2.65, df = 46, $p < 0.05$).

Caregiver dropout: considering 8 years as the cut off for the child age, it showed that parents of older children (33%) were more likely to leave the course than parents of young children (6%) (chi-square = 48.19, df = 1 $p < 0.000$). Similarly, the drop rate was higher for parents whose child had an additional diagnosis (29%) compared to those with a single diagnosis (9%) (chi-square = 26.08, df = 1, $p < 0.000$).

Fidelity checks: both the key person and caregiver fidelity in implementing the suggested practices were monitored using two specially developed rubrics. Parental fidelity scores were rated by the key person on each center on a four-scale rating, from weak to excellent. In all, 177 (42.4%) out of 336 caregivers were rated as excellent, and only 2 (0.5%) were rated as weak. The key person's fidelity on the same rating scale rated by the course supervisor showed no center staff was rated as weak, with 47% (14 daycare centers) rated as excellent. Caregivers' with higher fidelity ratings (81%) had more positive attitudes to the online course than those with lower fidelity scores (33%) (chi-square (6) = 74.18"df = 6, $p < 0.000$).

A significant relationship was also seen between levels of the key persons' fidelity score and previous participation in the ASD professional training course presented by ISWO (64% vs. 53% who did not participate and were cored as excellent based on the fidelity form), chi-square (2) = 8.32, $p = 0.016$. Although it was expected that key persons who scored higher in the fidelity rubric were more likely to have caregivers with higher scores of fidelity, the correlations between these fidelity ratings were not strong, although it was nearly statistically significant (Spearman correlation Rho = 0.33 $p < 054$.).

4. Discussion

This is one of the first studies to investigate the use of telepractice with families of children with ASD in a low resource country. Results indicating that a hybrid model of telepractice supervised by staff from daycare centers might be considered as useful support for children with ASD and their families in times of continuous caregiving due to situations, such as the COVID-19 pandemic. Caregivers can be guided to become effective teachers in the child's most natural environment of the home. Such an approach can enable ISWO to better fulfil its remit of supporting children with ASD and their families.

Regarding the question of the feasibility of the telepractice, the findings indicate that telepractice could be a feasible approach for certain caregivers of children with ASD in particular [34,35]. Findings indicate that updated and trained daycare staff using remote access via a smartphone can enter the caregivers' living places, and coach them while they are actively caregiving in their natural environments. Moreover, the telepractice services enabled the home environment to come under professional observation, at little expense, and without the time and effort involved in making visits to the family home.

Caregivers' overall satisfaction and positive attitudes to the online course allied to a relatively low level of dropouts also indicate the feasibility of this service. This engagement has also increased parental knowledge about the main challenges in taking care of their children, such as managing their child's behavior while also highlighting the difficulties around communication. This helped them to focus on increasing their nonverbal-communication skills in their interactions with the child [36].

However, there is a need for the daycare center staff to have training and support throughout the implementation of telepractice, as this approach requires them to have different skills, knowledge, and commitment. Those who participated in the previous ASD training course, provided by the course supervisor, were more successful in course implementation compared to those who did not. Hence, staff training and preparation should be considered as a key element in successful enactment of telepractice services.

Regarding the second question of this study which was searching for elements that contribute to caregivers' positive attitudes regarding the telepractice services, several factors contributed to the caregivers' satisfaction with online services. Younger caregivers were more optimistic about using telepractice; similar to that found in other services for children with ASD in Saudi Arabia: a similar culture to this sample [37]. Thus, telepractice might be targeted more at younger parents with younger children [38].

It was also found that having assistance at home is a good indicator of caregiver satisfaction with the online courses; presumably, because they had extra help at home and could devote more time to their child [31]. Consideration might then be given to the provision of more online support services directed at the carer's needs, such as sharing their parenting stresses and experiences with other parents involved with the course.

The third question of this study which was searching for ways to improve telepractice and boosting effectiveness of this service, some of which have been noted already. However, it is likely that hybrid approaches that combine face-to-face contacts alongside telepractice would be better suited to some parents, especially those unfamiliar or reluctant to use technology. Moreover, the lack of internet access, or its associated costs, are also factors that limit the use of telepractice, especially for less affluent families and those in rural areas. Moreover, although telepractice may seem a possible solution for families in more remote areas who receive no support, issues around the availability of smartphones and internet access will need to be resolved first.

Nevertheless, caregivers should be reassured that telepractice is not considered a substitute to in-person daycare services, as this was echoed in the comments from some parents who dropped out of the course. Rather, it provides a means for ensuring that the training presented in the daycare centers can be extended into home settings of children with ASD. Moreover, parents who had higher fidelity scores in implementing the advice they were given were more supportive of telepractice, a finding that has been previously noted [39]. A follow-up study over an extended data collection period is needed to monitor the level of fidelity in the implementation of the strategies used by the caregivers at home, after their involvement in an online course. This would also help to determine ways of sustaining their engagement in home-based activities.

Cost-benefit analyses need to be undertaken in terms of financial costs and staff time and to compare the outcomes with the cost-benefits of face-to-face support by therapists and day centers. In addition, the development of multi-media, telepractice support courses on specific topics should be considered as an efficient means of sharing knowledge with family caregivers.

Finally, there were some limitations to the present study. It had to be prepared in an emergency and it took place over a limited period. More parents might have dropped-out if it went on for a longer period. It was not possible to recruit a control group, which had received similar services in a face-to-face situation because of the lockdown. Moreover, this was a self-selected group of parents and the findings need to be replicated with a more representative group of families whose children attend the day centers.

Although this feasibility study demonstrated that telepractice applications hold promise as a way of addressing some of the caregivers' challenges during a time of a permanent caregiving situation, there is still lack of evidence for understanding the possible harms and limitations of the telepractice, and the way that various rehabilitation, assessments, and training protocols may be used through telepractice. Further studies needed to identify the caregivers and types of services in which a telepractice delivery system is appropriate or not. Such comparative studies will enable service providers to select a telepractice delivery model tailored to specific subgroups to maximize the benefit for them. Moreover, studies should focus on approaches to develop online support systems in developing countries, with the limitation of accessibility of services in remote areas, especially the rural parts in general [40].

It goes without saying that helping caregivers become capable members of the service intervention teams, involved with children with ASD, necessitates considerable specialized training in a wide range of domains for those leading the teams. The lack of highly trained professionals in different disciplines involved with children who have ASD is a major impediment in less affluent countries. Perhaps telepractice courses for clinicians developed internationally could help overcome this deficit.

5. Conclusions

With the increasing prevalence rate of ASD globally, service systems in less affluent countries face extra challenges in meeting the needs of caregivers and individuals with ASD. The telepractice model that has been tested with a sizeable number of families across Iran provides some basic evidence to support its potential to address some of the challenges associated with caregiving for children with ASD, even though it may not suit all parents. Telepractice, via telecommunication and mobile-based services, should be considered as a valuable adjunct to the current models of service provision in Iran and internationally. Further research is needed on the issue of COVID-19 and its impacts on children with ASD, their caregivers, support, and service, or possible alternative treatments not necessarily in the context of telepractice.

Author Contributions: Conceptualization, S.A.S.; methodology, S.A.S. and R.M.; validation, R.M. and S.A.S.; formal analysis, A.S.A.; investigation, S.B.-M., M.F., F.K., and M.P.-M.; resources, S.A.S.; data curation, S.A.S.,

S.B.-M., M.F., F.K., and M.P.-M.; writing—original draft preparation, S.A.S.; writing—review and editing, R.M.; supervision, S.A.S.; project administration, S.A.S. All authors have read and agreed to the published version of the manuscript.

Funding: This research received no external funding.

Acknowledgments: We wish to thank the caregivers and daycare centers who actively helped us in implementing this study.

Conflicts of Interest: The authors declare no conflict of interest.

References

1. Herschell, A.D.; McNeil, C.B.; McNeil, D.W. Clinical child psychology's progress in disseminating empirically supported treatments. *Clin. Psychol. Sci. Pract.* **2004**, *11*, 267–288. [CrossRef]
2. Cole-Lewis, H.; Kershaw, T. Text messaging as a tool for behavior change in disease prevention and management. *Epidemiol. Rev.* **2010**, *32*, 56–69. [CrossRef] [PubMed]
3. Mishra, S.R.; Lygidakis, C.; Neupane, D.; Gyawali, B.; Uwizihiwe, J.P.; Virani, S.S.; Kallestrup, P.; Miranda, J.J. Combating non-communicable diseases: Potentials and challenges for community health workers in a digital age, a narrative review of the literature. *Health Policy Plan.* **2019**, *34*, 55–66. [CrossRef] [PubMed]
4. Camden, C.; Pratte, G.; Fallon, F.; Couture, M.; Berbari, J.; Tousignant, M. Diversity of practices in telerehabilitation for children with disabilities and effective intervention characteristics: Results from a systematic review. *Disabil. Rehabil.* **2019**, *2019*, 1–13. [CrossRef] [PubMed]
5. Vismara, L.A.; McCormick, C.E.B.; Wagner, A.L.; Monlux, K.; Nadhan, A.; Young, G.S. Telehealth parent training in the early start Denver model: Results from a randomized controlled study. *Focus Autism Other Dev. Disabil.* **2016**, *33*, 67–79. [CrossRef]
6. Narzisi, A. Phase 2 and Later of COVID-19 Lockdown: Is it possible to perform remote diagnosis and intervention for autism spectrum disorder? An online-mediated approach. *J. Clin. Med.* **2020**, *9*, 1850. [CrossRef] [PubMed]
7. American Psychiatric Association. *Diagnostic and Statistical Manual of Mental Disorders (DSM-5®)*; American Psychiatric Association: Washington, DC, USA, 2013.
8. Parsons, D.; Cordier, R.; Vaz, S.; Lee, H. Parent-mediated intervention training delivered remotely for children with autism spectrum disorder living outside of urban areas: Systematic review. *J. Med. Internet Res.* **2017**, *19*, e198. [CrossRef]
9. Wilkes-Gillan, S.; Lincoln, M. Parent-mediated intervention training delivered remotely for children with autism spectrum disorder (ASD) has preliminary evidence for parent intervention fidelity and improving parent knowledge and children's social behaviour and communication skills. *Aust. Occup. Ther. J.* **2018**, *65*, 245. [CrossRef]
10. McConachie, H.; Diggle, T. Parent implemented early intervention for young children with autism spectrum disorder: A systematic review. *J. Eval. Clin. Pract.* **2007**, *13*, 120–129. [CrossRef]
11. Boisvert, M.; Lang, R.; Andrianopoulos, M.; Boscardin, M.L. Telepractice in the assessment and treatment of individuals with autism spectrum disorders: A systematic review. *Dev. Neurorehabil.* **2010**, *13*, 423–432. [CrossRef]
12. Sutherland, R.; Trembath, D.; Roberts, J. Telehealth and autism: A systematic search and review of the literature. *Int. J. Speech-Language Pathol.* **2018**, *20*, 324–336. [CrossRef] [PubMed]
13. Dudding, C. Reimbursement and telepractice. *Perspect. Telepractice* **2013**, *3*, 35–40. [CrossRef]
14. Samadi, S.A.; McConkey, R. Autism in developing countries: Lessons from Iran. *Autism Res. Treat.* **2011**, *2011*, 1–11. [CrossRef] [PubMed]
15. Samadi, S.A.; McConkey, R.; Kelly, G. Enhancing parental well-being and coping through a family-centred short course for Iranian parents of children with an autism spectrum disorder. *Autism* **2013**, *17*, 27–43. [CrossRef]
16. Samadi, S.A.; McConkey, R.; Bunting, B. Parental wellbeing of Iranian families with children who have developmental disabilities. *Res. Dev. Disabil.* **2014**, *35*, 1639–1647. [CrossRef]
17. Samadi, S.A.; Mahmoodizadeh, A. Omid early intervention resource kit for children with autism spectrum disorders and their families. *Early Child Dev. Care* **2013**, *184*, 354–369. [CrossRef]

18. Samadi, S.A.; Mahmoodizadeh, A. Parents' reports of their involvement in an Iranian parent-based early intervention programme for children with ASD. *Early Child Dev. Care* **2013**, *183*, 1720–1732. [CrossRef]
19. WHO. COVID-19: Vulnerable and High Risk Groups. Available online: https://www.who.int/westernpacific/emergencies/covid-19/information/high-risk-groups (accessed on 1 May 2020).
20. UNESCO. COVID-19 Educational Disruption and Response. Available online: https://en.unesco.org/covid19/educationresponse (accessed on 5 April 2020.).
21. Samadi, S.A.; Mahmoodizadeh, A.; McConkey, R. A national study of the prevalence of autism among five-year-old children in Iran. *Autism* **2011**, *16*, 5–14. [CrossRef]
22. Ghassemi, H.; Harrison, G.G.; Mohammad, K. An accelerated nutrition transition in Iran. *Public Health Nutr.* **2002**, *5*, 149–155. [CrossRef]
23. Javanparast, S.; Baum, F.; LaBonte, R.; Sanders, D. Community health workers' Perspectives on their contribution to rural health and well-being in Iran. *Am. J. Public Health* **2011**, *101*, 2287–2292. [CrossRef]
24. Gelvanovska, N.; Rogy, M.; Rossotto, C.M. *Broadband Networks in the Middle East and North Africa: Accelerating High-Speed Internet Access*; The World Bank: Washington, DC, USA, 2014.
25. Ghorbanzadeh, D.; Saeednia, H.R. Examining telegram users' motivations, technical characteristics, trust, attitudes, and positive word-of-mouth: Evidence from Iran. *Int. J. Electron. Mark. Retail.* **2018**, *9*, 344–365. [CrossRef]
26. Jalali, M.; Shahabi, S.; Lankarani, K.B.; Kamali, M.; Mojgani, P. COVID-19 and disabled people: Perspectives from Iran. *Disabil. Soc.* **2020**, *35*, 844–847. [CrossRef]
27. Vismara, L.A.; Young, G.S.; Stahmer, A.C.; Griffith, E.M.; Rogers, S.J. Dissemination of evidence-based practice: Can we train therapists from a distance? *J. Autism Dev. Disord.* **2009**, *39*, 1636–1651. [CrossRef] [PubMed]
28. Chorpita, B.F. Toward large-scale implementation of empirically supported treatments for children: A review and observations by the Hawaii empirical basis to services task force. *Clin. Psychol. Sci. Pract.* **2002**, *9*, 165–190. [CrossRef]
29. Chandran, H.; Jayanthi, K.; Prabavathy, S.; Renuka, K.; Bhargavan, R. Effectiveness of video assisted teaching on knowledge, attitude and practice among primary caregivers of children with autism spectrum disorder. *Adv. Autism* **2019**, *5*, 231–242. [CrossRef]
30. Flaspohler, P.D.; Meehan, C.; Maras, M.A.; Keller, K.E. Ready, willing, and able: Developing a support system to promote implementation of school-based prevention programs. *Am. J. Community Psychol.* **2012**, *50*, 428–444. [CrossRef]
31. Pickard, K.E.; Wainer, A.L.; Bailey, K.M.; Ingersoll, B.R. A mixed-method evaluation of the feasibility and acceptability of a telehealth-based parent-mediated intervention for children with autism spectrum disorder. *Autism* **2016**, *20*, 845–855. [CrossRef]
32. Miles, M.B.; Huberman, A.M. *Qualitative Data Analysis: An Expanded Sourcebook*; Sage: Thousand Oaks, CA, USA, 1994.
33. Samadi, S.A.; Nouparst, Z.; Mohammad, M.P.; Ghanimi, F.; McConkey, R. An Evaluation of a training course on autism spectrum disorders (ASD) for care centre personnel in Iran. *Int. J. Disabil. Dev. Educ.* **2018**, *67*, 280–292. [CrossRef]
34. Barkaia, A.; Stokes, T.F.; Mikiashvili, T. Intercontinental telehealth coaching of therapists to improve verbalizations by children with autism. *J. Appl. Behav. Anal.* **2017**, *50*, 582–589. [CrossRef]
35. Casale, E.G.; Stainbrook, J.A.; Staubitz, J.E.; Weitlauf, A.S.; Juárez, A.P. The promise of telepractice to address functional and behavioral needs of persons with autism spectrum disorder. In *International Review of Research in Developmental Disabilities*; Hodapp, R.M., Fidler, D.J., Eds.; Elsevier: Amsterdam, The Netherlands, 2017; pp. 235–295.
36. Coolican, J.; Smith, I.M.; Bryson, S.E. Brief parent training in pivotal response treatment for preschoolers with autism. *J. Child Psychol. Psychiatry* **2010**, *51*, 1321–1330. [CrossRef]
37. Alotaibi, F.; Almalki, N. Parents' perceptions of early interventions and related services for children with autism spectrum disorder in Saudi Arabia. *Int. Educ. Stud.* **2016**, *9*, 128. [CrossRef]
38. Knutsen, J.; Wolfe, A.; Burke, B.L.; Hepburn, S.; Lindgren, S.; Coury, D. A systematic review of telemedicine in autism spectrum disorders. *Rev. J. Autism Dev. Disord.* **2016**, *3*, 330–344. [CrossRef]

39. Wainer, A.L.; Ingersoll, B. Disseminating ASD interventions: A pilot study of a distance learning program for parents and professionals. *J. Autism Dev. Disord.* **2012**, *43*, 11–24. [CrossRef] [PubMed]
40. Vega, S.; Marciscano, I.; Holcomb, M.; Erps, K.A.; Major, J.; Lopez, A.M.; Barker, G.P.; Weinstein, R.S. Testing a top-down strategy for establishing a sustainable telemedicine program in a developing country: The Arizona telemedicine program–U.S. Army–Republic of Panama initiative. *Telemed. e-Health* **2013**, *19*, 746–753. [CrossRef] [PubMed]

Publisher's Note: MDPI stays neutral with regard to jurisdictional claims in published maps and institutional affiliations.

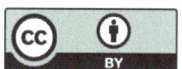

© 2020 by the authors. Licensee MDPI, Basel, Switzerland. This article is an open access article distributed under the terms and conditions of the Creative Commons Attribution (CC BY) license (http://creativecommons.org/licenses/by/4.0/).

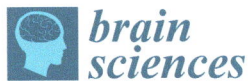

Review

Understanding Different Aspects of Caregiving for Individuals with Autism Spectrum Disorders (ASDs) a Narrative Review of the Literature

Hadi Samadi [1],* and Sayyed Ali Samadi [2]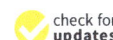

[1] Department of Philosophy, Faculty of Law, Theology and Political Science, Science and Research Branch, Islamic Azad University, Tehran 1477893855, Iran
[2] Institute of Nursing Research, University of Ulster, Newtownabbey BT37 0QB, Northern Ireland, UK; s.samadi@ulster.ac.uk
* Correspondence: samadiha@gmail.com

Received: 24 June 2020; Accepted: 11 August 2020; Published: 14 August 2020

Abstract: Background: There has been a considerable endeavor to understand associated challenges of caregiving for a child with Autism Spectrum Disorders (ASDs) and to develop the necessary skills and approaches to assist parents of children with ASD. Different studies have been stressed the importance and need for parental involvement in the intervention process to increase positive impacts. Methods: The process of caregiving and the associated challenges should be understood from different aspects to be able to facilitate parent involvement in intervention implementation. In a narrative literature review, ten selected reviews were considered and each review considered a special aspect of caregiving for an individual with ASD. Results: Five main different factors in the available literature and reviews were considered as different themes that needed to be reconsidered in the studies on the impacts of caregiving for an individual with ASD. Conclusions: It is concluded that to facilitate parental involvement in the intervention process, and to support caregivers of this group of individuals this review highlights the need for improved research in some proposed areas in this field and to bridge the gap between research and practice in this field.

Keywords: parental impact; caregiving; families living with ASD; autism spectrum disorders; parental engagement; narrative review; review of reviews

1. Introduction

Despite the recognition of Autism Spectrum Disorders for more than 75 years, the etiology, prognosis, and short or long term impacts of this diagnosis on caregivers have not yet been fully identified [1]. Present knowledge on ASD indicates that it is a lifelong neurodevelopmental disorder in which genes play a role but that environmental triggers likely contribute as well [2].

This lifelong disorder impacts sociocommunicational ability along with aspects of behavioral differences manifests itself through restricted interests or unusual behavioral repertoires [3].

The dominant contemporary idea is that children with disabilities such as children with ASD should not be separated from their parents [4] and families should play a more influential role in the treatment process [5]. Families who give care for a member with ASD can be referred to as families living with ASD [6] because generally, this is a lifelong process.

Understanding the impacts and psychological issues of the diagnosis of ASD on parents as the main caregivers have developed markedly in the last three decades [7]. Parents may experience emotional stress, anxiety, fear, and guilt, and based on the effectiveness of child-centered treatments they might simultaneously show some positive feelings [8].

There are only in some affluent countries and on some special occasions families given the opportunity of respite care or foster home or residential house [9]. Respite care is a break that parents in the affluent countries can have access to which involves a few hours/weekends that the child with special needs will be watched by someone else who will get paid by the state, but it is an underused service for several reasons such as difficulty to find a good respite worker. Foster care is a service available in affluent countries like the United States when parents are unable to care for children in their family homes and children have to be removed for a while until they can gain parenting skills or improve their socioeconomic status. Residential care (otherwise known as institutionalization) is mostly phased out in most states in the USA as disability advocates are moving towards in-home care with supports. Institutional care of children and adults with intellectual or developmental disabilities are more common in non-affluent countries. Therefore, it can be concluded that nearly all children with ASD like the rest of the children with other types of disabilities live at home and with their family members.

To develop and boost skills and approaches to assist parents of children with ASD considerable endeavor has been done. Parental involvement in the intervention process has been stressed in different studies. Involving parents in treatment implementation is advisable but to be able to facilitate this involvement different aspects of caregiving should be understood and taking into account.

This paper reviews key areas of existing literature focused on the parents of individuals with ASD to highlight different aspects of caregiving and the need for understanding the different impacts of caregiving. Therefore based on the Mayer [10] classification of different types of reviews, this paper is a narrative review in which few selected reviews are compared and summarized based on the authors' experience, existing theories, and models to understand the possible concerns, study trends, and ideas for future studies.

The ultimate goal of this review is to understand the potential of caregivers and caregiving process for an individual with ASD and to understand different aspects of caregiving for individuals with ASD in different societies and to recognize different impacts that caregiving might have on caregivers. This is done to answer the following questions;

Have the presented reviews covered the different aspects of caregiving for an individual with ASD?

How did the presented reviews on caregiving for an individual with ASD echo different theoretical frameworks to explain the phenomena that are considered to be investigated?

How did the presented reviews reveal the geographical distribution of the studies on the impacts of caregiving for an individual with ASD?

Based on the aims of the narrative review, which are described, and discussing the state of the science of a specific topic or theme from a theoretical and contextual point of view, this review also tries to highlight the research trends in the available literature and stresses the areas that are less studied through critical analysis of the literature published in books and electronic or paper-based journal articles.

1.1. Caregivers-Focused ASD Research

It has been long identified from previous studies that caregiving for a member with ASD are more at risk from psychiatric and/or stress disorders because of the range of distinct challenges they have [11,12].

The presence of a child with ASD seriously affects the family system as a whole [13,14]. It may have both negative and positive consequences for parents [15]. The majority of individuals with ASD require assistance with their daily routine activities, which is mainly provided by the caregivers who are family members. The activities are in a wide range and cover areas such as self-care, mobility, communication, and cognitive or emotional demands [16,17]. This is why many caregivers of individuals with ASD experience challenges with their general health compared to those who are caring for typically developing individuals or those who have other types of developmental disabilities [18–21].

1.2. Quality of Life and Sources of Stress among Family Members and Caregivers of Individuals with ASD.

To identify challenges associated with caregiving to a member with ASD in family settings many studies have been done and they mainly focused on the qualities of life and maternal stress as mothers are generally the main caregiver for individuals with ASD in the family.

Different factors are contributing to challenges associated with the caregivers' quality of life and general wellbeing. The level of functional impairment and the presence of challenging behavior appear to contribute specifically to parenting challenges [22]. For example sleep problems of children with ASD could be considered as a source of parental stress. The most common problems reported were "bedtime resistance" and parasomnias [23], which refer to any sleep disorder such as sleepwalking, teeth grinding, night terrors, rhythmic movement disorder, and restless legs syndrome [24].

To understand the contributing factors of challenges for parents of children with ASD investigation on other factors needs. Contributing factors might be coping strategies, available formal and informal supports, satisfaction with caregiving, and family functioning. It is concluded in many present studies that greater social supports for the caregivers, obtaining adaptive coping strategies and caring for an individual with a milder form of ASD related behaviors tend to adjust more easily to the caregiving demands and experience lower levels of stress [25–29]. The present findings extended the existing knowledge and instead of finding the sources of the distress of ASD caregivers inside the family system, we adopted a broader view and discovered that parents of this group of children were motivated to continue employment because of the extra expenses caregiving imposed on them [30], but there are serious burdens on the way of their employment such as a lack of proper childcare services and inflexible employment situations [31]. As a new threat to the general wellbeing and level of stress of caregivers of an individual with ASD unemployment has been added to the list [32].

The key phrases for this paper are parents of children with ASD and the care that they are providing to their child with ASD. To operationalize this phrase it should be defined as the caregiving and supports characterized by attention to the needs of their child; particularly for those unable to look after themselves sufficiently due to the diagnosis of ASD and involved in the provision of their health or social care. The focus of this narrative review is on the presented reviews on parental caregiving regardless of their age level and it covered both young and old caregivers.

2. Materials and Methods

In recruiting the review papers for this review, review papers published from 2010 to 2020 were considered, Google Scholar as the main base and publicly accessible source considered. The main focus was on recent review studies published in peer-reviewed journals to investigate the impact of ASD on parents in English language journal papers. The "Autism parents Review", "Autism caregivers' impacts review", and "family impacts and Autism review" were used as the keywords. The titles of the recruited studies are mentioned in the first column of Table 1. Several other keywords such as "parents", "family members", "caregivers", "mothers", and "fathers" also were used along with the backbone word of "review" to find desired review papers. The results are depicted in Table 1. Ten review papers in all were considered for this review.

The main purpose of this review was to find out what researchers have in mind when they review the impact of caregiving for an individual with ASD.

Table 1. Reviews about impacts of caregiving on parents of children with an Autism Spectrum Disorder (ASD).

The Review Title	Author(s)	Number of Reviewed Studies	Main Findings	The Geographical Area That the Study is Done	Considering Autism as a General Diagnosis/with Subtypes	Theoretical Framework Considered in the Review
The quality of life of parents of children with autism spectrum disorder: A systematic review	Vasilopoulou, and Nisbet (2016) [33]	88 studies	Compared to parents of typically developing children or population norms, parents of children with ASD show a poorer quality of life. Contributing factors of parental quality of life were discovered to be the behavioral challenge of the child with ASD, parental unemployment, mother caregivers, and lack of social support for parents.	UK	Autism Spectrum Disorders (ASD) considered as one main diagnosis	TF in the reviewed studies was not considered
Mindfulness, Stress, and Well-Being in Parents of Children with Autism Spectrum Disorder: A Systematic Review	Cachia, Anderson, Moore (2010) [34]	10 Studies	Reviewing the efficacy of interventions in reducing stress and increasing parental psychological wellbeing indicates that all included studies contributed to the efficacy of mindfulness interventions in reducing stress and increasing parental self-reported psychological wellbeing	Australia	Autism as a general diagnosis is mentioned	TF in the reviewed studies was not considered
Couple relationships among parents of children and adolescents with Autism Spectrum Disorder: Findings from a scoping review of the literature	Saini, M., Stoddart, K.P., Gibson, M., Morris, R., Barrett, D., Muskat, B. and Zwaigenbaum, L. (2015) [35]	59 studies	Factors that support the development and maintenance of positive couple and co-parenting marital relationship are strategies such as developing common goals, increasing partner respect, securing social support, reducing stress, and instilling hope and service providers and parents of individuals with ASD benefited in receiving information about all the mentioned factors	Canada	The severity of autism as a main diagnosis is considered	TF in the reviewed studies was not considered
Parent and Family Impact of Autism Spectrum Disorders: A Review and Proposed Model for Intervention Evaluation	Karst, and Van Hecke, (2012). [36]	Not Mentioned	Most reviews on ASD intervention considered children as the main focus; parent and family factors are ignored. It is not possible to assume that even significant improvements in the diagnosed child will improve parental distress, especially as the time and expense of intervention might increase family disruption.	USA	Contribution of the different levels of severity of ASD is considered	TF in the reviewed studies is considered
Coping in Parents and Caregivers of Children with Autism Spectrum Disorders (ASD): a Review	Lai and Oei, (2014).) [37]	37 studies	Parental use of coping strategies determined by (1) demographical characteristics (such as gender, age, education, income, and language) and psychological and personal factors (such as personality, cultural values, optimism, sense of coherence, benefit-finding and sense-making abilities, emotional health, and coping styles). It is also concluded that child characteristics (i.e., age, gender, medical conditions, cognitive and adaptive functioning abilities, language difficulties, and behavior problems) and also situational factors (such as treatment availability, family function, and clinician referrals to support resources) are all important determinants.	Singapore	ASD as a general term and main diagnosis	TF in the reviewed studies is considered

Table 1. *Cont.*

The Review Title	Author(s)	Number of Reviewed Studies	Main Findings	The Geographical Area That the Study is Done	Considering Autism as a General Diagnosis/with Subtypes	Theoretical Framework Considered in the Review
A Review of Parent Education Programs for Parents of Children With Autism Spectrum Disorders	Schultz, Schmidt and Stichter (2011) [38]	30 studies	Studies mainly included descriptions of programs for parents of young children with ASD. They are generally focused on a one-on-one training approach. They moderately considered a manual or curriculum. Mostly included data on parent and child outcomes. A majority considered single-case designs to evaluate program affectivity. No data on fidelity of implementation reported in the reviewed studies	USA	The severity of symptoms not mentioned and ASD considered a general diagnostic term.	TF in the reviewed studies was not considered
The Need for More Effective Father Involvement in Early Autism Intervention. A Systematic Review and Recommendations	Flippin and Crais (2011). [39]	27 studies	Considering communication and play as a focal point for the interventions that support fathers' communication styles and learning needs will likely attract fathers and make them feel more influential in their reciprocity with their child with ASD. Involving fathers effectively in communication and play interventions may reduce maternal stress and boost family cohesion.	USA	ASD has generally used as a diagnostic term	TF in the reviewed studies was not considered
Family-focused autism spectrum disorder research: A review of the utility of family systems approaches	Cridland, Jones, Magee, and Caputi, (2014). [40]	Not mentioned	The theoretical and methodological directions for family-focused ASD research indicates that family systems approaches as a common theoretical framework needs to be more considered in future family-focused ASD research. Considering theoretical concepts such as boundaries, ambiguous loss, resilience, and traumatic growth are all different aspects of family systems TF.	Australia	ASD has generally been used as a diagnostic term	TF in the reviewed studies is considered
Fathers of Youth with Autism Spectrum Disorder: A Systematic Review of the Impact of Fathers' Involvement on Youth, Families, and Intervention.	Rankin, Paisley, Tomeny, and Eldred (2019). [41]	18 studies	There is a dearth of studies on fathers and ASD. this review suggests that fathers of individuals with ASD play an important role in the life of children with ASD and the family as a whole and should be included in future research on children with ASD.	USA	ASD as a general diagnostic label is considered	TF in the reviewed studies was not considered
Siblings and family environments of persons with autism spectrum disorder: A review of the literature	Smith, and Elder (2010). [42]	12 studies	Factors such as biological, psychological, sociological, and ecological aspects impacted families and siblings are influenced by the context of their families that has already been under the influence of the mentioned factors. To identify people who are at risk of adjustment problem assessment of siblings is necessary.	USA	Autism as a general diagnosis is used	TF in the reviewed studies is considered

3. Results

Out of ten reviewed reviews, four of them considered the theoretical framework (TF) as one main factor in their review and some others reviews although TF was named or mentioned hence, it was not considered in the review as a factor. Although the wealth of data out of the considerable amount of studies reviewed it was mentioned that studies mainly recruited mothers and fathers are rarely investigated. The recruited sample of fathers in those studies that considered both parents was far lower than the number of mothers. Available studies rarely focused on the positive side of caregiving. Additionally, only one review (in Singapore) was done in non-western societies and considered the cultural factor as a factor to consider in the review. There was only one review that considered the impacts of the level of functioning of ASD as a factor. The rest of the other reviews although tried to consider the level of the functioning or severity of the symptoms in some of the recruited studies, but mainly considered ASD as a general diagnostic term regardless of the level of functioning based on the formal diagnostic procedure.

The following part based on the narrative review aims to find important topics on different general findings of the reviewed reviews presented under the different extracted subtitles. Therefore this narrative review of the reviews will give a detailed explanation of the important findings of the recruited reviews.

3.1. Impacts of Adopting a Theoretical Framework

The theoretical framework acts as a guide or plan for a study. According to philosophers of science like Thomas Kuhn [43], observations are "theory-laden" and impacted by the theoretical presuppositions considered by the researcher. That is an inevitable part of every research that needs data collection, so degrees of contamination of data by background assumptions are unavoidable. However, the explicit mention of the theoretical work acts as a caveat for the reader. The reviews reviewed for the current paper have been based on a range of theoretical models. In some reviews these theories were explicit but often the theories were not considered as independent under the review factor. Based on the World Health Organization [44] suggestion any theoretical framework that is adopted for studies on impacts on caregiving for individuals with ASD should consider at least the following three criteria:

- Cultural issues: the theories had to consider the impact of the social context, cultural influences, and attitudes.
- Compatibility with the family-centered approach: theories had to be compatible with family-centered approaches.
- Conceptions of disability: the theories needed to reflect modern thinking about disability, such as is reflected in the International Classification of Functioning (ICF).

Set against these considerations, the two most promising frameworks were ecological approaches to the family [45] and family systems theory [46]. Having a review of the present studies also highlights the limitations of basic research designs adopted from the considered theoretical framework in an attempt to understand the complex interplay between contributing factors of the challenges associated with caregiving for individuals with ASD. As an example to depict the impacts of adopting different theoretical frameworks is that as Turnbull, et al. [47] say, while some theoretical frameworks try to "fix" the individual with a disability and having him/her fit into different levels of family, community, and society, the ecological model's [48] main endeavor is on "fixing" the multiple ecological environments. Therefore, according to an ecological model, the focus is on a transformed ecology in which children with different types of disabilities can develop through the interaction of their skills with a responsive context [47]. Therefore, in this TF "passive change" as an important factor is taken into account in which a person is not entirely passive and can cause changes in his/her context [49]. Another used TF is the Double ABCX model [50,51], which consists of three components: demands, capabilities, and meanings (situational appraisals) and has been employed to understand the psychosocial impact of children's chronic conditions in parenting and the factors affecting their adjustment to the child's diagnosis. In sum, the different and changing nature of the under investigation caregiving factors urged the researcher to adopt different TFs. To bridge the existing gap between research and practice, it became evident that there is a need to expand TF through adopted TF conceptual models that are consistent with each other, and could cover conceptual shortcomings and generalize findings [52]

3.2. Impacts of Recruiting Convenient Samples

Most of the studies considered mothers and research on the impact of caregiving for a child with different types of developmental disabilities such as ASD on fathers has been infrequent [53,54]. One of the obvious limitations with the present data is that they are skewed towards mothers and in most of the present studies the mothers' perspective is considered to be the perspective of all the caregivers in the family [55,56]. Although mothers are considered to be the main caregivers in most cultures, different caregivers in the family might have a different experience in the process of caregiving for an individual with ASD at home [57]. Although the word "parents" is in the title of most of the studies in the files of caregivers' impacts, the research often was undertaken exclusively or mainly on mothers. Nevertheless, recognizing fathers and their needs has received more attention in recent studies [58]. While available reviews suggest that fathers of children with ASD are not often included in research on individuals with ASD, American Counseling Association [59] proposed special counseling for fathers with counselors deeply considering the fathers' cultural context. Researchers in the field of developmental disabilities have identified fathers with different words and adjectives, words such as "hard to reach" [60], or "just a shadow" [61]. One main justification is that mothers are generally the main caregivers of their children with special needs globally. Bailey and Powell [53] suggest that mothers tend to spend more time with their children with developmental disabilities and they are more available to participate in studies. According to Altiere and Kluge [62], although the experience and behavior of fathers of children with ASD were considered important, it has not been evaluated consistently. A review of the available literature on child and family psychopathology revealed that 48% of the studies assessed mothers exclusively and 1% assessed fathers. Traustadottir [63] believed that this is because in families of children with developmental disabilities mothers are less likely to be employed in paid jobs and they are expected to take the major caring responsibilities for the child.

3.3. Focusing on Negative Aspects Of Caregiving

In one of the reviews it mentioned that only a small number of parents highlighted the positive impacts of caregiving for a child with ASD on parents/caregivers [35]. There is substantial evidence that the presence of a child with ASD seriously affects the family system as a whole with both negative and positive impacts [14]. There is a considerable amount of studies on the stress and wellbeing of families who have a child with ASD [64,65]. However, only a small number of the available existing research also recognizes some positive influences of ASD on caregivers and their overall functioning, including psychological and emotional strength, improved communication skills, and higher levels of empathy and patience [66] reported positive impacts associated with bringing up a child with ASD such as increased spirituality or increased compassion and acceptance of differences reported by Pakenham, et al., [67] or Hastings and Taunt [68] found that positive perception of parents of children with different severe forms of disabilities such as ASD could help parents to cope with high levels of stress and serve as an adaptive function.

In a review of the available literature on the impact of caregiving for a child with disabilities, which has been done by Savage and Bailey [69] in Australia, they found that generally researchers found less satisfaction with life and caring among parents of this group of children. They also found some other studies about the positive impact of caring of a child with disabilities on parents, in which factors such as giving pleasure to the care recipient, maintaining the dignity and maximizing the potential of the care recipient were mentioned by parents [68].

3.4. The Dearth of Cross-Cultural Studies

Internationally, most studies were done in the west research on parents of children with ASD and the effects of having a child with ASD to date have been limited largely to families in western countries, and there is a dearth of studies in non-western counties [70]. Bailey and Powell [51] reported that different cultures have different opinions about ASD. Nonetheless, in addition to the World Autism Organization, national organizations for children and families with autism now exist in over 80 countries, suggesting that at least the diagnostic category has traveled around the world. Hence even inside multicultural countries, there are tendencies toward focusing on research interest towards special groups such as White Euro-American families [71]. Unfortunately, there is a dearth of studies regarding the impact of the condition on parents of children with ASD in less affluent countries.

In sum, although there is an appreciable amount of literature on families of children with different types of disabilities, including ASD, in western countries, little is known about the experience of parents in non-western societies. A small group of the reviewed studies investigated the impacts of cross-cultural factors on caregiving for an individual with ASD as a process in different contexts. Due to the possible impact of cultural factors on parental adjustment to the demands of this special type of caregiving, it is recommended that future studies consider the effects of cultural values through adopting cross-cultural studies.

3.5. Considering ASD as a Single Diagnosis with Similar Impacts

Individuals with ASD are a very heterogeneous group with different types of abilities and challenges and some studies attributed this heterogeneity to different factors such as genetic heterogeneity among the members of this group [72]. A hallmark of ASD and different needs is due to heterogeneity in etiology, phenotype, and outcome. Different support and services and a variety of impacts on caregivers might be an inevitable output of this heterogeneity. Hence, most of the reviewed studies combine different levels of ASD into one general class of diagnosis. Some studies stress the need to investigate a different type of ASD separately. As an example, the impacts on caregiving for the high functioning group are less studied [73] and most of the available considered the severe forms of ASDs. In a concise review of the literature, it was concluded that understanding of ASD subgroups, their associated markers of pathological states, and different cross-cultural factors such as impacts on the family are imperative to advancing this field of research [74].

4. Discussion

There is a growing interest in studying the impact of caregiving for children with ASD on parents. Hence, there are aspects of the available literature that needs revision.

It cannot be neglected that there is a need for studies that reflect on the bigger picture and create linkages rather than perpetuating the highly specific compartments in which much of the present knowledge and understanding about ASD is imperfectly created.

Instead of reviewing the studies, we believed that highlighting the present concern in the available literature as an aim might be better achieved by undertaking a narrative review of the various literature reviews that have been published in the past decade through a 'review of reviews' that is rarely undertaken and they lend themselves well to a narrative review.

We believe that this type of review would provide a stronger basis to identify the different levels of theoretical frameworks; for example, a high-level TF such as ecological approaches provides an over-arching framework in which other frameworks such as family systems theory or stress/coping could be defined.

TF as a guiding base for the research in this field was considered as one of the main factors in this review. The theory is defined as an expression of knowledge, a creative and rigorous structuring of ideas that project a tentative, purposeful, and systematic view of phenomena [75]. As Waterhouse [76] suggests, without adopting an appropriate theoretical framework, studies are more likely to be influenced by extraneous factors such as social consensus, convenience samples, opportunities for immediate applications, and researcher preferences. To limit the probability of these risks there is a need for adopting a generic theoretical framework. The reason for considering the common theoretical frameworks in any scientific field is to provide an explanation for the connections among the phenomena under investigation and to provide insights to discover new relationships between phenomena [77]. Swanson [78] concluded that the benefits of a theoretically driven body of work include the utilization of common terminology to improve communication of findings, research methodologies grounded in theoretically sound concepts, and a greater synthesis of results from various individual research studies allowing for detection of emerging patterns.

The review also revealed ambivalence between different negative and positive sides of caregiving. Parents who have a child with disabilities are not automatically under stress [79]. Some studies [66] found that some families have been able to cope successfully and control stress conditions. In other words, there are several studies on the positive impact of having a family member with a disability on their quality of life and strengthening of the family members as a unit [80,81]. Having a member with ASD in the family may have both negative and positive consequences for parents [82] For example, concepts such as "benefit finding" and "sense-making" was explored as the perception of parents of children with ASD [67]. They found that there are parents who are trying to understand the way that their children with ASD perceive the world around them and this endeavor might improve the parent–child relationship. This was considered a positive consequence of having a child with ASD. This aspect might be worth exploring further with parental caregiving to a child with ASD globally. For example, many caregivers report various positive psychological outcomes attributed to parenting their offspring with ASD including selflessness, compassion, and peace during hardship such as a time of uncertainty and a refocus of energy [40,66]. Research into the positive impacts of ASD on families is encouraging but is only relatively recent. Additionally, there are areas such as parental resilience, traumatic growth, family relationship, different aspects of development, and appreciation of life and enrichment of relationships that would benefit further research [83–85]. Positive psychology has already recommended similar approaches within the field of developmental disabilities research [66–68]. At present, there are mixed results and opposite findings with some reporting positive effects in areas such as self-concept and self-competence of the family members [86,87] and mainly negative impacts on areas such as stigma mainly in the form of social embarrassment [88,89] and psychological distress [90]. On the other hand, some findings indicated no differential impact in areas such as self-concept, self-efficacy, and locus of control [91,92]. The presented work is justified differently, hence, it reflects different impacts of caregiving on caregivers. The findings also revealed the dynamic nature of caregiving, which prohibits any "cause–effect" and direct simple relationship between the under investigating phoneme [57]. Furthermore, the mixed findings of the studies might be an indicator of the attributing factors that are not investigated, understood, or taken into account in previously implemented research designs; factors such as level and sources of parents and caregivers information, family type (extended or non-extended), caregiving at different stages of life, and a range of cultural and demographic factors such as socioeconomic status, nationality, and locality and the severity of a specific diagnosis such as ASD [40]. It is concluded that present inconsistencies in the interpretation of the findings of the available wealth of data are due to considering the contributing factors in isolation and away from other possibly related causative issues [78,93,94].

It is also an important factor to conclude this review with, although ASD is considered as a global public health concern [95], it is estimated that approximately 90% of individuals with ASD live in low/middle-income countries [96]. Hence most of the studies are done in high-income countries and the resulting data due to a significantly different situation may result in very different consequences. There is a growing urge for doing cross-cultural studies in this field because culturally adapted parental services for ethnic minorities could also contribute to the diversity of the parental support and training services in the countries in which immigrants live. This is also relevant to high-income countries that admit immigrants from different cultures, to offer more culturally sensitive services concerning the supports provided to parents as caregivers. The main extracted findings from the reviewed reviews in this paper are not unique to the level of the development of the countries and there are particular challenges for parents of these children, which is global and of relevance to different nations. Furthermore, additional cross-cultural research, albeit within a local context in different countries, is essential if the international understanding of ASD is to be boosted globally.

In sum, it is reported that impacts of caregiving for an individual with ASD is multifaceted and pervasive [97] the main reason for this justification is that approximately 85% of individuals with ASD present with different types limitations and disabilities such as cognitive and/or adaptive in a degree that reduced their possibility of living independently. This lifelong condition caused livelong supervision or assistance in different degrees from their parents or a family member as the main caregivers [98]. Longitudinal studies revealed that almost 50% of over fifty parents of an individual with ASD indicated that they are still caregiving for their offspring with ASD [99]. Caregiving of a child with ASD might have different impacts on different family members and all members deserve to be taken into account in the studies on impacts of caregiving. Parents and caregivers should receive adequate attention and services. It seems that providing opportunities to both parents in a balanced way and considering the ideas and impacts of ASD on both parents and also giving the opportunity of hearing their voices through their own words may produce more generalizable and reliable results.

Not only parents of children with ASD consisting of a diverse group of people with different backgrounds and needs, but individuals with ASD also are a very heterogeneous group with different levels of abilities or functioning that makes it difficult to consider an individual with this diagnosis as an equal group with similar impacts on caregivers. Underrating the level of functioning and severity of symptoms might yield less trustful results. Proposed changes to the DSM-5 in 2013 include dimensional assessments intended to allow clinicians to rate both the presence and severity of psychiatric and related symptoms in a clear way within diagnostic categories [100]. The proposed revisions about the diagnosis of an Autism Spectrum Disorder (ASD) include a severity marker based on the degree of impairment in the domains of social communication and restricted and repetitive behaviors as the dyad of impaired core symptoms. The most recent revision of the Autism Diagnostic Observation Scale—Second Edition (ADOS-2) [101] provides guidelines for calculating the overall level of autism symptoms relative to individuals with ASD of the same age and language level using a rubric called Comparison Scores (CS).

Another possible source for classification following the level of abilities is the International Classification of Functioning, Disability, and Health (ICF), which is a classification and description of functioning, disability, and health using a biopsychosocial theoretical concept that classifies information into four components to classify individuals with a different type of disabilities such as ASD. These components are (1) body functions and body structures, (2) activities and participation, (3) environmental factors, and (4) personal factors. These factors interact with each other to influence the functioning and are classified and described in the ICF manual [102]. These systems might be able to be used for classifying the level of functioning and degree of severities of individuals with ASD.

Although considering that the methodology and data analysis approaches were out of the coverage of this review, most of the available studies adopted a quantitative approach and the mixed approaches or qualitative method is rarely used. Most of the studies adopted a voluntary survey approach in which sampling bias is more possible to happen. This group of participants is more active and open to share their experiences and they do not necessarily echo the existing ideas of all caregivers of the ASD population.

The role of the cultural components can be considered in qualitative studies in more depth. Participants of the qualitative or mixed approaches studies get the opportunity of expressing their ideas through their own words.

5. Conclusions

The present review of the reviews highlighted a lack of strong empirical evidence on the structure of studies that considered impacts of caregiving for an individual with ASD on parents/caregivers.

ASD implies a very heterogeneous group of individuals and this is a multifaceted diagnosis with a range of severity and levels of abilities. Individuals place a range of demands on their caregivers, and parents have varying challenges that need to be responded to reduce any additional pressures associated with caregiving. To be able to prepare caregivers of individuals with ASD different aspects of caregiving should be understood.

This review also cautions against the acceptance of the impacts of caregiving at face value and recommends that at the beginning the context and structure of caregiving should be established, before determining links between different aspects of under investigated contributing factors.

In this note, future evaluations need to be done to understand different aspects of caregiving in different cultural contexts to facilitate issues such as parental presence in the intervention process and to provide effective parental support and services packages.

Author Contributions: Both H.S. and S.A.S. conceived of the presented idea. H.S. developed the theory and performed the search. S.A.S verified the analytical methods and prepared the table. H.S. extracted the main themes and encouraged S.A.S. to reanalyze the extracted themes. H.S. supervised the findings of this work. S.A.S. prepared the first and final draft of the paper. Both authors discussed the results and contributed to the final manuscript before the submission. All authors have read and agreed to the published version of the manuscript.

Funding: This research received no external funding.

Acknowledgments: The authors appreciate Roy McConkey's kind guidance and comments on the first draft of this review paper.

Conflicts of Interest: The authors declare no conflict of interest.

References

1. Harris, J. Leo Kanner and autism: A 75-year perspective. *Int. Rev. Psychiatry* **2018**, *30*, 3–17. [CrossRef] [PubMed]
2. Inglese, M.D.; Elder, J.H. Caring for children with autism spectrum disorder, part I: Prevalence, etiology, and core features. *J. Pediatric Nurs.* **2009**, *24*, 41–48. [CrossRef] [PubMed]
3. American Psychiatric Association. *Diagnostic and Statistical Manual of Mental Disorders (DSM-5®)*; American Psychiatric Pub: Washington, DC, USA, 2013.
4. Benderix, Y.; Nordstrom, B.; Sivberg, B. Parents, experience of having a child with autism and learning disabilities living in a group home. *Autism* **2007**, *10*, 629–641. [CrossRef]
5. Matson, J.L.; Mahan, S.; LoVullo, S.V. Parent training: A review of methods for children with developmental disabilities. *Res. Dev. Disabil.* **2009**, *30*, 961–968. [CrossRef]
6. Neely-Barnes, S.L.; Hall, H.R.; Roberts, R.J.; Graff, J.C. Parenting a Child with an Autism Spectrum Disorder: Public Perceptions and Parental Conceptualizations. *J. Fam. Soc. Work.* **2011**, *14*, 208–225. [CrossRef]
7. Levy, S.E.; Mandell, D.S.; Schultz, R.T. Autism. *Lancet* **2009**, *374*, 1627–1638. [CrossRef]
8. Remington, B.; Hastings, R.P.; Kovshoff, K.; degli Espinosa, F.; Jahr, E.; Brown, T.; Alsford, P.; Lemaic, M.; Ward, N. Early intensive behavioral intervention: Outcomes for children with autism and their parents after two years. *Am. J. Ment. Retard.* **2007**, *112*, 418–438. [CrossRef]
9. Grunewald, K. *Close the Institutions for the Intellectually Disabled Everyone Can. Live in the Open Society*; Independent Living Institute: Duvnas, Sweden, 2003.
10. Mayer, P. *Guidelines for Writing a Review Article*; Zurich-Basel Plant Science Center (PSC): Zürich, Switzerland, 2009; pp. 443–446.
11. Attwood, T. *The Complete Guide to Asperger's Syndrome*; Jessica Kingsley Publishers: London, UK, 2007.
12. Pakenham, K.I.; Samios, C.; Sofronoff, K. Adjustment in mothers of children with Asperger syndrome. *Autism* **2005**, *9*, 191–212. [CrossRef]
13. Sivberg, B. Family System and Coping Behaviours: A Comparison between Parents of Children with Autistic Spectrum Disorders and Parents with Non-Autistic Children. *Autism* **2002**, *6*, 397–409. [CrossRef] [PubMed]

14. Sivberg, B. Coping Strategies and Parental Attitudes: A Comparison of Parents with Children with Autistic Spectrum Disorders and Parents with Non Autistic Children. *Int. J. Circumpolar Health* **2002**, *61*, 36–50. [CrossRef] [PubMed]
15. Baker-Ericzén, M.J.; Brookman-Frazee, L.; Stahmer, A.; Baker-Ericzn, M.J. Stress Levels and Adaptability in Parents of Toddlers with and without Autism Spectrum Disorders. *Res. Pr. Pers. Sev. Disabil.* **2005**, *30*, 194–204. [CrossRef]
16. World Health Organization. *Child and Adolescent Mental Health Policies and Plans*; World Health Organization: Geneva, Switzerland, 2005.
17. Salomone, E.; Leadbitter, K.; Aldred, C.; Barrett, B.; Byford, S.; Charman, T. The association between child and family characteristics and the mental health and wellbeing of parents of children with autism in mid-childhood. *J. Autism Dev. Disord.* **2018**, *48*, 1189–1198. [CrossRef] [PubMed]
18. Samadi, S.A.; McConkey, R.; Bunting, B. Parental wellbeing of Iranian families with children who have developmental disabilities. *Res. Dev. Disabil.* **2014**, *35*, 1639–1647. [CrossRef] [PubMed]
19. Hastings, R.P. Child behaviour problems and partner mental health as correlates of stress in mothers and fathers of children with autism. *J. Intellect. Disabil. Res.* **2003**, *47*, 231–237. [CrossRef]
20. Miodrag, N.; Hodapp, R.M. Chronic stress and health among parents of children with intellectual and developmental disabilities. *Curr. Opin. Psychiatry* **2010**, *23*, 407–411. [CrossRef]
21. Ashum, G.; Singhal, N. Psychological support for families of children with Autism. *Asia Pacific Disabil. Rehabilitation J.* **2005**, *16*, 62–83.
22. Tobing, L.E.; Glenwick, D.S. Relation of the childhood autism rating scale parent version to diagnosis, stress and age. *Res. Dev. Disabil.* **2002**, *23*, 211–223. [CrossRef]
23. Doo, S.; Wing, Y.K. Sleep problems of children with a pervasive developmental disorders: Correlation with parental stress. *Dev. Med. Child Neurol.* **2006**, *48*, 650–655. [CrossRef]
24. Corsini, R. *Dictionary of Psychology*; Routledge: London, UK, 2001.
25. Baghdadli, A.; Pry, R.; Michelon, C.; Rattaz, C. Impact of autism in adolescents on parental quality of life. *Qual. Life Res.* **2014**, *23*, 1859–1868. [CrossRef]
26. Benson, P.R. Network characteristics, perceived social support, and psychological adjustment in mothers of children with autism spectrum disorder. *J. Autism Dev. Disord.* **2012**, *42*, 2597–2610. [CrossRef]
27. Boehm, T.L.; Carter, E.W.; Taylor, J.L. Family quality of life during the transition to adulthood for individuals with intellectual disability and/or autism spectrum disorders. *Am. J. Intellect. Dev. Disabil.* **2015**, *120*, 395–411. [CrossRef]
28. Lu, M.-H.; Wang, G.; Lei, H.; Shi, M.-L.; Zhu, R.; Jiang, F. Social Support as Mediator and Moderator of the Relationship Between Parenting Stress and Life Satisfaction Among the Chinese Parents of Children with ASD. *J. Autism Dev. Disord.* **2018**, *48*, 1181–1188. [CrossRef]
29. Pozo, P.; Sarriá, E.; Brioso, A. Family quality of life and psychological well-being in parents of children with autism spectrum disorders: A double ABCX model. *J. Intellect. Disabil. Res.* **2013**, *58*, 442–458. [CrossRef]
30. Barrett, B.; Mosweu, I.; Jones, C.R.G.; Charman, T.; Baird, G.; Simonoff, E.; Pickles, A.; Happe, F.; Byford, S. Comparing service use and costs among adolescents with autism spectrum disorders, special needs and typical development. *Autism* **2014**, *19*, 562–569. [CrossRef] [PubMed]
31. Hill, E.L.; Jones, A.P.; Lang, J.; Yarker, J.; Patterson, A. Employment experiences of parents of children with ASD or ADHD: An exploratory study. *Int. J. Dev. Disabil.* **2014**, *61*, 166–176. [CrossRef]
32. Stoner, C.R.; Stoner, J.B. How can we make this work? Understanding and responding to working parents of children with autism. *Bus. Horizons* **2014**, *57*, 85–95. [CrossRef]
33. Vasilopoulou, E.; Nisbet, J. The quality of life of parents of children with autism spectrum disorder: A systematic review. *Res. Autism Spectr. Disord.* **2016**, *23*, 36–49. [CrossRef]
34. Cachia, R.L.; Anderson, A.; Moore, D.W. Mindfulness, Stress and Well-Being in Parents of Children with Autism Spectrum Disorder: A Systematic Review. *J. Child Fam. Stud.* **2015**, *25*, 1–14. [CrossRef]
35. Saini, M.; Stoddart, K.P.; Gibson, M.; Morris, R.; Barrett, D.; Muskat, B.; Nicholas, D.; Rampton, G.; Zwaigenbaum, L. Couple relationships among parents of children and adolescents with Autism Spectrum Disorder: Findings from a scoping review of the literature. *Res. Autism Spectr. Disord.* **2015**, *17*, 142–157. [CrossRef]
36. Karst, J.S.; Van Hecke, A.V. Parent and Family Impact of Autism Spectrum Disorders: A Review and Proposed Model for Intervention Evaluation. *Clin. Child Fam. Psychol. Rev.* **2012**, *15*, 247–277. [CrossRef]

37. Lai, W.W.; Oei, T.P. Coping in Parents and Caregivers of Children with Autism Spectrum Disorders (ASD): A Review. *Rev. J. Autism Dev. Disord.* **2014**, *1*, 207–224. [CrossRef]
38. Schultz, T.R.; Schmidt, C.T.; Stichter, J.P. A Review of Parent Education Programs for Parents of Children With Autism Spectrum Disorders. *Focus Autism Other Dev. Disabil.* **2011**, *26*, 96–104. [CrossRef]
39. Flippin, M.; Crais, E.R. The Need for More Effective Father Involvement in Early Autism Intervention. *J. Early Interv.* **2011**, *33*, 24–50. [CrossRef]
40. Cridland, E.K.; Jones, S.C.; Magee, C.; Caputi, P. Family-focused autism spectrum disorder research: A review of the utility of family systems approaches. *Autism* **2013**, *18*, 213–222. [CrossRef] [PubMed]
41. Rankin, J.A.; Paisley, C.A.; Tomeny, T.S.; Eldred, S.W. Fathers of Youth with Autism Spectrum Disorder: A Systematic Review of the Impact of Fathers' Involvement on Youth, Families, and Intervention. *Clin. Child Fam. Psychol. Rev.* **2019**, *22*, 458–477. [CrossRef]
42. Smith, L.O.; Elder, J.H. Siblings and family environments of persons with autism spectrum disorder: A review of the literature. *J. Child Adolesc. Psychiatr. Nurs.* **2010**, *23*, 189–195. [CrossRef]
43. Kuhn, T.S. *The Structure of Scientific Revolutions*; University of Chicago press: Chicago, IL, USA, 2012.
44. Fekri, O.; Macarayan, E.R.; Klazinga, N. *Health System Performance Assessment in the WHO European Region: Which Domains and Indicators have been Used by Member States for its Measurement*; WHO Regional Office for Europe: Copenhagen, Denmark, 2018.
45. Hornby, G. *Improving Parental Involvement*; Bloomsbury Publishing: London, UK, 2000.
46. Turnbull, A.P.; Turnbull, H.R. *Families, Professionals and Exceptionality: A Special Parentship*; Merrill Publishing Company: Columbia, OH, USA, 1990.
47. Turnbull, A.P.; Blue-Banning, M.; Turbiville, V.; Park, J. From Parent Education to Partnership Education: A Call for a Transformed Focus. *Top. Early Child. Spéc. Educ.* **1999**, *19*, 164–172. [CrossRef]
48. Bronfenbrenner, U. Contexts of child rearing: Problems and prospects. *Am. Psychol.* **1979**, *34*, 844. [CrossRef]
49. Tudge, J.R.H.; Mokrova, I.; Hatfield, B.; Karnik, R.B. Uses and misuses of Bronfenbrenner's bioecological theory of human development. *J. Fam. Theory Rev.* **2009**, *1*, 198–210. [CrossRef]
50. McCubbin, H.I.; Patterson, J.M. The family stress process: The Double ABCX Model of family adjustment and adaptation. In *Social Stress and the Family: Advances and Developments in Family Stress Theory and Research*; McCubbin, H.I., Sussman, M., Patterson, J.M., Eds.; Haworth: New York, NY, USA, 1983; pp. 7–37.
51. Manning, M.M.; Wainwright, L.; Bennett, J. The Double ABCX Model of Adaptation in Racially Diverse Families with a School-Age Child with Autism. *J. Autism Dev. Disord.* **2010**, *41*, 320–331. [CrossRef]
52. Samadi, S.A.; Samadi, H.; McConkey, R. A Conceptual Model for Empowering Families in Less Affluent Countries Who Have a Child With Autism. In *Autism Spectrum Disorder—Recent Advances*; IntechOpen: London, UK, 2015.
53. Bailey, D.B.; Powell, T. Assessing the information needs of families in early intervention. In *The Developmental System Approach to Early Intervention*; Paul H Brookes Publishing: Baltimore, MD, USA, 2005; pp. 151–183.
54. Gavidia-Payne, S.; Stoneman, Z. Family predictors of maternal and paternal involvement in programmes for young children with disabilities. In *Early Intervention: The Essential Readings*; Feldman, M.A., Ed.; Blackwell Oxford: Oxford, UK, 2004.
55. Hannon, M.D.; Hannon, L.V. Fathers' Orientation to their Children's Autism Diagnosis: A Grounded Theory Study. *J. Autism Dev. Disord.* **2017**, *47*, 2265–2274. [CrossRef] [PubMed]
56. Prendeville, P.; Kinsella, W. The role of grandparents in supporting families of children with autism spectrum disorders: A family systems approach. *J. Autism. Dev. Disord.* **2019**, *49*, 738–749. [CrossRef] [PubMed]
57. Seligman, M.; Darling, R.B. *Ordinary Families, Special Children: A Systems Approach to ChildhoodDisability*; Guilford Publications: New York, NY, USA, 2017.
58. Carpenter, B.; Towers, C. Recognising fathers: The needs of the fathers of children with disabilities. *Support Learn.* **2008**, *23*, 118–125. [CrossRef]
59. American Counseling Association. Code of ethics. Available online: https://www.counseling.org/resources/aca-code-of-ethics.pdf (accessed on 5 March 2019).
60. McConkey, R. Early Intervention: Planning Futures, Shaping Years. *Ment. Handicap. Res.* **2010**, *7*, 4–15. [CrossRef]
61. West, S. *Just a Shadow: A Review of Support for the Fathers of Children with Disabilities*; The Handsel Trust: Birmingham, AL, USA, 2000.

62. Altiere, M.J.; Von Kluge, S. Family Functioning and Coping Behaviors in Parents of Children With Autism. *PsycEXTRA Dataset* **2013**, *18*, 83. [CrossRef]
63. Traustadottir, R. Mothers who *care: Gender disability* and family life. *J. Fam. Issues* **1991**, *12*, 211–228. [CrossRef]
64. McKinney, B.; Peterson, R.A.; McKINNEY, B. Predictors of Stress in Parents of Developmentally Disabled Children. *J. Pediatr. Psychol.* **1987**, *12*, 133–150. [CrossRef]
65. Dunn, M.; Burbine, T.; Bowers, C.; Tantleff-Dunn, S. Moderators of Stress in Parents of Children with Autism. *Community Ment. Health J.* **2001**, *37*, 39–52. [CrossRef]
66. Bayat, M. Evidence of resilience in families of children with autism. *J. Intellect. Disabil. Res.* **2007**, *51*, 702–714. [CrossRef]
67. Pakenham, K.I.; Sofronoff, K.; Samios, C. Finding meaning in parenting a child with Asperger syndrome: Correlates of sense making and benefit finding. *Res. Dev. Disabil.* **2004**, *25*, 245–264. [CrossRef]
68. Hastings, R.P.; Taunt, H.M. Positive perceptions in families of children with developmental disabilities. *Am. J. Ment. Retard.* **2002**, *107*, 116–127. [CrossRef]
69. Savage, S.; Bailey, S. The impact of caring on caregivers' mental health: A review of the literature. *Aust. Heal. Rev.* **2004**, *27*, 111–117. [CrossRef] [PubMed]
70. Daley, T.C. From symptom recognition to diagnosis: Children with autism in urban India. *Soc. Sci. Med.* **2004**, *58*, 1323–1335. [CrossRef]
71. Dyches, T.T.; Wilder, L.K.; Sudweeks, R.R.; Obiakor, F.E.; Algozzine, B. Multicultural issues in autism. *J. Autism Dev. Disord.* **2004**, *34*, 211–222. [CrossRef]
72. Van Eylen, L.; Ceulemans, E.; Steyaert, J.; Wagemans, J.; Legius, E.; Noens, I. Does the cognitive heterogeneity within autism spectrum disorder reflect the underlying genetic heterogeneity? Available online: file:///C:/Users/Ali%20Samadi/Downloads/Van%20Eylen%20et%20al%20_2016_final%20(1).pdf (accessed on 12 December 2019).
73. Kasari, C.; Rotheram-Fuller, E. Current trends in psychological research on children with high-functioning autism and Asperger disorder. *Curr. Opin. Psychiatry* **2005**, *18*, 497–501. [CrossRef]
74. Masi, A.; DeMayo, M.M.; Glozier, N.; Guastella, A.J. An Overview of Autism Spectrum Disorder, Heterogeneity and Treatment Options. *Neurosci. Bull.* **2017**, *33*, 183–193. [CrossRef]
75. Chinn, P.L.; Kramer, M.K. *Theory and Nursing: Integrated Knowledge Development*; Mosby: St. Louis, MO, USA, 1999.
76. Waterhouse, L. Autism overflows: Increasing prevalence and proliferating theories. *Neuropsychol. Rev.* **2008**, *18*, 273–286. [CrossRef]
77. Ntoimo, L.F.C.; Odimegwu, C.O. Theoretical perspectives on family research. In *Family demography and post-2015 development agenda in Africa*; Odimegwu, C.O., Ed.; Springer: New York, NY, USA, 2020; pp. 75–82.
78. Swanson, H.L. Toward a Metatheory of Learning Disabilities. *J. Learn. Disabil.* **1988**, *21*, 196–209. [CrossRef]
79. Yau, M.K.; Li-Tsang, C.W. Adjustment and Adaptation in Parents of Children with Developmental Disability in Two-Parent Families: A Review of the Characteristics and Attributes. *Br. J. Dev. Disabil.* **1999**, *45*, 38–51. [CrossRef]
80. Summers, J.A.; Behr, S.K.; Turnbull, A.P. Positive adaptation and coping strengths of families who have children with disabilities. In *Support for Caregiving Families: Enabling Positive Adaptation to Disability*; Singer, G.H.S., Irvin, L.K., Eds.; Paul H Brookes Publishing Co: Baltimore, MD, USA, 1989; pp. 27–40.
81. Winzer, M. *Children with Exceptionalities: A Canadian Perspective*, 2nd ed.; Prentice Hall: Upper Saddle River, NJ, USA, 1990.
82. Estes, A.; Swain, D.M.; MacDuffie, K.E. The effects of early autism intervention on parents and family adaptive functioning. *Pediatr. Med.* **2019**, *2*, 21. [CrossRef]
83. Brewin, B.J.; Renwick, R.; Schormans, A.F. Parental Perspectives of the Quality of Life in School Environments for Children With Asperger Syndrome. *Focus Autism Other Dev. Disabil.* **2008**, *23*, 242–252. [CrossRef]
84. Phelps, K.W.; Hodgson, J.; McCammon, S.L.; Lamson, A.L. Caring for an individual with autism disorder: A qualitative analysis. *J. Intellect. Dev. Disabil.* **2009**, *34*, 27–35. [CrossRef] [PubMed]
85. Schlebusch, L.; Dada, S. Positive and negative cognitive appraisal of the impact of children with autism spectrum disorder on the family. *Res. Autism Spectr. Disord.* **2018**, *51*, 86–93. [CrossRef]
86. Barnett, R.A.; Hunter, M. Adjustment of Siblings of Children with Mental Health Problems: Behaviour, Self-Concept, Quality of Life and Family Functioning. *J. Child Fam. Stud.* **2011**, *21*, 262–272. [CrossRef]

87. Kinnear, S.H.; Link, B.G.; Ballan, M.S.; Fischbach, R.L. Understanding the Experience of Stigma for Parents of Children with Autism Spectrum Disorder and the Role Stigma Plays in Families' Lives. *J. Autism Dev. Disord.* **2015**, *46*, 942–953. [CrossRef]
88. Ahmadina, S.; Sherafat, S.; Taghikhant, K.; Tavakoli, S. The Experience of Social Stigma and the Spoiled Identity of Mothers with Autistic Children. *Iranian J. Soc. Problems* **2017**, *8*, 103–117.
89. Yorke, I.; White, P.; Weston, A.; Rafla, M.; Charman, T.; Simonoff, E. The Association Between Emotional and Behavioral Problems in Children with Autism Spectrum Disorder and Psychological Distress in Their Parents: A Systematic Review and Meta-analysis. *J. Autism Dev. Disord.* **2018**, *48*, 3393–3415. [CrossRef]
90. Salomone, E.; Settanni, M.; Ferrara, F.; Salandin, A.; Team, C.I. The CST Italy Team The Interplay of Communication Skills, Emotional and Behavioural Problems and Parental Psychological Distress. *J. Autism Dev. Disord.* **2019**, *49*, 4365–4374. [CrossRef]
91. Frantzen, K.K.; Lauritsen, M.B.; Jørgensen, M.; Tanggaard, L.; Fetters, M.D.; Aikens, J.E.; Bjerrum, M. Parental Self-perception in the Autism Spectrum Disorder Literature: A Systematic Mixed Studies Review. *Rev. J. Autism Dev. Disord.* **2015**, *3*, 18–36. [CrossRef]
92. O'Brien, Z.K.; Cuskelly, M.; Slaughter, V. Social Behaviors of Children with ASD during Play with Siblings and Parents: Parental Perceptions. *Res. Dev. Disabil.* **2020**, *97*, 103525. [CrossRef]
93. Meadan, H.; Stoner, J.B.; Angell, M.E. Review of Literature Related to the Social, Emotional, and Behavioral Adjustment of Siblings of Individuals with Autism Spectrum Disorder. *J. Dev. Phys. Disabil.* **2009**, *22*, 83–100. [CrossRef]
94. Ludlow, A.; Skelly, C.; Rohleder, P. Challenges faced by parents of children diagnosed with autism spectrum disorder. *J. Heal. Psychol.* **2011**, *17*, 702–711. [CrossRef] [PubMed]
95. Daniels, A.M.; Como, A.; Hergüner, S.; Kostadinova, K.; Stosic, J.; Shih, A. Autism in southeast europe: A survey of caregivers of children with autism spectrum disorders. *J. Autism. Dev. Disord.* **2017**, *47*, 2314–2325. [CrossRef] [PubMed]
96. De Vries, P.J. Thinking globally to meet local needs. *Curr. Opin. Neurol.* **2016**, *29*, 130–136. [CrossRef]
97. Söderqvist, H.; Kajsa, E.; Ahlström, B.H.; Wentz, E. The caregivers' perspectives of burden before and after an internet-based intervention of young persons with ADHD or autism spectrum disorder. *Scand. J. Occup. Ther.* **2017**, *24*, 383–392.
98. Volkmar, F.; Koenig, K.; McCarthy, M. Autism. *Autism Spectrum Disorders* **2003**, *362*, 1–14. [CrossRef]
99. Seltzer, M.; Greenberg, J.S.; Floyd, F.J.; Pettee, Y.; Hong, J. Life course impacts of parenting a child with a disability. *Am. J. Ment. Retard.* **2001**, *106*, 265. [CrossRef]
100. American Psychiatric Association. DSM-5. Frequently asked questions: Can you describe the dimensional assessments that are being considered for DSM-5? Available online: http://www.dsm5.org/about/Pages/faq.aspx#3 (accessed on 10 March 2019).
101. Lord, C.; Rutter, M.; DiLavore, P.; Risi, S.; Gotham, K.; Bishop, S.L. *Autism Diagnostic Observation Schedule (ADOS-2): Manual*, 2nd ed.; Western Psychological Services: Los Angeles, CA, USA, 2012.
102. World Health Organization. *International Classification of Functioning, Disability and Health: ICF: Children and Youth Version*; World Health Organization: Geneva, Switzerland, 2007.

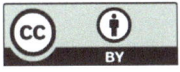

© 2020 by the authors. Licensee MDPI, Basel, Switzerland. This article is an open access article distributed under the terms and conditions of the Creative Commons Attribution (CC BY) license (http://creativecommons.org/licenses/by/4.0/).

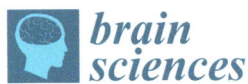

Article

Reward Responsiveness in the Adolescent Brain Cognitive Development (ABCD) Study: African Americans' Diminished Returns of Parental Education

Shervin Assari [1,*], Shanika Boyce [2], Golnoush Akhlaghipour [3], Mohsen Bazargan [1,4] and Cleopatra H. Caldwell [5,6]

1. Department of Family Medicine, Charles R Drew University of Medicine and Science, Los Angeles, CA 90059, USA; mohsenbazargan@cdrewu.edu
2. Department of Pediatrics, Charles R Drew University of Medicine and Science, Los Angeles, CA 90059, USA; ShanikaBoyce@cdrewu.edu
3. Department of Neurology, University of California Los Angeles, Los Angeles, CA 90095, USA; Golnoush.akhlaghi@gmail.com
4. Department of Family Medicine, University of California Los Angeles, Los Angeles, CA 90095, USA
5. Center for Research on Ethnicity, Culture, and Health (CRECH), School of Public Health, University of Michigan, Ann Arbor, MI 48104, USA; cleoc@umich.edu
6. Department of Health Behavior and Health Education, School of Public Health, University of Michigan, Ann Arbor, MI 48104, USA
* Correspondence: assari@umich.edu; Tel.: + (734)-232-0445; Fax: +734-615-8739

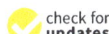

Received: 22 May 2020; Accepted: 16 June 2020; Published: 19 June 2020

Abstract: (1) Background: Reward responsiveness (RR) is a risk factor for high-risk behaviors such as aggressive behaviors and early sexual initiation, which are all reported to be higher in African American and low socioeconomic status adolescents. At the same time, parental education is one of the main drivers of reward responsiveness among adolescents. It is still unknown if some of this racial and economic gap is attributed to weaker effects of parental education for African Americans, a pattern also called minorities' diminished returns (MDRs). (2) Aim: We compared non-Hispanic White and African American adolescents for the effects of parent education on adolescents RR, a psychological and cognitive construct that is closely associated with high-risk behaviors such as the use of drugs, alcohol, and tobacco. (3) Methods: This was a cross-sectional analysis that included 7072 adolescents from the adolescent brain cognitive development (ABCD) study. The independent variable was parent education. The main outcome as adolescents' RR measured by the behavioral inhibition system (BIS) and behavioral activation system (BAS) measure. (4) Results: In the overall sample, high parent education was associated with lower levels of RR. In the overall sample, we found a statistically significant interaction between race and parent education on adolescents' RR. The observed statistical interaction term suggested that high parent education is associated with a weaker effect on RR for African American than non-Hispanic White adolescents. In race-stratified models, high parent education was only associated with lower RR for non-Hispanic White but not African American adolescents. (5) Conclusion: Parent education reduces RR for non-Hispanic White but not African American adolescents. To minimize the racial gap in brain development and risk-taking behaviors, we need to address societal barriers that diminish the returns of parent education and resources in African American families. We need public and social policies that target structural and societal barriers, such as the unequal distribution of opportunities and resources. To meet such an aim, we need to reduce the negative effects of social stratification, segregation, racism, and discrimination in the daily lives of African American parents and families. Through an approach like this, African American families and parents can effectively mobilize their resources and utilize their human capital to secure the best possible tangible outcomes for their adolescents.

Keywords: race; education; parenting; socioeconomic status; adolescents; reward; brain development; risk behaviors; cognition; brain; inhibitory control

---

1. Introduction

Reward responsiveness (RR) [1], a trait closely linked to impulsivity and risk taking [2], is a major driver of high-risk behaviors such as tobacco use [3–8], alcohol use [9–12], emotional eating [13], obesity [14], aggression [15], and sexual risk [16,17]. High RR is also associated with a wide range of psychiatric disorders such as depression, bipolar disorder, anxiety, and post-traumatic stress disorder (PTSD) [18]. Similar to the evidence that high-risk behaviors [19] and impulsivity [20,21] may be linked to race and socioeconomic status (SES), youth and adults with African American and low SES backgrounds may report higher RR than individuals from non-Hispanic White and high SES backgrounds [22].

Based on Gray's reinforcement sensitivity theory (RST) [23], RR is one of the two neurobiological bases that guide human's emotions, motivations, and behaviors. Rooted in the behavioral approach system (BAS) developed by the Carver and White [14], high RR reflects individuals' high sensitivity to conditioned cues, which signal them about a higher-than-luck probability of reward. Individuals with a high score on the RR trait are more likely to act on any cues that may generate internal or external reward. In the recent version of the same theory [24], Gray and McNaughton have discussed BAS-based RR as well as approach-related behaviors and stimuli that contribute to human decisions, choices, and behaviors. Many investigators have found evidence linking the RR trait to a wide range of health and behavioral outcomes in clinical [22,25,26] as well as community [27] samples. RR is also highly relevant to adolescents' behaviors and risk-taking [9,13,28].

Relative to their non-Hispanic White counterparts, African American adolescents are at an increased risk of high-risk behaviors. For example, African American adolescents are more likely than non-Hispanic White adolescents to be at risk of aggression [29], early sexual debut [30], and poor school performance [31]. As these early risk taking behaviors operate as a barrier against positive and desired health and economic outcomes later in life [32–35], it is essential to study environmental and psychological factors that explain high RR (and associated risky behaviors) of African American adolescents. Such knowledge may inform public and social policies as well as interventions that can be implemented during adolescence to eliminate later racial inequalities [32–35].

Given the close overlap between race and parental education in the US [36], researchers have shown immense interest in understanding the combined effects of race and parental education on adolescents' inequalities [37–39]. As both racial minority status and low parental education reflect food and housing insecurity, economic adversities, stress, and financial difficulties [40–43], some of the effects of race may be in fact due to low parental education in African American families. Thus, low parental education may carry some of the effects of race on adolescents' outcomes [36]. Recent data, however, show that the effects of race and parental education are more complex as they show both mediation and moderation effects on health inequalities [44–47]. While parental education is also a proxy of access to risk and protective factors [44–47], the protective effects of parental education seem to be weaker for African American than non-Hispanic White adolescents.

There are at least two complementary theories that provide an explanation for how race and parental education jointly impact adolescents' outcomes. The first theory, dominant in the literature, and more commonly used as an explanation of the inequalities, attributes the observed racial gap in adolescents' outcomes to the observed differences in parental education and other family SES indicators across racial groups [36,48–50]. In a statistical term, this theory conceptualizes parental education as the mediator (why) for racial differences in adolescents' outcomes [51–53]. If this theory is followed, then the strategic goal for closing the racial gap in adolescents' health would be to close the racial gap in family SES. Some example policy modalities in line with this strategy include income redistribution policies, minimum wage policies, or an earned income tax credit that help racial minorities to earn higher income and accumulate more wealth [54,55].

Minorities' diminished returns (MDRs) [56,57], the second theory, however, argues that the effects of parental education and other family SES indicators tend to be weaker for racial minority groups such as African Americans, when compared to non-Hispanic Whites. This line of view is not against the traditional mediational model but provides an additional explanation for why, despite years of investment and the decline in the gap between races in terms of family SES, the racial and economic health gaps are still sustained and in some cases, widened [58–62]. The MDRs theory has been supported by a large number of papers showing that parental education [63], family income [64,65], and marital status [66] generate less health and well-being for African American than non-Hispanic White adolescents. This literature is repeatedly shown for emotional and behavioral outcomes [63–65,67,68]. For example, high family SES showed a smaller effect as a preventive factor on impulsivity [64], depression [67], anxiety [69], aggression [63], low grade point average (GPA) [63,70,71], and substance use [63] for African American than non-Hispanic White adolescents. Similarly, high SES African American youth are found to be at high risk of attention deficit hyperactive disorder (ADHD) [72] and obesity [73]. Given the existing MDRs, it would be too optimistic and unrealistic to expect racial inequities to disappear even if we could fully eliminate SES inequalities. In this view, SES indicators such as parental education are seen as both a remedy and also a source of inequalities across racial groups. While it is essential to eliminate the SES gap, we should complement our policy responses in a specific way that particularly empowers African American families to mobilize their resources and secure better health outcomes [56,57].

As described above, the MDR literature suggests that the educational attainment of oneself [74] and one's parents [75–77] generate fewer tangible outcomes for racial minorities such as African Americans. This might be because African Americans and non-Hispanic Whites differ in getting chances and opportunities to mobilize their education and secure high paying jobs in the presence of high education [57,64,69,76,78,79]. As a result of these MDRs of parental education, compared to their non-Hispanic White counterparts, African American adolescents with highly educated parents show worse than expected outcomes that are disproportionate to their family SES [56,57,64,65,68]. Although these findings may be similar to what may be expected due regression to the mean, in a recent paper, we published and showed that MDRs are not due to such a superfluous association [80].

Aims

To extend the science on what we already know about the role of RR as a mechanism for explaining MDRs for high-risk behaviors such as aggression, tobacco use, and impulsivity, in this study, we explored the combined effects of race and parent education on adolescents' RR. Thus, we compared African American and non-Hispanic White adolescents for the effect of parent education, a strong family SES determinant of adolescents' various behaviors, and RR. We expected a weaker effect of parent education on RR for African American than non-Hispanic White adolescents.

2. Methods

2.1. Design and Settings

We performed a secondary analysis of data from the adolescent brain cognitive development (ABCD) study [81–85], a landmark adolescents brain development study in the United States. Detailed information on the ABCD study is available elsewhere [81,86].

2.2. Participants and Sampling

Participants of the ABCD study were adolescents ages 9–10 years old. Adolescents in the ABCD study were recruited from multiple cities across states. Overall, there were 21 sites that recruited adolescents to the ABCD study. The recruitment of the ABCD sample was mainly done through school systems. A detailed description of the ABCD sampling is available here [87]. Four thousand one hundred eighty-eight participants entered our analysis. Eligibility for our analysis had valid data on race, parental education, marital status, RR, and being African American or non-Hispanic White. The analytical sample of this paper consisted of 7072 participants.

2.3. Study Variables

The study variables included race, demographic factors, parent education, parental marital status, and RR.

2.4. Outcome

Reward responsiveness (RR). In this study, RR was measured using the behavioral approach system (BAS) [1] developed by the Carver and White [14]. They define RR as a trait closely linked to impulsivity and risk taking [2], with a significant relevance to high-risk behaviors such as tobacco use [3–8], alcohol use [9–12], emotional eating [13], obesity [14], aggression [15], and sexual risk [16,17]. Based on Gray's reinforcement sensitivity theory (RST) [23], a high score on the RR trait reflects individuals' high sensitivity to conditioned cues, which signal the individual about a higher-than-luck probability of reward. We operationalized a BAS-based RR score, which was a continuous measure. Although BAS had other measures such as drive and fun seeking, we only used RR. This was because we built this study to examine effects on RR, not all BAS measures.

2.4.1. Moderator: Race

Race was self-identified. Race was a categorical variable and coded 1 for African Americans and 0 for non-Hispanic Whites (reference category). All people of a Hispanic background were excluded. We used the one drop rule to handle people who identified as both White and African American. That means individuals would be considered African American if they identify as both African American and White.

2.4.2. Independent Variable: Parent Education

Participants were asked, "What is the highest grade or level of school you have completed or the highest degree you have received?". Responses were 0 = never attended/kindergarten only; 1 = 1st grade; 2 = 2nd grade; 3 = 3rd grade; 4 = 4th grade 4; 5 = 5th grade; 6 = 6th grade 6; 7 = 7th grade 7; 8 = 8th grade; 9 = 9th grade; 10 = 10th grade 10; 11 = 11th grade; 12 = 12th grade; 13 = high school graduate; 14 = GED or equivalent diploma; 15 = some college; 16 = associate degree: occupational; 17 = associate degree: academic program; 18 = Bachelor's degree (ex. BA); 19 = Master's degree (ex. MA); 20 = professional school degree (ex. MD); and 21 = Doctoral degree. This variable was coded in two distinct ways. First, it was coded as measured. This was an interval measure with a range between 1 and 21. Second, we adopted the Jaeger [88] coding approach with a range from 31 to 46. For both variables, a higher score indicated higher educational attainment.

2.4.3. Confounders: Demographic Factors

Age, sex, parental marital status, and household size were the confounders. Parents reported the age of their adolescents. Age (years) was calculated as the difference between the date of birth to the date of the enrollment to the study. Sex was a dichotomous variable: males = 1, females = 0. Parental marital status was a dichotomous variable. This variable was self-reported by the parent who was interviewed. This variable was coded as married = 1 vs. other = 0. Household size, reported by the parent, was a continuous measure.

2.5. Data Analysis

We used the statistical package SPSS to perform our data analysis. Mean (standard deviation (SD)) and frequency (%) were described depending on the variable type. We also performed a Chi square and independent sample *t* test to test bivariate associations between race and study variables. For our multivariable modeling, we performed four linear regression models. Our first two models were performed in the overall sample. *Model 3* was performed without the interaction terms. *Model 4* added an interaction term between race and parental education attainment. Then we performed two additional models specifically to race (race-stratified models). *Model 3* was tested in non-Hispanic White and *Model 4* was tested in African American adolescents. Our models used age, sex, marital status, and household size as the covariates. We ran identical models using various coding of educational variable. Our first model used the census and our second variable used the Jaeger [88] code of educational attainment. Unstandardized regression coefficient (b), standardized regression coefficient, SE, 95% CI, *t* value, and *p* value were reported for each model. *p* value equal or less 0.05 were statistically significant.

2.6. Ethical Aspect

The ABCD study received an Institutional Review Board (IRB) approval from the University of California, San Diego (UCSD). Each adolescent provided assent. Each parent signed an informed consent [86]. As this analysis was performed on fully de-identified data, the study was found to be non-human subject research. Thus, our analysis was exempt from a full IRB review.

3. Results

3.1. Descriptives

As shown in Table 1, 7072, 8–11-year-old adolescents entered to this analysis. From this number, most were non-Hispanic Whites (*n* = 5099; 72.1%) and the rest were African Americans (*n* = 1973; 27.9%). Table 1 presents a summary of the descriptive statistics for the pooled sample.

Table 1. Data overall and by race ($n = 7072$).

Characteristics	All		Non-Hispanic Whites		African Americans	
	n	%	n	%	n	%
Race						
Non-Hispanic Whites	5099	72.1	5099	100.0	-	-
African Americans	1973	27.9	-	-	1973	100.0
Sex						
Male	3417	48.3	2432	47.7	985	49.9
Female	3655	51.7	2667	52.3	988	50.1
Marital Status *						
Other	2257	31.9	908	17.8	1349	68.4
Married	4815	68.1	4191	82.2	624	31.6
	Mean	SD	Mean	SD	Mean	SD
Age (Year)	9.47	0.51	9.47	0.50	9.47	0.52
Household Size	4.70	1.52	4.72	1.40	4.63	1.81
Parent education (Census Coding) *	16.92	2.40	17.55	2.00	15.30	2.57
Parent education (Jager Coding) *	42.06	2.20	42.61	1.87	40.58	2.23
Reward Responsiveness (RR) *	8.78	2.41	8.58	2.37	9.29	2.44

Note: SD = Standard deviation, * $p < 0.05$ for comparison of African American and non-Hispanic White adolescents.

3.2. Multivariate Analysis (Pooled Sample)

Table 2 shows the results of two linear regression models in the overall (pooled) sample. *Model 1* (the main effect model) showed a protective effect of high parent education against RR. *Model 2* (the interaction model) showed a statistically significant interaction between race and parent education on RR, which was suggestive of a weaker protective effect of high parent education on RR for African American adolescents relative to non-Hispanic White adolescents.

3.3. Multivariate Analysis (Race-Stratified Models)

Table 3 shows the results of two linear regression models in racial groups. *Model 3* (non-Hispanic Whites) showed protective effects of high parent education on RR of non-Hispanic White adolescents. *Model 4* (African Americans) did not show any protective effects of high parent education on RR for African American adolescents.

Table 2. Summary of linear regressions overall ($n = 7072$).

Characteristics	Model 1 Main Effects						Model 2 Interaction Effects					
	b	SE	95% CI		T	p	B	SE	95% CI		t	p
Education (Jager Code)												
Race (African Americans)	0.61	0.09	0.43	0.79	6.53	<0.001	-2.67	1.56	-5.74	0.39	-1.71	0.087
Sex (Male)	0.31	0.07	0.17	0.45	4.44	<0.001	0.31	0.07	0.17	0.45	4.40	<0.001
Age	-0.02	0.07	-0.16	0.11	-0.31	0.760	-0.02	0.07	-0.16	0.11	-0.35	0.727
Married Household	-0.14	0.09	-0.33	0.04	-1.52	0.129	-0.15	0.09	-0.34	0.03	-1.64	0.101
Household Size	-0.03	0.02	-0.08	0.01	-1.37	0.171	-0.03	0.02	-0.08	0.01	-1.37	0.171
Parent Education	-0.07	0.02	-0.11	-0.04	-3.85	<0.001	-0.10	0.02	-0.14	-0.05	-4.37	<0.001
Parent Education × African Americans	-	-	-	-	-	-	0.08	0.04	0.01	0.15	2.10	0.035
Constant	14.12	1.04	12.08	16.16	13.57	<0.001	15.28	1.18	12.97	17.59	12.99	<0.001
Education (Census Code)												
Race (African Americans)	0.53	0.08	0.38	0.68	6.98	<0.001	-0.34	0.45	-1.23	0.55	-0.75	0.454
Sex (Male)	0.33	0.06	0.21	0.44	5.69	<0.001	0.32	0.06	0.21	0.44	5.65	<0.001
Age	-0.05	0.06	-0.16	0.06	-0.88	0.381	-0.05	0.06	-0.16	0.06	-0.91	0.361
Married Household	-0.11	0.08	-0.26	0.04	-1.43	0.153	-0.12	0.08	-0.27	0.03	-1.51	0.131
Household Size	-0.03	0.02	-0.06	0.01	-1.33	0.185	-0.03	0.02	-0.07	0.01	-1.34	0.181
Parent Education	-0.05	0.01	-0.08	-0.03	-3.79	<0.001	-0.07	0.02	-0.11	-0.04	-4.22	<0.001
Parent Education × African Americans	-	-	-	-	-	-	0.05	0.03	0.00	0.11	1.95	0.050
Constant	10.03	0.59	8.86	11.19	16.90	<0.001	10.40	0.62	9.18	11.62	16.69	<0.001

Note: Unstandardized Regression Coefficient (b); Standard Error (SE); Confidence Interval (CI); Outcome: Reward Responsiveness (RR); $p \leq 0.050$ considered significant.

Table 3. Summary of linear regressions between parental education and reward responsiveness (RR) by race (n = 7072).

Characteristics	Model 1 non-Hispanic Whites						Model 2 African Americans					
	B	SE	95% CI		T	p	b	SE	95% CI		t	p
Education (Jager Code)												
Sex (Male)	0.47	0.08	0.31	0.62	5.74	<0.001	−0.13	0.14	−0.40	0.14	−0.95	0.345
Age	−0.08	0.08	−0.23	0.08	−0.94	0.349	0.12	0.13	−0.14	0.39	0.91	0.365
Married Household	−0.23	0.11	−0.45	0.00	−2.00	0.0	−0.01	0.16	−0.33	0.31	−0.07	0.944
Household Size	−0.02	0.03	−0.08	0.04	−0.57	0.566	−0.06	0.04	−0.14	0.02	−1.48	0.138
Parent Education	−0.09	0.02	−0.14	−0.05	−4.10	<0.001	−0.03	0.03	−0.10	0.04	−0.91	0.364
Constant	15.42	1.25	12.97	17.87	12.35	<0.001	11.98	1.87	8.30	15.66	6.39	<0.001
Education (Census Code)												
Sex (Male)	0.47	0.07	0.34	0.60	7.18	<0.001	−0.09	0.11	−0.32	0.13	−0.83	0.405
Age	−0.09	0.07	−0.22	0.04	−1.42	0.157	0.07	0.11	−0.15	0.29	0.61	0.539
Married Household	−0.17	0.09	−0.35	0.01	−1.80	0.072	−0.02	0.13	−0.28	0.25	−0.14	0.892
Household Size	−0.01	0.02	−0.06	0.04	−0.54	0.592	−0.05	0.03	−0.11	0.02	−1.47	0.141
Parent Education	−0.07	0.02	−0.10	−0.03	−3.97	<0.001	−0.03	0.02	−0.07	0.02	−1.05	0.296
Constant	10.62	0.70	9.24	11.99	15.14	<0.001	9.31	1.12	7.12	11.50	8.33	<0.001

Note: Unstandardized Regression Coefficient (b); Standard Error (SE); Confidence Interval (CI); Outcome: Reward Responsiveness (RR).

4. Discussion

In this study, while high parent education was associated with lower RR overall, this was only true for non-Hispanic White but not African American adolescents, as shown by the pooled sample as well as by race-stratified models. This suggests racial minority status limits the boosting effect of parent education on RR for American adolescents.

The observed diminished returns of parental education on RR is very similar to the previous publications on the MDRs of parental education and income on impulsivity [64], ADHD [72], and inhibitory control [89], social problems, emotional problems, behavioral problems [90], anxiety [69], depression [67], aggression [63], GPA [63,70,71], and substance use [63]. These are all examples of diminishing returns of parental education for African American youth when compared with non-Hispanic White youth [74,78,91,92].

MDRs are not specific to a specific resource or age group, outcome, or even marginalizing identities [56,57]. Education [74], income [64], employment [93], and marital status [69] show weaker effects on adolescents [64,65,68], adults [78], and older adults [94] who are African Americans [65], Hispanics [74,95–97], Asian Americans [98], Native Americans [99], lesbian, gay, bisexual, transgender, and queer (LGBTQ) [91], immigrants [100], or even marginalized non-Hispanic Whites [101].

Various sociological, economic, and behavioral mechanisms are involved in explaining the MDRs of parent education for African American families. African American parents and families experience high levels of economic, social, general, and race-related stress in their daily lives at all SES levels [102]. Racial groups do not have the same chance of upward social mobility in the US [103]. High SES African American families show an increase in exposure [104–108] and vulnerability [109] to discrimination, which may reduce the protective effects of SES on health. African American families with high SES are frequently surrounded by non-Hispanic Whites, which increases their exposure to discrimination [104,105]. Discrimination results in poor health across domains and limits the health gains that follow improving SES [107,109,110].

Residential segregation results in differences in African American and non-Hispanic White environmental and contextual exposures. Due to segregation, school options are different for high SES African American and Hispanic families. As a result, children of high SES African American families attend highly segregated schools with low resources [70,71,111]. That means there are differential effects of SES on education and schooling of non-Hispanic White and African American. While high SES non-Hispanic White adolescents attend schools in suburban areas with more funding and higher-quality teachers, African Americans go to schools that are of less quality [112].

While lower SES of African Americans is one type of disadvantage, MDRs reflect another class of disadvantage [56,57]. While the first one is about a lack of access to SES resources, MDRs are reflective of unequal outcomes despite access to SES. Thus, researchers and policymakers should not only address inequality in SES, but they should also address inequality in the returns of SES. African Americans are at a double disadvantage because they are affected by low SES and low return of the existing SES resources [56,113].

Multilevel economic, psychological, and societal mechanisms may be involved in explaining racial gaps in the returns of parental education [56,113]. MDRs may be due to racism across multiple societal institutions and social structures [56,113]. Racial prejudice interferes with the processes that are needed to gain benefits from available SES resources [114–116]. MDRs of educational attainment may be in part due to a history of childhood poverty [117]. The current study, however, did not explore societal and contextual processes that could explain such MDRs.

African American families are more likely to stay in poor neighborhoods despite high SES. Highly educated African Americans are more likely to stay poor than non-Hispanic Whites [77,118]. Similarly, African American families from high SES backgrounds are more likely to remain at risk of negative environmental exposures than non-Hispanic Whites with similar SES [104,105,107,119–123]. Similarly, high SES African American adolescents spend time with peers with higher risk and behavioral problems than non-Hispanic Whites with the same SES [63,98].

As this study showed, health disparities are not all due to SES differences, and some can be seen across all SES spectrum. This means, it is not race or SES but race and SES that shape health disparities [124–126]. The implication of these MDRs is that merely equalizing access to SES is not enough to tackle racial inequalities. Beyond attempts to eliminate or reduce SES gaps, there is a need to increase the degree to which SES can result in outcomes for African American families. To do so, policymakers should think about societal, environmental, and structural barriers that generate MDRs by reducing African Americas' ability to leverage their resources. A real solution to MDRs-related disparities should be different from a solution to those who are caused by the SES-gaps. While the policy solution to health disparities due to SES gap is to increase African Americans' access to SES resources, a true and sustainable remedy to the MDRs-related inequalities is to reduce structural barriers so African American families can efficiently and effectively translate their SES and human capital and secure tangible outcomes. This is not possible unless we equalize the daily living conditions of African Americans and non-Hispanic Whites.

While this study's main association of interest was the effect of parental education on RR, we also found auxiliary results. We found results considering gender. In the pooled sample, boys showed a higher RR than girls. In Whites but not Blacks, males had higher RR. A higher reward responsiveness of males than females is known. This is also related to the higher impulsivity [127–131], reward dependence [16,132–139], and novelty seeking [140–143] of males than females. The result is a higher risk taking of males than females [127,144–146]. However, as mentioned before, this was not an exploratory study on correlates of RR. We were specifically interested in knowing if Black and White youth differ in the contribution of their parental educational attainment on their RR.

We also want to make it clear that MDRs are not due to Kelly's Paradox [147] or regression toward the mean [148–152]. Under certain conditions, statistical artifacts, like regression to the mean or Kelly's paradox, can produce similar results. However, in previous research [80], we showed that the MDRs were not attributable to statistical artifacts. While we do not verify that this is the case in the present study, we would argue, based on past results, that these MDRs represent the effects of the social environment. Kelly's paradox [147], closely related to the regression to the mean [148–152], may occur when multiple groups with different starting points are compared. As described by Wainer and Brown (2007) [147], when a person from the poor-performing group exceeds the expectations, that person is expected to continue to overachieve, meaning he/she would perform even better. The opposite is also relevant to an underperformer in a high-performing group. In both cases, in reality, and opposite to the expectation, the individuals would regress toward their group means. That means, underperformers in a high-performing group and overperformers in a low-performing group are all more likely to have the average outcome rather than the expected outcome. In a recent paper, we have shown that MDRs are not due to regression toward the mean or Kelley's paradox [147]. In fact, MDRs are not exclusively to the high-achiever or high-performance individuals, but any incremental increase in the resource generates less increase in the outcome for Blacks than Whites.

5. Limitations

This study, like any other studies, comes with a specific set of methodological limitations. As our data were cross-sectional in nature, we could not draw any causal inference between race, parent education, and adolescents' RR. Similarly, we only tested the MDRs of parent education. Future research should test if MDRs go beyond parent education and hold for other SES indicators such as income, wealth, class, occupational prestige, and neighborhood SES indicators. Finally, this study only described the MDRs of parent education on RR and did not seek to understand the contextual factors that cause such MDRs.

In this study, RR [1] was measured using the behavioral approach, using BAS, which was developed by the Carver and White. We are unaware of any studies on the psychometric properties of this scale by race. So, we are not confident that the applied item measures identically the very same constructs in our race groups. So, there is a need to study if this measure is invariant across groups. As expected, we found a main effect of race on RR, suggesting that in line with the literature on associated traits such as impulsivity [64], RR is higher in Black than White youth. Future research should assess racial variation in measurement aspects of the BAS-based RR variable. Such effort would increase our confidence in comparing the results across groups and the observed means.

6. Conclusions

Relative to their non-Hispanic White counterparts, African American adolescents show lower parent education and higher RR. This adversity in African American youth is compounded by another profound and systemic disadvantage, weaker effects of parent education on adolescents RR. As a result of the latter disadvantage, African American adolescents show low RR across all parental education levels. That means some of the racial inequalities in RR remains across all educational levels. In other terms, racial inequalities in RR show a spill-over effect in middle-class people. As a result of high RR, African American adolescents engage in a high risk of behaviors across all levels of parental education. This is in contrast to the pattern for non-Hispanic White adolescents who show a social patterning of their RR. That is, for non-Hispanic White youth, RR is lowest when parental education is highest.

Author Contributions: S.A. conceptualization, data analysis, first draft, and revision. S.B., G.A., M.B., and C.H.C. conceptualization and revision. All authors have read and agreed to the published version of the manuscript.

Funding: Shervin Assari is supported by the National Institutes of Health (NIH) grants D084526-03, 5S21MD000103, CA201415 02, DA035811-05, U54MD008149, U54MD007598, and U54CA229974.

Conflicts of Interest: The authors declare no conflict of interest.

References

1. Van den Berg, I.; Franken, I.H.; Muris, P. A new scale for measuring reward responsiveness. *Front. Psychol.* **2010**, *1*, 239. [CrossRef] [PubMed]
2. Johnson, P.L.; Potts, G.F.; Sanchez-Ramos, J.; Cimino, C.R. Self-reported impulsivity in Huntington's disease patients and relationship to executive dysfunction and reward responsiveness. *J. Clin. Exp. Neuropsychol.* **2017**, *39*, 694–706. [CrossRef] [PubMed]
3. Powell, J.; Dawkins, L.; Davis, R.E. Smoking, reward responsiveness, and response inhibition: Tests of an incentive motivational model. *Biol. Psychiatry* **2002**, *51*, 151–163. [CrossRef]
4. Barr, R.S.; Pizzagalli, D.A.; Culhane, M.A.; Goff, D.C.; Evins, A.E. A single dose of nicotine enhances reward responsiveness in nonsmokers: Implications for development of dependence. *Biol. Psychiatry* **2008**, *63*, 1061–1065. [CrossRef] [PubMed]
5. Cummings, J.R.; Gearhardt, A.N.; Miller, A.L.; Hyde, L.W.; Lumeng, J.C. Maternal nicotine dependence is associated with longitudinal increases in child obesogenic eating behaviors. *Pediatr. Obes.* **2019**, *14*, e12541. [CrossRef] [PubMed]
6. Pergadia, M.L.; Der-Avakian, A.; D'Souza, M.S.; Madden, P.A.F.; Heath, A.C.; Shiffman, S.; Markou, A.; Pizzagalli, D.A. Association between nicotine withdrawal and reward responsiveness in humans and rats. *JAMA Psychiatry* **2014**, *71*, 1238–1245. [CrossRef]
7. Snuggs, S.; Hajek, P. Responsiveness to reward following cessation of smoking. *Psychopharmacology* **2013**, *225*, 869–873. [CrossRef]
8. Janes, A.C.; Pedrelli, P.; Whitton, A.E.; Pechtel, P.; Douglas, S.; Martinson, M.A.; Huz, I.; Fava, M.; Pizzagalli, D.A.; Evins, A.E. Reward Responsiveness Varies by Smoking Status in Women with a History of Major Depressive Disorder. *Neuropsychopharmacology* **2015**, *40*, 1940–1946. [CrossRef]
9. Aloi, J.; Blair, K.S.; Crum, K.I.; Bashford-Largo, J.; Zhang, R.; Lukoff, J.; Carollo, E.; White, S.F.; Hwang, S.; Filbey, F.M.; et al. Alcohol Use Disorder, But Not Cannabis Use Disorder, Symptomatology in Adolescents Is Associated With Reduced Differential Responsiveness to Reward Versus Punishment Feedback During Instrumental Learning. *Biol. Psychiatry Cogn. Neurosci. Neuroimaging* **2020**. [CrossRef]
10. Black, A.C.; Rosen, M.I. A money management-based substance use treatment increases valuation of future rewards. *Addict. Behav.* **2011**, *36*, 125–128. [CrossRef]

11. Boger, K.D.; Auerbach, R.P.; Pechtel, P.; Busch, A.B.; Greenfield, S.F.; Pizzagalli, D.A. Co-Occurring Depressive and Substance Use Disorders in Adolescents: An Examination of Reward Responsiveness During Treatment. *J. Psychother. Integr.* **2014**, *24*, 109–121. [CrossRef] [PubMed]
12. Enoch, M.A.; Gorodetsky, E.; Hodgkinson, C.; Roy, A.; Goldman, D. Functional genetic variants that increase synaptic serotonin and 5-HT3 receptor sensitivity predict alcohol and drug dependence. *Mol. Psychiatry* **2011**, *16*, 1139–1146. [CrossRef] [PubMed]
13. Cummings, J.R.; Lumeng, J.C.; Miller, A.L.; Hyde, L.W.; Siada, R.; Gearhardt, A.N. Parental substance use and child reward-driven eating behaviors. *Appetite* **2020**, *144*, 104486. [CrossRef]
14. Carver, C.S.; White, T.L. Behavioral inhibition, behavioral activation, and affective responses to impending reward and punishment: The BIS/BAS scales. *J. Personal. Soc. Psychol.* **1994**, *67*, 319. [CrossRef]
15. Harmon-Jones, E. Anger and the behavioral approach system. *Personal. Individ. Differ.* **2003**, *35*, 995–1005. [CrossRef]
16. Balda, M.A.; Anderson, K.L.; Itzhak, Y. Adolescent and adult responsiveness to the incentive value of cocaine reward in mice: Role of neuronal nitric oxide synthase (nNOS) gene. *Neuropharmacology* **2006**, *51*, 341–349. [CrossRef] [PubMed]
17. Opel, N.; Redlich, R.; Grotegerd, D.; Dohm, K.; Haupenthal, C.; Heindel, W.; Kugel, H.; Arolt, V.; Dannlowski, U. Enhanced neural responsiveness to reward associated with obesity in the absence of food-related stimuli. *Hum. Brain Mapp.* **2015**, *36*, 2330–2337. [CrossRef]
18. Johnson, S.L.; Turner, R.J.; Iwata, N. BIS/BAS levels and psychiatric disorder: An epidemiological study. *J. Psychopathol. Behav. Assess.* **2003**, *25*, 25–36. [CrossRef]
19. Blum, R.W.; Beuhring, T.; Shew, M.L.; Bearinger, L.H.; Sieving, R.E.; Resnick, M.D. The effects of race/ethnicity, income, and family structure on adolescent risk behaviors. *Am. J. Public Health* **2000**, *90*, 1879.
20. Zalot, A.; Jones, D.J.; Kincaid, C.; Smith, T. Hyperactivity, impulsivity, inattention (HIA) and conduct problems among African American youth: The roles of neighborhood and gender. *J. Abnorm. Child Psychol.* **2009**, *37*, 535–549. [CrossRef]
21. Weiss, N.H.; Tull, M.T.; Davis, L.T.; Dehon, E.E.; Fulton, J.J.; Gratz, K.L. Examining the association between emotion regulation difficulties and probable posttraumatic stress disorder within a sample of African Americans. *Cogn. Behav. Ther.* **2012**, *41*, 5–14. [CrossRef] [PubMed]
22. Alloy, L.B.; Bender, R.E.; Whitehouse, W.G.; Wagner, C.A.; Liu, R.T.; Grant, D.A.; Jager-Hyman, S.; Molz, A.; Choi, J.Y.; Harmon-Jones, E.; et al. High Behavioral Approach System (BAS) sensitivity, reward responsiveness, and goal-striving predict first onset of bipolar spectrum disorders: A prospective behavioral high-risk design. *J. Abnorm. Psychol.* **2012**, *121*, 339–351. [CrossRef] [PubMed]
23. Gray, J. Neural systems of motivation, emotion and affect. In *Neurobiology of Learning, Emotion and Affect*; Maden, J., Ed.; Raven Press: New York, NY, USA, 1991.
24. McNaughton, N.; Gray, J.A. Anxiolytic action on the behavioural inhibition system implies multiple types of arousal contribute to anxiety. *J. Affect. Disord.* **2000**, *61*, 161–176. [CrossRef]
25. Fletcher, K.; Parker, G.; Manicavasagar, V. Behavioral Activation System (BAS) differences in bipolar I and II disorder. *J. Affect. Disord.* **2013**, *151*, 121–128. [CrossRef]
26. Keough, M.T.; Wardell, J.D.; Hendershot, C.S.; Bagby, R.M.; Quilty, L.C. Fun Seeking and Reward Responsiveness Moderate the Effect of the Behavioural Inhibition System on Coping-Motivated Problem Gambling. *J. Gambl. Stud.* **2017**, *33*, 769–782. [CrossRef] [PubMed]
27. Tsypes, A.; Gibb, B.E. Time of day differences in neural reward responsiveness in children. *Psychophysiology* **2020**, *57*, e13550. [CrossRef] [PubMed]
28. Kujawa, A.; Burkhouse, K.L.; Karich, S.R.; Fitzgerald, K.D.; Monk, C.S.; Phan, K.L. Reduced Reward Responsiveness Predicts Change in Depressive Symptoms in Anxious Children and Adolescents Following Treatment. *J. Child Adolesc. Psychopharmacol.* **2019**, *29*, 378–385. [CrossRef] [PubMed]
29. Cotten, N.U.; Resnick, J.; Browne, D.C.; Martin, S.L.; McCarraher, D.R.; Woods, J. Aggression and fighting behavior among African-American adolescents: Individual and family factors. *Am. J. Public Health* **1994**, *84*, 618–622. [CrossRef]
30. Cavazos-Rehg, P.A.; Krauss, M.J.; Spitznagel, E.L.; Schootman, M.; Bucholz, K.K.; Peipert, J.F.; Sanders-Thompson, V.; Cottler, L.B.; Bierut, L.J. Age of sexual debut among US adolescents. *Contraception* **2009**, *80*, 158–162. [CrossRef]

31. Bumpus, J.P.; Umeh, Z.; Harris, A.L. Social Class and Educational Attainment: Do Blacks Benefit Less from Increases in Parents' Social Class Status? *Sociol. Race Ethn.* **2020**. [CrossRef]
32. Cohen, G.L.; Sherman, D.K. Stereotype threat and the social and scientific contexts of the race achievement gap. *Am. Psychol.* **2005**, *60*, 270–271. [CrossRef]
33. Burchinal, M.; McCartney, K.; Steinberg, L.; Crosnoe, R.; Friedman, S.L.; McLoyd, V.; Pianta, R.; Network, N.E.C.C.R. Examining the Black-White achievement gap among low-income children using the NICHD study of early child care and youth development. *Child Dev.* **2011**, *82*, 1404–1420. [CrossRef]
34. Gorey, K.M. Comprehensive School Reform: Meta-Analytic Evidence of Black-White Achievement Gap Narrowing. *Educ. Policy Anal. Arch.* **2009**, *17*, 1. [CrossRef] [PubMed]
35. Hair, N.L.; Hanson, J.L.; Wolfe, B.L.; Pollak, S.D. Association of Child Poverty, Brain Development, and Academic Achievement. *JAMA Pediatr.* **2015**, *169*, 822–829. [CrossRef] [PubMed]
36. Kaufman, J.S.; Cooper, R.S.; McGee, D.L. Socioeconomic status and health in blacks and whites: The problem of residual confounding and the resiliency of race. *Epidemiology* **1997**, *8*, 621–628. [CrossRef] [PubMed]
37. Valencia, M.L.C.; Tran, B.T.; Lim, M.K.; Choi, K.S.; Oh, J.K. Association Between Socioeconomic Status and Early Initiation of Smoking, Alcohol Drinking, and Sexual Behavior Among Korean Adolescents. *Asia Pac. J. Public Health* **2019**, *31*, 443–453. [CrossRef]
38. Ahmad, A.; Zulaily, N.; Shahril, M.R.; Syed Abdullah, E.F.H.; Ahmed, A. Association between socioeconomic status and obesity among 12-year-old Malaysian adolescents. *PLoS ONE* **2018**, *13*, e0200577. [CrossRef]
39. Merz, E.C.; Tottenham, N.; Noble, K.G. Socioeconomic Status, Amygdala Volume, and Internalizing Symptoms in Children and Adolescents. *J. Clin. Child Adolesc. Psychol.* **2018**, *47*, 312–323. [CrossRef]
40. Dismukes, A.; Shirtcliff, E.; Jones, C.W.; Zeanah, C.; Theall, K.; Drury, S. The development of the cortisol response to dyadic stressors in Black and White infants. *Dev. Psychopathol.* **2018**, *30*, 1995–2008. [CrossRef]
41. Hanson, J.L.; Nacewicz, B.M.; Sutterer, M.J.; Cayo, A.A.; Schaefer, S.M.; Rudolph, K.D.; Shirtcliff, E.A.; Pollak, S.D.; Davidson, R.J. Behavioral problems after early life stress: Contributions of the hippocampus and amygdala. *Biol. Psychiatry* **2015**, *77*, 314–323. [CrossRef]
42. Miller, B.; Taylor, J. Racial and socioeconomic status differences in depressive symptoms among black and white youth: An examination of the mediating effects of family structure, stress and support. *J. Youth Adolesc.* **2012**, *41*, 426–437. [CrossRef] [PubMed]
43. DeSantis, A.S.; Adam, E.K.; Doane, L.D.; Mineka, S.; Zinbarg, R.E.; Craske, M.G. Racial/ethnic differences in cortisol diurnal rhythms in a community sample of adolescents. *J. Adolesc. Health* **2007**, *41*, 3–13. [CrossRef] [PubMed]
44. Alvarado, S.E. The impact of childhood neighborhood disadvantage on adult joblessness and income. *Soc. Sci. Res.* **2018**, *70*, 1–17. [CrossRef]
45. Barreto, S.M.; de Figueiredo, R.C.; Giatti, L. Socioeconomic inequalities in youth smoking in Brazil. *BMJ Open* **2013**, *3*, e003538. [CrossRef] [PubMed]
46. Schreier, H.M.; Chen, E. Socioeconomic status and the health of youth: A multilevel, multidomain approach to conceptualizing pathways. *Psychol. Bull.* **2013**, *139*, 606–654. [CrossRef] [PubMed]
47. Hemovich, V.; Lac, A.; Crano, W.D. Understanding early-onset drug and alcohol outcomes among youth: The role of family structure, social factors, and interpersonal perceptions of use. *Psychol. Health Med.* **2011**, *16*, 249–267. [CrossRef] [PubMed]
48. Bell, C.N.; Sacks, T.K.; Thomas Tobin, C.S.; Thorpe, R.J., Jr. Racial Non-equivalence of Socioeconomic Status and Self-rated Health among African Americans and Whites. *SSM Popul. Health* **2020**, *10*, 100561. [CrossRef]
49. Samuel, L.J.; Roth, D.L.; Schwartz, B.S.; Thorpe, R.J.; Glass, T.A. Socioeconomic Status, Race/Ethnicity, and Diurnal Cortisol Trajectories in Middle-Aged and Older Adults. *J. Gerontol. B Psychol. Sci. Soc. Sci.* **2018**, *73*, 468–476. [CrossRef]
50. Fuentes, M.; Hart-Johnson, T.; Green, C.R. The association among neighborhood socioeconomic status, race and chronic pain in black and white older adults. *J. Natl. Med. Assoc.* **2007**, *99*, 1160–1169.
51. Assari, S.; Khoshpouri, P.; Chalian, H. Combined Effects of Race and Socioeconomic Status on Cancer Beliefs, Cognitions, and Emotions. *Healthcare* **2019**, *7*, 17. [CrossRef]
52. Assari, S. Number of Chronic Medical Conditions Fully Mediates the Effects of Race on Mortality; 25-Year Follow-Up of a Nationally Representative Sample of Americans. *J. Racial Ethn. Health Disparities* **2017**, *4*, 623–631. [CrossRef] [PubMed]

53. Assari, S. Distal, intermediate, and proximal mediators of racial disparities in renal disease mortality in the United States. *J. Nephropathol.* **2016**, *5*, 51–59. [CrossRef] [PubMed]
54. Williams, D.R.; Costa, M.V.; Odunlami, A.O.; Mohammed, S.A. Moving upstream: How interventions that address the social determinants of health can improve health and reduce disparities. *J. Public Health Manag. Pract.* **2008**, *14*, S8–S17. [CrossRef]
55. Williams, D.R. Race, socioeconomic status, and health the added effects of racism and discrimination. *Ann. N. Y. Acad. Sci.* **1999**, *896*, 173–188. [CrossRef] [PubMed]
56. Assari, S. Health Disparities due to Diminished Return among Black Americans: Public Policy Solutions. *Soc. Issues Policy Rev.* **2018**, *12*, 112–145. [CrossRef]
57. Assari, S. Unequal Gain of Equal Resources across Racial Groups. *Int. J. Health Policy Manag.* **2018**, *7*, 1–9. [CrossRef]
58. Bleich, S.N.; Jarlenski, M.P.; Bell, C.N.; LaVeist, T.A. Health inequalities: Trends, progress, and policy. *Annu. Rev. Public Health* **2012**, *33*, 7–40. [CrossRef]
59. Homma, Y.; Saewyc, E.; Zumbo, B.D. Is it getting better? An analytical method to test trends in health disparities, with tobacco use among sexual minority vs. heterosexual youth as an example. *Int J. Equity Health* **2016**, *15*, 79. [CrossRef]
60. Lorant, V.; de Gelder, R.; Kapadia, D.; Borrell, C.; Kalediene, R.; Kovacs, K.; Leinsalu, M.; Martikainen, P.; Menvielle, G.; Regidor, E.; et al. Socioeconomic inequalities in suicide in Europe: The widening gap. *Br. J. Psychiatry* **2018**, *212*, 356–361. [CrossRef]
61. Mackenbach, J.P.; Bos, V.; Andersen, O.; Cardano, M.; Costa, G.; Harding, S.; Reid, A.; Hemstrom, O.; Valkonen, T.; Kunst, A.E. Widening socioeconomic inequalities in mortality in six Western European countries. *Int. J. Epidemiol.* **2003**, *32*, 830–837. [CrossRef]
62. Whitehead, M.M. Where do we stand? Research and policy issues concerning inequalities in health and in healthcare. *Acta Oncol.* **1999**, *38*, 41–50. [CrossRef] [PubMed]
63. Assari, S.; Caldwell, C.H.; Bazargan, M. Association Between Parental Educational Attainment and Youth Outcomes and Role of Race/Ethnicity. *JAMA Netw. Open* **2019**, *2*, e1916018. [CrossRef]
64. Assari, S.; Caldwell, C.H.; Mincy, R. Family Socioeconomic Status at Birth and Youth Impulsivity at Age 15; Blacks' Diminished Return. *Children* **2018**, *5*, 58. [CrossRef] [PubMed]
65. Assari, S.; Thomas, A.; Caldwell, C.H.; Mincy, R.B. Blacks' Diminished Health Return of Family Structure and Socioeconomic Status; 15 Years of Follow-up of a National Urban Sample of Youth. *J. Urban. Health* **2018**, *95*, 21–35. [CrossRef]
66. Assari, S.; Bazargan, M. Being Married Increases Life Expectancy of White but Not Black Americans. *J. Fam. Reprod Health* **2019**, *13*, 132–140. [CrossRef]
67. Assari, S.; Caldwell, C.H. High Risk of Depression in High-Income African American Boys. *J. Racial Ethn. Health Disparities* **2018**, *5*, 808–819. [CrossRef]
68. Assari, S.; Caldwell, C.H.; Mincy, R.B. Maternal Educational Attainment at Birth Promotes Future Self-Rated Health of White but Not Black Youth: A 15-Year Cohort of a National Sample. *J. Clin. Med.* **2018**, *7*, 93. [CrossRef] [PubMed]
69. Assari, S.; Caldwell, C.H.; Zimmerman, M.A. Family Structure and Subsequent Anxiety Symptoms; Minorities' Diminished Return. *Brain Sci.* **2018**, *8*, 97. [CrossRef]
70. Assari, S. Parental Educational Attainment and Academic Performance of American College Students; Blacks' Diminished Returns. *J. Health Econ. Dev.* **2019**, *1*, 21–31.
71. Assari, S.; Caldwell, C.H. Parental Educational Attainment Differentially Boosts School Performance of American Adolescents: Minorities' Diminished Returns. *J. Fam. Reprod Health* **2019**, *13*, 7–13. [CrossRef]
72. Assari, S.; Caldwell, C.H. Family Income at Birth and Risk of Attention Deficit Hyperactivity Disorder at Age 15: Racial Differences. *Children* **2019**, *6*, 10. [CrossRef] [PubMed]
73. Assari, S.; Boyce, S.; Bazargan, M.; Mincy, R.; Caldwell, C.H. Unequal Protective Effects of Parental Educational Attainment on the Body Mass Index of Black and White Youth. *Int. J. Environ. Res. Public Health* **2019**, *16*, 3641. [CrossRef] [PubMed]
74. Assari, S.; Farokhnia, M.; Mistry, R. Education Attainment and Alcohol Binge Drinking: Diminished Returns of Hispanics in Los Angeles. *Behav. Sci.* **2019**, *9*, 9. [CrossRef] [PubMed]
75. Assari, S. Parental Education Attainment and Educational Upward Mobility; Role of Race and Gender. *Behav. Sci.* **2018**, *8*, 107. [CrossRef] [PubMed]

76. Assari, S. Parental Educational Attainment and Mental Well-Being of College Students; Diminished Returns of Blacks. *Brain Sci.* **2018**, *8*, 193. [CrossRef]
77. Assari, S. Parental Education Better Helps White than Black Families Escape Poverty: National Survey of Children's Health. *Economies* **2018**, *6*, 30. [CrossRef]
78. Assari, S. Blacks' Diminished Return of Education Attainment on Subjective Health; Mediating Effect of Income. *Brain Sci.* **2018**, *8*, 176. [CrossRef]
79. Assari, S.; Hani, N. Household Income and Children's Unmet Dental Care Need; Blacks' Diminished Return. *Dent. J.* **2018**, *6*, 17. [CrossRef]
80. Assari, S.; Boyce, S.; Bazargan, M.; Caldwell, C.H. Diminished Returns of Parental Education in Terms of Youth School Performance: Ruling Out Regression Toward the Mean. *Children* **2020**, in press.
81. Alcohol Research: Current Reviews Editorial. NIH's Adolescent Brain Cognitive Development (ABCD) Study. *Alcohol. Res.* **2018**, *39*, 97.
82. Casey, B.J.; Cannonier, T.; Conley, M.I.; Cohen, A.O.; Barch, D.M.; Heitzeg, M.M.; Soules, M.E.; Teslovich, T.; Dellarco, D.V.; Garavan, H.; et al. The Adolescent Brain Cognitive Development (ABCD) study: Imaging acquisition across 21 sites. *Dev. Cogn. Neurosci.* **2018**, *32*, 43–54. [CrossRef] [PubMed]
83. Karcher, N.R.; O'Brien, K.J.; Kandala, S.; Barch, D.M. Resting-State Functional Connectivity and Psychotic-like Experiences in Childhood: Results From the Adolescent Brain Cognitive Development Study. *Biol. Psychiatry* **2019**, *86*, 7–15. [CrossRef] [PubMed]
84. Lisdahl, K.M.; Sher, K.J.; Conway, K.P.; Gonzalez, R.; Feldstein Ewing, S.W.; Nixon, S.J.; Tapert, S.; Bartsch, H.; Goldstein, R.Z.; Heitzeg, M. Adolescent brain cognitive development (ABCD) study: Overview of substance use assessment methods. *Dev. Cogn. Neurosci.* **2018**, *32*, 80–96. [CrossRef] [PubMed]
85. Luciana, M.; Bjork, J.M.; Nagel, B.J.; Barch, D.M.; Gonzalez, R.; Nixon, S.J.; Banich, M.T. Adolescent neurocognitive development and impacts of substance use: Overview of the adolescent brain cognitive development (ABCD) baseline neurocognition battery. *Dev. Cogn. Neurosci.* **2018**, *32*, 67–79. [CrossRef] [PubMed]
86. Auchter, A.M.; Hernandez Mejia, M.; Heyser, C.J.; Shilling, P.D.; Jernigan, T.L.; Brown, S.A.; Tapert, S.F.; Dowling, G.J. A description of the ABCD organizational structure and communication framework. *Dev. Cogn. Neurosci.* **2018**, *32*, 8–15. [CrossRef]
87. Garavan, H.; Bartsch, H.; Conway, K.; Decastro, A.; Goldstein, R.Z.; Heeringa, S.; Jernigan, T.; Potter, A.; Thompson, W.; Zahs, D. Recruiting the ABCD sample: Design considerations and procedures. *Dev. Cogn. Neurosci.* **2018**, *32*, 16–22. [CrossRef]
88. Jaeger, D.A. Reconciling the old and new census bureau education questions: Recommendations for researchers. *J. Bus. Econ. Stat.* **1997**, *15*, 300–309.
89. Assari, S. Parental Education on Youth Inhibitory Control in the Adolescent Brain Cognitive Development (ABCD) Study: Blacks' Diminished Returns. *Brain Sci.* **2020**, *10*, 312. [CrossRef] [PubMed]
90. Assari, S.; Boyce, S.; Caldwell, C.H.; Bazargan, M. Minorities' Diminished Returns of Parental Educational Attainment on Adolescents' Social, Emotional, and Behavioral Problems. *Children* **2020**, *7*, 49. [CrossRef]
91. Assari, S. Education Attainment and Obesity Differential Returns Based on Sexual Orientation. *Behav. Sci.* **2019**, *9*, 16. [CrossRef]
92. Assari, S. Family Income Reduces Risk of Obesity for White but Not Black Children. *Children* **2018**, *5*, 73. [CrossRef] [PubMed]
93. Assari, S. Life Expectancy Gain Due to Employment Status Depends on Race, Gender, Education, and Their Intersections. *J. Racial Ethn. Health Disparities* **2018**, *5*, 375–386. [CrossRef] [PubMed]
94. Assari, S.; Lankarani, M.M. Education and Alcohol Consumption among Older Americans; Black-White Differences. *Front. Public Health* **2016**, *4*, 67. [CrossRef]
95. Shervin, A.; Ritesh, M. Diminished Return of Employment on Ever Smoking Among Hispanic Whites in Los Angeles. *Health Equity* **2019**, *3*, 138–144. [CrossRef]
96. Assari, S. Socioeconomic Determinants of Systolic Blood Pressure; Minorities' Diminished Returns. *J. Health Econ. Dev.* **2019**, *1*, 1. [PubMed]
97. Assari, S. Socioeconomic Status and Self-Rated Oral Health; Diminished Return among Hispanic Whites. *Dent. J.* **2018**, *6*, 11. [CrossRef]
98. Assari, S.; Boyce, S.; Bazargan, M.; Caldwell, C.H. Mathematical Performance of American Youth: Diminished Returns of Educational Attainment of Asian-American Parents. *Educ. Sci.* **2020**, *10*, 32. [CrossRef]

99. Assari, S.; Bazargan, M. Protective Effects of Educational Attainment Against Cigarette Smoking; Diminished Returns of American Indians and Alaska Natives in the National Health Interview Survey. *Int. J. Travel Med. Glob. Health* **2019**, *7*, 105. [CrossRef]
100. Assari, S. Income and Mental Well-Being of Middle-Aged and Older Americans: Immigrants' Diminished Returns. *Int. J. Travel Med. Glob. Health* **2020**, *8*, 37–43. [CrossRef]
101. Assari, S.; Boyce, S.; Bazargan, M.; Caldwell, C.H.; Zimmerman, M.A. Place-Based Diminished Returns of Parental Educational Attainment on School Performance of Non-Hispanic White Youth. *Front. Educ.* **2020**, *5*. [CrossRef]
102. Bowden, M.; Bartkowski, J.; Xu, X.; Lewis, R., Jr. Parental occupation and the gender math gap: Examining the social reproduction of academic advantage among elementary and middle school students. *Soc. Sci.* **2017**, *7*, 6. [CrossRef]
103. Chetty, R.; Hendren, N.; Kline, P.; Saez, E. Where is the land of opportunity? The geography of intergenerational mobility in the United States. *Q. J. Econ.* **2014**, *129*, 1553–1623. [CrossRef]
104. Assari, S.; Gibbons, F.X.; Simons, R. Depression among Black Youth; Interaction of Class and Place. *Brain Sci.* **2018**, *8*, 108. [CrossRef] [PubMed]
105. Assari, S.; Gibbons, F.X.; Simons, R.L. Perceived Discrimination among Black Youth: An 18-Year Longitudinal Study. *Behav. Sci.* **2018**, *8*, 44. [CrossRef]
106. Assari, S. Does School Racial Composition Explain Why High Income Black Youth Perceive More Discrimination? A Gender Analysis. *Brain Sci.* **2018**, *8*, 140. [CrossRef]
107. Assari, S.; Lankarani, M.M.; Caldwell, C.H. Does Discrimination Explain High Risk of Depression among High-Income African American Men? *Behav. Sci.* **2018**, *8*, 40. [CrossRef]
108. Assari, S.; Moghani Lankarani, M. Workplace Racial Composition Explains High Perceived Discrimination of High Socioeconomic Status African American Men. *Brain Sci.* **2018**, *8*, 139. [CrossRef]
109. Assari, S.; Preiser, B.; Lankarani, M.M.; Caldwell, C.H. Subjective Socioeconomic Status Moderates the Association between Discrimination and Depression in African American Youth. *Brain Sci.* **2018**, *8*, 71. [CrossRef]
110. Assari, S.; Caldwell, C.H. Social Determinants of Perceived Discrimination among Black Youth: Intersection of Ethnicity and Gender. *Children* **2018**, *5*, 24. [CrossRef]
111. Assari, S.; Boyce, S.; Bazargan, M.; Caldwell, C.H. African Americans' Diminished Returns of Parental Education on Adolescents' Depression and Suicide in the Adolescent Brain Cognitive Development (ABCD) Study. *Eur. J. Investig. Health Psychol. Educ.* **2020**, *10*, 48. [CrossRef]
112. Jefferson, A.L.; Gibbons, L.E.; Rentz, D.M.; Carvalho, J.O.; Manly, J.; Bennett, D.A.; Jones, R.N. A life course model of cognitive activities, socioeconomic status, education, reading ability, and cognition. *J. Am. Geriatr. Soc.* **2011**, *59*, 1403–1411. [CrossRef] [PubMed]
113. Assari, S.; Nikahd, A.; Malekahmadi, M.R.; Lankarani, M.M.; Zamanian, H. Race by Gender Group Differences in the Protective Effects of Socioeconomic Factors Against Sustained Health Problems Across Five Domains. *J. Racial Ethn. Health Disparities* **2017**, *4*, 884–894. [CrossRef]
114. Hudson, D.L.; Bullard, K.M.; Neighbors, H.W.; Geronimus, A.T.; Yang, J.; Jackson, J.S. Are benefits conferred with greater socioeconomic position undermined by racial discrimination among African American men? *J. Mens. Health* **2012**, *9*, 127–136. [CrossRef] [PubMed]
115. Hudson, D.L.; Neighbors, H.W.; Geronimus, A.T.; Jackson, J.S. The relationship between socioeconomic position and depression among a US nationally representative sample of African Americans. *Soc. Psychiatry Psychiatr. Epidemiol.* **2012**, *47*, 373–381. [CrossRef] [PubMed]
116. Hudson, D.; Sacks, T.; Irani, K.; Asher, A. The Price of the Ticket: Health Costs of Upward Mobility among African Americans. *Int. J. Environ. Res. Public Health* **2020**, *17*, 1179. [CrossRef]
117. Bartik, T.J.; Hershbein, B. *Degrees of Poverty: The Relationship between Family Income Background and the Returns to Education*; WE Upjohn Institute for Employment Research: Kalamazoo, MI, USA, 2018.
118. Assari, S.; Preiser, B.; Kelly, M. Education and Income Predict Future Emotional Well-Being of Whites but Not Blacks: A Ten-Year Cohort. *Brain Sci.* **2018**, *8*, 122. [CrossRef]
119. Assari, S.; Bazargan, M. Second-hand exposure home Second-Hand Smoke Exposure at Home in the United States; Minorities' Diminished Returns. *Int. J. Travel Med. Glob. Health* **2019**, *7*, 135. [CrossRef]

120. Assari, S.; Bazargan, M. Unequal Effects of Educational Attainment on Workplace Exposure to Second-Hand Smoke by Race and Ethnicity; Minorities' Diminished Returns in the National Health Interview Survey (NHIS). *J. Med. Res. Innov.* **2019**, *3*, e000179. [CrossRef]
121. Assari, S. Family Socioeconomic Status and Exposure to Childhood Trauma: Racial Differences. *Children* **2020**, *7*, 57. [CrossRef]
122. Race Assari, S. Intergenerational Social Mobility and Stressful Life Events. *Behav. Sci.* **2018**, *8*, 86. [CrossRef]
123. Assari, S.; Bazargan, M. Unequal Associations between Educational Attainment and Occupational Stress across Racial and Ethnic Groups. *Int. J. Environ. Res. Public Health* **2019**, *16*, 3539. [CrossRef] [PubMed]
124. Navarro, V. Race or class or race and class: Growing mortality differentials in the United States. *Int. J. Health Serv.* **1991**, *21*, 229–235. [CrossRef] [PubMed]
125. Navarro, V. Race or class versus race and class: Mortality differentials in the United States. *Lancet* **1990**, *336*, 1238–1240. [CrossRef]
126. Navarro, V. Race or class, or race and class. *Int. J. Health Serv.* **1989**, *19*, 311–314. [CrossRef]
127. Bajaj, S.; Killgore, W.D.S. Sex differences in limbic network and risk-taking propensity in healthy individuals. *J. Neurosci. Res.* **2020**, *98*, 371–383. [CrossRef]
128. Bjork, J.M.; Straub, L.K.; Provost, R.G.; Neale, M.C. The ABCD study of neurodevelopment: Identifying neurocircuit targets for prevention and treatment of adolescent substance abuse. *Curr. Treat. Options Psychiatry* **2017**, *4*, 196–209. [CrossRef]
129. Chowdhury, T.G.; Wallin-Miller, K.G.; Rear, A.A.; Park, J.; Diaz, V.; Simon, N.W.; Moghaddam, B. Sex differences in reward- and punishment-guided actions. *Cogn. Affect. Behav. Neurosci.* **2019**, *19*, 1404–1417. [CrossRef]
130. Navas, J.F.; Martin-Perez, C.; Petrova, D.; Verdejo-Garcia, A.; Cano, M.; Sagripanti-Mazuquin, O.; Perandres-Gomez, A.; Lopez-Martin, A.; Cordovilla-Guardia, S.; Megias, A.; et al. Sex differences in the association between impulsivity and driving under the influence of alcohol in young adults: The specific role of sensation seeking. *Accid. Anal. Prev.* **2019**, *124*, 174–179. [CrossRef]
131. Silveri, M.M.; Rohan, M.L.; Pimentel, P.J.; Gruber, S.A.; Rosso, I.M.; Yurgelun-Todd, D.A. Sex differences in the relationship between white matter microstructure and impulsivity in adolescents. *Magn. Reson. Imaging* **2006**, *24*, 833–841. [CrossRef]
132. Barrett, S.T.; Thompson, B.M.; Emory, J.R.; Larsen, C.E.; Pittenger, S.T.; Harris, E.N.; Bevins, R.A. Sex Differences in the Reward-Enhancing Effects of Nicotine on Ethanol Reinforcement: A Reinforcer Demand Analysis. *Nicotine Tob. Res.* **2020**, *22*, 238–247. [CrossRef]
133. Hammerslag, L.R.; Gulley, J.M. Age and sex differences in reward behavior in adolescent and adult rats. *Dev. Psychobiol.* **2014**, *56*, 611–621. [CrossRef] [PubMed]
134. Harden, K.P.; Mann, F.D.; Grotzinger, A.D.; Patterson, M.W.; Steinberg, L.; Tackett, J.L.; Tucker-Drob, E.M. Developmental differences in reward sensitivity and sensation seeking in adolescence: Testing sex-specific associations with gonadal hormones and pubertal development. *J. Pers. Soc. Psychol.* **2018**, *115*, 161–178. [CrossRef] [PubMed]
135. Richard, J.M. Female Rodents Yield New Insights into Compulsive Alcohol Use and the Impact of Dependence: Commentary on Xie et al., 2019, "Sex Differences in Ethanol Reward Seeking Under Conflict in Mice". *Alcohol. Clin. Exp. Res.* **2019**, *43*, 1648–1650. [CrossRef] [PubMed]
136. Wallin-Miller, K.G.; Chesley, J.; Castrillon, J.; Wood, R.I. Sex differences and hormonal modulation of ethanol-enhanced risk taking in rats. *Drug Alcohol. Depend.* **2017**, *174*, 137–144. [CrossRef] [PubMed]
137. Wang, J.; Fan, Y.; Dong, Y.; Ma, M.; Ma, Y.; Dong, Y.; Niu, Y.; Jiang, Y.; Wang, H.; Wang, Z.; et al. Alterations in Brain Structure and Functional Connectivity in Alcohol Dependent Patients and Possible Association with Impulsivity. *PLoS ONE* **2016**, *11*, e0161956. [CrossRef]
138. Westbrook, S.R.; Hankosky, E.R.; Dwyer, M.R.; Gulley, J.M. Age and sex differences in behavioral flexibility, sensitivity to reward value, and risky decision-making. *Behav. Neurosci.* **2018**, *132*, 75–87. [CrossRef]
139. Xie, Q.; Buck, L.A.; Bryant, K.G.; Barker, J.M. Sex Differences in Ethanol Reward Seeking Under Conflict in Mice. *Alcohol. Clin. Exp. Res.* **2019**, *43*, 1556–1566. [CrossRef]
140. Davis, B.A.; Clinton, S.M.; Akil, H.; Becker, J.B. The effects of novelty-seeking phenotypes and sex differences on acquisition of cocaine self-administration in selectively bred High-Responder and Low-Responder rats. *Pharmacol. Biochem. Behav.* **2008**, *90*, 331–338. [CrossRef]

141. Palanza, P.; Morley-Fletcher, S.; Laviola, G. Novelty seeking in periadolescent mice: Sex differences and influence of intrauterine position. *Physiol Behav* **2001**, *72*, 255–262. [CrossRef]
142. Pitychoutis, P.M.; Pallis, E.G.; Mikail, H.G.; Papadopoulou-Daifoti, Z. Individual differences in novelty-seeking predict differential responses to chronic antidepressant treatment through sex- and phenotype-dependent neurochemical signatures. *Behav. Brain Res.* **2011**, *223*, 154–168. [CrossRef]
143. Ray, J.; Hansen, S. Temperament in the rat: Sex differences and hormonal influences on harm avoidance and novelty seeking. *Behav. Neurosci.* **2004**, *118*, 488–497. [CrossRef] [PubMed]
144. Cobey, K.D.; Stulp, G.; Laan, F.; Buunk, A.P.; Pollet, T.V. Sex differences in risk taking behavior among Dutch cyclists. *Evol. Psychol.* **2013**, *11*, 350–364. [CrossRef]
145. Cross, C.P.; Cyrenne, D.L.; Brown, G.R. Sex differences in sensation-seeking: A meta-analysis. *Sci. Rep.* **2013**, *3*, 2486. [CrossRef] [PubMed]
146. Killgore, W.D.; Grugle, N.L.; Killgore, D.B.; Balkin, T.J. Sex differences in self-reported risk-taking propensity on the Evaluation of Risks scale. *Psychol. Rep.* **2010**, *106*, 693–700. [CrossRef] [PubMed]
147. Listed, A.N. Three statistical paradoxes in the interpretation of group differences: Illustrated with medical school admission and licensing data. In *Handbook of Statistics*; Rao, C.R., Sinharay, S., Eds.; North-Holland: Amsterdam, The Netherlands, 2006; Volume 26, pp. 893–918.
148. Gmel, G.; Wicki, M.; Rehm, J.; Heeb, J.L. Estimating regression to the mean and true effects of an intervention in a four-wave panel study. *Addiction* **2008**, *103*, 32–41. [CrossRef] [PubMed]
149. Stout, R.L. Regression to the mean in addiction research. *Addiction* **2008**, *103*, 53. [CrossRef]
150. Novack, G.D.; Crockett, R.S. Regression to the mean. *Ocul. Surf.* **2009**, *7*, 163–165. [CrossRef]
151. Furrow, R.E. Regression to the Mean in Pre-Post Testing: Using Simulations and Permutations to Develop Null Expectations. *CBE Life Sci. Educ.* **2019**, *18*, le2. [CrossRef]
152. Moore, M.N.; Atkins, E.R.; Salam, A.; Callisaya, M.L.; Hare, J.L.; Marwick, T.H.; Nelson, M.R.; Wright, L.; Sharman, J.E.; Rodgers, A. Regression to the mean of repeated ambulatory blood pressure monitoring in five studies. *J. Hypertens* **2019**, *37*, 24–29. [CrossRef]

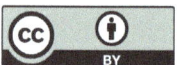

© 2020 by the authors. Licensee MDPI, Basel, Switzerland. This article is an open access article distributed under the terms and conditions of the Creative Commons Attribution (CC BY) license (http://creativecommons.org/licenses/by/4.0/).

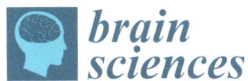

Article

Promoting the Social Inclusion of Children with ASD: A Family-Centred Intervention

Roy McConkey [1,*], Marie-Therese Cassin [2] and Rosie McNaughton [2]

1. Institute of Nursing and Health Research, Ulster University, Newtownabbey BT37 0QB, UK
2. Cedar Foundation, Belfast BT6 8RB, UK; mt.cassin@cedar-foundation.org (M.-T.C.); r.mcnaughton@cedar-foundation.org (R.M.)
* Correspondence: r.mcconkey@ulster.ac.uk; Tel.: +44-289-085-2537

Received: 23 April 2020; Accepted: 15 May 2020; Published: 25 May 2020

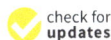

Abstract: The social isolation of children with autism spectrum disorder (ASD) is well documented. Their dearth of friends outside of the family and their lack of engagement in community activities places extra strains on the family. A project in Northern Ireland provided post-diagnostic support to nearly 100 families and children aged from 3 to 11 years. An experienced ASD practitioner visited the child and family at home fortnightly in the late afternoon into the evening over a 12-month period. Most children had difficulty in relating to other children, coping with change, awareness of dangers, and joining in community activities. Likewise, up to two-thirds of parents identified managing the child's behaviour, having time to spend with other children, and taking the child out of the house as further issues of concern to them. The project worker implemented a family-centred plan that introduced the child to various community activities in line with their learning targets and wishes. Quantitative and qualitative data showed improvements in the children's social and communication skills, their personal safety, and participation in community activities. Likewise, the practical and emotional support provided to parents boosted their confidence and reduced stress within the family. The opportunities for parents and siblings to join in fun activities with the child with ASD strengthened their relationships. This project underscores the need for, and the success of, family-based, post-diagnostic support to address the social isolation of children with ASD and their families.

Keywords: ASD; autism; families; social inclusion: home-based; Ireland

1. Introduction

Internationally, there has been a marked rise in the number of children diagnosed with an autism spectrum disorder (ASD) [1]. Early intervention is an agreed priority to ameliorate the main symptoms as soon as the condition is identified, especially in early childhood [2]. Even so, a national UK survey of more than 1000 parents found that nearly half (46%) received no follow-up appointment after the diagnosis was made and only 21% of parents received a direct offer of help/assistance. Additionally, more than 60% of parents expressed dissatisfaction with post-diagnostic support and only 5% were very satisfied with it [3].

A particular concern of parents is the lack of social and communication skills experienced by children with autism [4]. This often results in difficulties in interacting with their peers and isolation from community activities. Interventions aimed at promoting community participation have proved effective and a systematic review identified the factors that contributed to their success. This included facilitating "friendships alongside recreational participation, include typically developing peers, consider the activity preferences of children and adolescents in developing programmes, and accommodate individual impairments and needs through grading and adaptive leisure activities" [5] (p. 825).

Families are the primary caregivers of children with ASD. Tint & Weiss [6] in their scoping review noted that considerable research had detailed the correlates of the chronic physical, emotional, social, and financial stressors these families experience. They concluded that "a better understanding of family well-being of individuals with ASD is essential for effective policy and practice" (p. 262). A review of international research to date has identified promising strategies for supporting families [7] as well as targeting parental challenges such as stress, depression, and self-efficacy. "It may be especially constructive to provide wraparound services for families, in which resources and supports are provided (i.e., parent training, therapeutic services, respite care, social services, family counselling) in addition to developmental and behavioural services for the child" (p. 72).

Moreover, the impact on non-disabled siblings is worthy of attention given the increasing evidence that they fared worse in terms of psychological functioning, internalized behaviour problems, social functioning, and sibling relationships while also showing increased anxiety and depression [8].

A Canadian study into family quality of life (FQOL) who have a child with ASD found that opportunities to engage in leisure and recreation activities for the family as a whole was associated with an increased FQOL [9]. However, many families are not engaging in these activities on a regular basis. These researchers recommended that: "service providers could offer leisure and therapeutic recreation options to families, while they wait for other therapeutic services in order to provide additional options to families with a child with ASD." (p. 340).

Tint & Weiss [6] also identified the value of parents meeting other parents. Research studies indicate that socially isolated mothers may experience greater stress and have fewer socially satisfying interactions with their children. "Participating in group interventions may be beneficial for parents of children with ASD because it provides them with an opportunity to connect with other parents who are having similar experiences" (p. 94).

To date, most research studies have been undertaken with better educated, more affluent parents and little attention has been paid as to how 'under-resourced' families (those with low incomes and limited education) can be better supported when a child has ASD. A small-scale study in the USA found that "specific strategies to increase participant retention and decrease attrition included providing sessions in home, reducing travel requirements... and providing community resource support. One of the strengths was the presence of a strong referral system... and a team committed to helping patients access ASD-specific services" [10] (p. 94). More generally, a systematic review of home visiting programs for disadvantaged families concluded that: "home visitation by paraprofessionals is an intervention that holds promise for socially high-risk families with young children" [11] (p. 1).

The foregoing review provided the rationale for the family-centred, post-diagnostic support service to families and children aged 4 to 11 years with ASD in rural counties of Northern Ireland. The main focus was on promoting the social inclusion of the child and family within their local communities.

2. Materials and Methods

The project was conceived and delivered by the Cedar Foundation, which is a voluntary, non-profit organisation with a long history of delivering services to people with disabilities and their families. Charitable funding was obtained from the UK Big Lottery Fund for a five-year period.

A logic model was developed to guide the design and implementation of the service as well as its evaluation (see Figure 1). The model summarises the theory of change as to how the intervention would produce the intended outcomes in the short term and the possible longer-term consequences for the child and family [12].

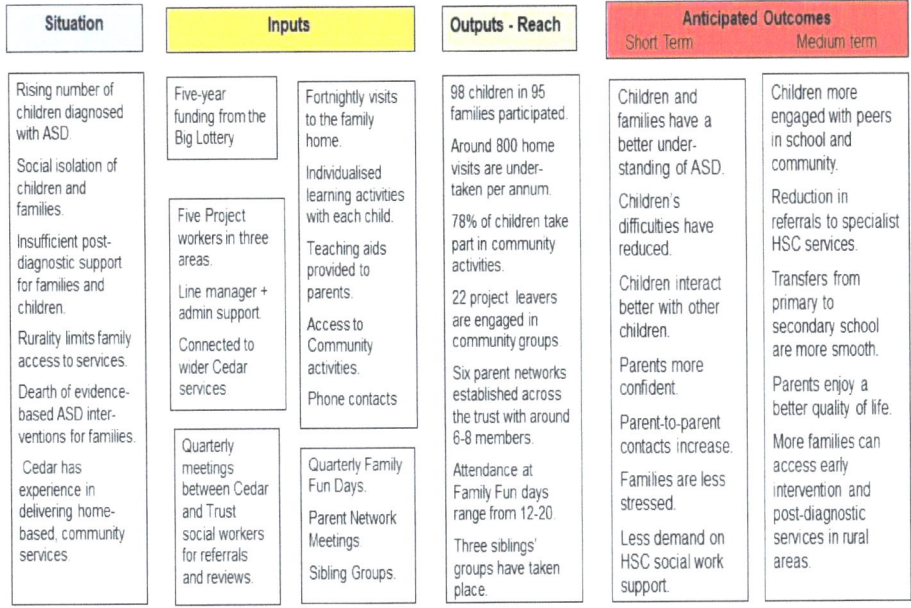

Figure 1. The logic model for the family-centred intervention.

2.1. Description of Inputs and Activities

Five project workers including one full-time and two part-time job shares each covered one of three counties in the western part of Northern Ireland, which is largely rural with a higher proportion of under-resourced families. All staff had a bachelor's degree in psychology plus a minimum of one year of paid experience. In addition to their qualifications and experience in autism, they received further training in ASD during the course of the project. Fortuitously, the appointed workers lived in the county in which they worked and were familiar with the community resources available there.

The project workers were line managed through Cedar's Community Services Manager who also managed Cedar's other projects in the western area. Links with these projects provided project workers with further support and training.

Each family received fortnightly visits for a 12-month period. However, all families were given opportunities to maintain contact with the project and to participate in all future group activities.

Quarterly meetings were held in each county between Cedar staff and the social workers from the children's ASD multi-disciplinary team of the statutory Health and Social Care Trust who undertake assessment and diagnosis of ASD. Potential referrals of families to the project were discussed with the social workers and the ongoing case load of families and children reviewed. An extension of time on the project was agreed for those families who had continuing needs. Similarly, families deemed to have higher needs were given priority when a place became available on the project.

A project worker visited the child and family at home in the late afternoon into the evening once every two weeks on average. The first visits were used to assess the child and family needs and agree on an individual plan for meeting those needs. The project worker devised and implemented learning activities to address the children's needs. These occurred within the family home or on outings to community locations and activities. The aim was to embed the learning in real-life settings, which schools are often unable to do.

Project staff made learning aids, such as visual schedules or story books. These resources were left for the families to use.

The visits also provided opportunities to advise and guide the families on managing the child's behaviour as well as furthering their learning. As the relationship with the project worker developed, families became more open about further issues and worries they had. As well as providing emotional support, the workers signposted families to other services in their locality.

The home visits were at a time when the project workers met other family members such as siblings and fathers. If appropriate, siblings were also invited to join in the activities the project worker undertook with the child, with the goal of enhancing the child's inclusion in family activities.

The project worker introduced the child to community activities in line with their learning targets and wishes. These provided opportunities to teach road safety or social interactions with other children as well as introducing the child to leisure activities such as swimming, horse-riding, football, and youth clubs.

Project workers also made contact with schools if required but especially for children with ASD who were soon to transfer from primary to secondary school. This gave opportunities for devising common approaches across home and school settings. These visits have led to increased contact between the schools and families.

Family Fun days were organized in each county four times a year and families were invited to attend. Siblings were especially welcome along with the fathers and mothers. They were held in community locations such as leisure centres or soft-play facilities with a range of activities organized to provide social interactions among the children and among the parents. The intention was also to introduce families to locations to which they could take their children in the future.

Parent Networking meetings were organized in two counties since there was less interest in a third county where parents already had access to other parent groups. An invited speaker talked on a topic of interest or else 'pampering sessions' for mothers took place.

Sibling groups were also provided in one county as a trial that brought together the brothers and sisters for play activities, but they also provided opportunities for them to learn more about autism and how they could respond to their sibling's behaviours.

2.2. The Characteristics of Families and Children Involved with the Project

In all, 92 families with 96 children with ASD were involved with the project over a four-year period.

One quarter of families (25%) had a lone parent, which is higher than the Northern Ireland average of 18%. More than two-thirds had a wage earner in the family but more than one-quarter were dependent on social security benefits. This is also higher than the average for Northern Ireland, which is 16.1%. Around half of the families (51%) lived in the top 30% of socially deprived areas in Northern Ireland with very few families coming from more affluent areas. Thus, the project had recruited and retained under-resourced families, which was its intention.

Of the 96 children, 76 (79.2%) were male and 20 (20.8%) were female. The median age when they joined the project was 7.7 years (range of 3.4 to 11.8 years).

A small proportion of the children were enrolled in a special school or special unit attached to a mainstream school (14.5%) but most attended their local primary school (85.5%). However, 79 children (82.3%) had a statement of special educational needs and others were in the process of being assessed for such. Seven children (7.3%) had an additional learning difficulty. This group were enrolled at the start of the project but, in later years, children with a learning disability and autism were not referred to the project.

More than one-third of the children (35.5%) were an only child. Three families had two children with ASD who also participated in the project.

Further details of the difficulties experienced by the children with ASD are given below.

2.3. Evaluation of Project Outcomes

The first author was the external evaluator and a mix of qualitative and quantitative descriptive data was collected. The qualitative data was obtained through face-to-face interviews conducted with all the project staff and their managers (seven in all) and the three social workers who referred families to the project. Seven parents were interviewed at one of two family events. In addition, telephone interviews were conducted with 10 parents chosen by project staff to represent the range of children and families involved in the project across the three counties. Self-completion questionnaires requesting their views on the project and perceived outcomes were completed by a further 15 families who responded to an invitation sent to all parents by project staff as a text message.

The quantitative data was obtained through two rating scales that were developed in association with the project staff with one relating to the child and another relating to the family (see Tables 1 and 2 in the results section). They provided a means for assessing each child's difficulties at the start of their involvement and the outcomes achieved as a result of their involvement. Similarly, family needs could be identified and outcomes could be assessed. The project staff completed both rating scales based on their records for all the families with whom they had been involved and the reviews they had undertaken with them during and at the end of the home visits.

Formal ethical approval was not required since this study was deemed an evaluation of an ongoing service and not a research project according to Guidance from the UK Health Research Authority. Families gave consent for the information they provided directly or indirectly to be used anonymously in any reports on the project internally and externally, such as to project funders.

The evaluation was completed at the end of December 2019.

Due to time and resource constraints, information was not obtained from the children about the project nor were any external assessments available of their developmental progress. Moreover, there was no comparable group of children and families who did not receive the service since this was not ethically feasible for Cedar Foundation to undertake.

3. Results

3.1. Children's Difficulties and Outcomes

The project staff who had been involved with the children and families helped to devise a summary tool for assessing each child's difficulties at the start of their involvement and the outcome achieved in relation to them. Table 1 lists the items and the ratings provided by the project worker across the 96 children, but some items were omitted for some individuals due to uncertainty or irrelevance for the child or family. Hence, the totals do not add to 96. The percentages are calculated on the number of ratings made.

The first column of Table 1 describes the issues that were of concern to families about their child with ASD at the start of their involvement with the project. The lower the percentage, the more children for whom the difficulty was identified. In all, eight of the sixteen listed difficulties were ones affecting the majority of families.

Difficulties in relating to other children affected all of the children in the project. The next most common cluster of difficulties related to awareness of dangers, difficulty with change, and joining in community activities with over seven in eight children affected by them. A cluster of emotional reactions was the next most common and this included anxiety, extreme fear and nervousness, anger, and meltdowns. In addition, more than 50% of children had problems with following instructions.

By contrast, some difficulties were identified by fewer than one in five children even though they include behaviours commonly associated with ASD such as an unusual response to something new, unusual interest in toys or objects, problems with play, and keeping themselves occupied.

Overall, the median number of issues identified as being a difficulty for the child was eight (range of 3 to 14).

Table 1. The number and percentage of children rated by staff on outcomes achieved.

Child Difficulties	Never Had a Problem	Was a Problem— Getting Better since Start of Project	Still a Problem at End of Project
Difficulty in relating to other children and in making friends	0 (0%)	68 (81.0%)	16 (19.0%)
Awareness of dangers, road safety	8 (9.6%)	58 (69.9%)	17 (20.5%)
Difficulty with change	10 (12.0%)	56 (67.5%)	17 (20.5%)
Joining in community activities	12 (14.3%)	59 (70.2%)	13 (15.5%)
Anxious, agitated, nervous	18 (22.8%)	53 (64.6%)	10 (12.7%)
Extreme fear and nervousness, lack of confidence, depressed	33 (39.3%)	45 (53.6%)	6 (7.1%)
Anger, temper tantrums, meltdowns	34 (40.5%)	40 (47.65%)	10 (11.9%)
Problem with following instructions	36 (42.9%)	38 (45.2%)	10 (11.9%)
Personal care (toileting, dressing)	50 (59.5%)	23 (27.4%)	11 (13.1%)
Difficulties in communication: speech and/or language	51 (62.2%)	21 (25.6%)	10 (12.2%)
Issues with school, homework, etc.	53 (63.1%)	25 (29.8%)	6 (7.1%)
Problem with bedtime, sleeping	58 (69.0%)	15 (17.9%)	11 (13.1%)
Unusual interest in toys or objects	66 (78.6%)	10 (11.9%)	8 (9.5%)
Problems with play, keeping self-occupied	67 (79.8%)	14 (16.7%)	3 (3.6%)
Eating	69 (82.1%)	5 (6.0%)	10 (11.9%)
Unusual response to something new	69 (83.1%)	13 (15.7%)	1 (1.2%)

3.2. Changes in the Children

Columns 2 and 3 in Table 1 indicate the outcomes from the help provided by the project. On all items, the difference in the ratings was significantly different from what would be expected by chance (Chi Square tests $p < 0.001$). Column 2 indicates difficulties that had improved since participating in the project and which were now considered less of a problem. The majority of children had improved on the six most commonly mentioned difficulties including relating to other children, awareness of dangers, coping with change, joining in community activities, and managing anxieties and fears. In all the median number of difficulties on which children were deemed to have improved was seven (range 1 to 13).

Column 3 indicates the difficulties that remained a problem even though project staff had addressed it and, as such, they represent a continuing need for children and families. The most common – albeit for only one in five children or less - were the top three items listed in Table 1, which include notable difficulty in relating to other children, in awareness of danger, and in managing change. Overall, most children had no difficulties that were a continuing problem, but others had up to 10 difficulties that continued.

3.3. Issues for Families and Outcomes

The issues that commonly face families who have a child with ASD were listed in a similar rating scale to that used for the child's difficulties. Table 2 lists the items and the ratings provided by the project worker.

The first column of Table 2 indicates the issues that were of concern to families at the start of their involvement with the project. The lower the percentage, the more families for whom the issue was identified. In all, nine of the 14 were issues that affected the majority of families. Having knowledge about the services and supports available was the most common and identified in 96% of families. Up to two-thirds of families identified managing the child's behaviour, having time to spend with other children, and taking the child out of the house as the main issues.

By contrast, three issues affected 20% of parents or less including family quality of life, main caregiver being anxious or depressed, and having people to turn to if a problem arose. Overall, families were presented with a median of seven different issues (range from 0 to 11 issues identified).

Table 2. The number and percentage of families rated by staff on outcomes achieved.

Issues Families Can Face	Issues that were NOT a Concern	Project Helped and No Longer an Issue	Project Gave Some Help but Still an Issue
Knowing what services and supports are available to parents and children	3 (3.5%)	70 (82.4%)	11 (12.9%)
Managing the child's behaviour, temper tantrums, and meltdowns	23 (27.7%)	38 (45.8%)	22 (26.5%)
Having time to spend with my other children	25 (29.1%)	50 (58.1%)	11 (12.8%)
Taking the child out of the house, joining in community activities	28 (32.6%)	40 (46.5%)	17 (19.8%)
Communicating with schools	36 (41.9%)	41 (47.7%)	9 (10.5%)
Relationships with siblings (or other children)	36 (42.9%)	32 (38.1%)	16 (19.0%)
Finding activities all the families can join in	37 (43.0%)	34 (39.5%)	15 (17.4%)
Worries about the child's future	41 (47.7%)	7 (8.1%)	37 (43.0%)
Lack of confidence in how to manage my child	46 (47.9%)	20 (23.8%)	18 (21.4%)
Meeting other parents and sharing experiences	44 (51.2%)	38 (44.2%)	4 (4.7%)
Understanding what it means to have Autism/ASD	51 (59.3%)	29 (33.7%)	6 (7.0%)
Family quality of life	65 (79.3%)	12 (14.6%)	5 (6.1%)
Main caregiver often feels anxious or depressed	70 (81.4%)	3 (3.5%)	13 (15.1%)
Main caregiver has people to turn to if s/he has a problem	74 (86.0%)	7 (8.1%)	5 (5.8%)

3.4. Outcomes for Families

Columns 2 and 3 of Table 2 indicate the outcomes from the help provided by the project. On all items, the difference in the ratings was significantly different from what would be expected by chance (Chi Square tests, $p < 0.001$). The second column indicates issues that were deemed to be no longer an issue for families. The two issues that a majority of families (50% and over) benefited from were: knowing the supports and services available and having time to spend with other children. In addition, more than two in five families also gained from communication with schools, the child going out of the house, meeting other parents, and finding activities that the whole family can join in. In all, families had a median of five issues resolved (range from 0 to 11).

3.5. Perceptions of Project Outcomes and Impact

The perceptions of three groups of stakeholders were sought regarding the outcomes of the project for the children and for the families as a whole: namely parents ($n = 16$), project staff ($n = 7$), and social workers who had referred children to the project ($n = 4$). This information was obtained mostly through one-to-one interviews, which were audio-recorded and transcribed and were supplemented by self-completed questionnaires. A thematic content analysis using the framework proposed by Braun & Clarke [13] was undertaken. The initial codes derived from the responses were grouped under two core themes: the impact on the child and the impact on families. Table 3 summarises the subthemes along with supporting quotations from parents that the other respondents confirmed. The person quoted is noted in brackets.

Table 3. The themes and subthemes reported as outcomes of the project by parents.

Main Themes	Subthemes	Supporting Quotes
Impact on the children	Social Interaction	N is an only child and his social skills were lacking. But whenever she would have taken him out and interacted him with other children as well, we could see a very big change in the social skills (Mother S).
	Improved behaviour	He was very frustrated, would have lashed out a lot, he would have cried and screamed a lot. So over time, she built up taking him out for like for a half an hour at one of the wee local centres ... where anybody could come in with their children. And he actually started interacting with the kids. (Mother TR)
	Acquisition of new skills	The project helped my child to understand a lot of topics including personal safety, peer pressure, and safe strangers (Mother TA)
Impact on families	New learning for parents	The project was a massive help to my son and our whole family, to help us understand his condition and work together as a family to help him. (Mother DH)
	Increased confidence	They give us the confidence to think that you're not doing a bad job ... you're doing your best. They were able to make people feel more confident in themselves that 'I can do this'. (Mother H).
	Free time	I have a little six-year-old too. It's very difficult for her when you have a little autistic child so, it gave me a bit of time with her. And she also went out too with the Cedar person at times, which also gave me a bit of time to do things about the house or go and do a bit of shopping and stuff like that. (Father).
	Meeting other parents	There was a family day and then a thing at Halloween and ... you're meeting other parents there as well with children who are similar, you know, so that's quite good so it is. (Mother JO).

All the stakeholders recounted various impacts that the project had on the children, which elaborated the changes noted in Table 1. Enhanced social interactions were a common outcome since the children learned to overcome their difficulties in interacting with their siblings and other children. Improvements in the children's behaviours were also noted with fewer meltdowns and less anger. The acquisition of new skills was confirmed especially those needed when accessing community facilities.

The stake-holders also confirmed the impact of the project on families. Parents had learned new ways of interacting with their child from the project workers. The changes they saw in their child boosted their confidence and this, coupled with the opportunity to have some free time to spend with their other children, resulted in them feeling less stressed. They also appreciated the opportunity to meet with other parents.

3.5.1. The Most Successful Aspects of the Project

Not surprisingly, the stake-holders identified different aspects of the project that they considered to be particularly successful. To some extent, this reflects the diversity of needs that families and children present and the flexibility of the project in meeting their needs. For most though, the one-to-one work with the children were the most frequently cited.

She had a great rapport with him, you know, she really met him at his level and he never said I don't want her coming, never, never did. She has a fantastic rapport with him.

(Mother JU)

Listening to families and addressing their concerns was seen as vital.

They were very good at consulting with the parents in what we wanted and what we needed and then they would have done their plans around that.

(Mother T)

The social aspects were also valued for both the child and the family.

They got a wee buddy system as well where he was going out with his friend, he met a wee friend a couple of days and the two of them went out together.

(Mother T.)

The most successful aspect of the project is seeing families come together and be able to participate in family activities which all family members can be included in.

(Project staff)

The trusted relationship between the project and the social workers who had referred families brought benefits to both.

There's brilliant relationships with us and Cedar... there's a two-way flow of communication. When a family is known to Cedar... that family does not need to contact us. They do not seem to need us. Their issues have been dealt with it. That really allows our social workers to deal with families with even more complex needs. It's been a real resource to us in that way: to staff as well as to the families.

(Trust staff 4)

3.5.2. Improvements for the Project

Parents would have liked the project to have continued for longer and for more family days to be provided. Reduced waiting times for a place on the project was also noted. Project staff would welcome more contact with schools so that the strategies used in school and at home could be shared and closer links nurtured between schools and parents.

4. Discussion

This project is unique in a number of respects and the lessons from it can inform the provision of post-diagnostic support services for families whose children have ASD.

The project focused on promoting the social inclusion of children within their families and the local community. These two settings —the family and the community—provided the context in which children's skills could be enhanced and practical support could be provided to families. Yet this approach stands in contrast with the focus on therapeutic approaches often used with children who have ASD [2]. Nevertheless, the focus on social inclusion brought about other specific gains to the child and to families as shown by the issues that were resolved during the project. Moreover, equipping children and families with the skills needed to function socially has potentially longer-term gains for the child as the Logic Model for the project identified (see Figure 1).

The project aimed to support families as well as the child especially 'low-resource' parents that the project had targeted. The most commonly expressed need was for information about available services and supports. This needs to be provided on an ongoing basis as parents' needs will change over time. Regular home-based contact with parents created a trusted and more intimate relationship between staff and parents, which clinic visits or occasional parent-teacher meetings would find hard to replicate. Two outcomes are worth underlining. Parents' self-confidence was boosted, which is a necessary prelude for them to instigate new ways of interacting with their child and trying new approaches. Additionally, many parents reported a reduction in stress within the family as they became more adept at managing the child's behaviour and meltdowns. Hence, interventions solely focused on the child will not necessarily bring about the practical and emotional supports that parents need [7].

The choice of home-based supports was not just for practical reasons. Although, in rural areas, it overcame the lack of transport options available to low resourced families in particular. Rather, having project staff coming to the child's home ensured that all the project work was personalised to the individual needs of the child and family [14]. Although children with ASD may share some common features, there were marked differences in how ASD was manifested in even this relatively homogenous sample of children. When the diversity found among families is added in, then the need for individualised interventions become ever more apparent. Admittedly, home visits are a more costly option than group-based parent training sessions. Yet, this is the only alternative presently offered to most parents in Northern Ireland and likely elsewhere. However, the uptake of group-based training is low especially for low resourced families and, to date, there is limited evidence as to the effectiveness of such training [15].

The project aimed to address the needs of siblings of the child with ASD who are often overlooked in ASD interventions. By contrast, parents are very aware of the impact the child with ASD has on their other children. Going to the family home meant that the staff could include the siblings in activities designed to help the child. The organisation of family days was another means of involving siblings in play and recreational activities. Both of the foregoing were arguably more successful that organising sessions for groups of unrelated siblings, which had been tried even though other studies have shown sibling support groups to be effective [16]. These may work better for teenage siblings whereas the siblings of the children in the project were mostly under 12 years of age. Nonetheless, the main message is that family interventions have to extend beyond parents to embrace siblings as well.

As with any innovative project, there are inevitably improvements that could be made to the service. Currently, the demand for it exceeds the places that can be available at any one time and, with increasing numbers of children being identified, this situation will worsen [17]. One option would be to reduce the length of time families are visited by the project or to increase the time between visits. Both options would allow more families to be accommodated for the same cost. Future research and evaluation could test out these options even though the solution is more likely for projects to become adept at adjusting their service to family needs and outcomes rather than having equivalent service inputs across all families.

The longer-term impact of the service also bears further study. There is evidence that early preschool intervention for children with developmental delays does result in longer term legacies [18], but this has yet to be determined for older children with ASD as well as for their families.

Evaluation methods could also be improved if the necessary resources were made available by the commissioners of new services. Pre-test and post-test measures of the children and parents would provide more robust evidence of change, as would the recruitment of a 'waiting list' control group to identify the improvements that might occur over a period of time even without any intervention.

5. Conclusions

In conclusion, post-diagnostic support for children with ASD and their families is vital. Providing cost-effective ways is a priority as is gathering evidence to show its impact. Staff trained in ASD but from non-clinical backgrounds, such as in this project, are an effective means of providing home-based community support to children and families.

Author Contributions: M.-T.C. and R.M. (Rosie McNaughton) designed the service, obtained funding for it, and provided managerial support and leadership throughout. R.M. (Roy McConkey) was commissioned by the Cedar Foundation to evaluate the project and he undertook the data analysis and initial drafts of the paper. All authors have read and agreed to the published version of the manuscript.

Funding: The UK Big Lottery and the evaluation by the Cedar Foundation funded the project.

Acknowledgments: Our thanks to the project staff, parents, and colleagues in the Western Health and Social Care Trust for their active participation.

Conflicts of Interest: R.M. (Roy McConkey) received a fee from the Cedar Foundation and M.-T.C. and R.M. (Rosie McNaughton) are employed by the Cedar Foundation. However, neither the project funders or the Cedar Foundation had any influence on the evaluation of the project and the reporting of the findings.

References

1. Elsabbagh, M.; Divan, G.; Koh, Y.-J.; Kim, Y.S.; Kauchali, S.; Marcin, C.; Montiel-Nava, C.; Patel, V.; Paula, C.S.; Wang, C.; et al. Global Prevalence of Autism and Other Pervasive Developmental Disorders. *Autism Res.* **2012**, *5*, 160–179. [CrossRef] [PubMed]
2. Vivanti, G.; Kasari, C.; Green, J.; Mandell, D.; Maye, M.; Hudry, K. Implementing and evaluating early intervention for children with autism: Where are the gaps and what should we do? *Autism Res.* **2017**, *11*, 16–23. [CrossRef] [PubMed]
3. Crane, L.; Chester, J.W.; Goddard, L.; Henry, L.; Hill, E. Experiences of autism diagnosis: A survey of over 1000 parents in the United Kingdom. *Autism* **2015**, *20*, 153–162. [CrossRef] [PubMed]
4. Lai, J.; Weiss, J.A. Priority service needs and receipt across the lifespan for individuals with autism spectrum disorder. *Autism Res.* **2017**, *10*, 1436–1447. [CrossRef] [PubMed]
5. Andrews, J.; Falkmer, M.; Girdler, S. Community participation interventions for children and adolescents with a neurodevelopmental intellectual disability: A systematic review. *Disabil. Rehabil.* **2014**, *37*, 825–833. [CrossRef] [PubMed]
6. Tint, A.; Weiss, J.A. Family wellbeing of individuals with autism spectrum disorder: A scoping review. *Autism* **2015**, *20*, 262–275. [CrossRef] [PubMed]
7. Frantz, R.; Hansen, S.; Machalicek, W. Interventions to Promote Well-Being in Parents of Children with Autism: A Systematic Review. *Rev. J. Autism Dev. Disord.* **2017**, *5*, 58–77. [CrossRef]
8. Shivers, C.; Jackson, J.B.; McGregor, C. Functioning Among Typically Developing Siblings of Individuals with Autism Spectrum Disorder: A Meta-Analysis. *Clin. Child Fam. Psychol. Rev.* **2018**, *22*, 172–196. [CrossRef]
9. Jones, S.; Bremer, E.; Lloyd, M. Autism spectrum disorder: Family quality of life while waiting for intervention services. *Qual. Life Res.* **2016**, *26*, 331–342. [CrossRef]
10. Carr, T.; Lord, C. A Pilot Study Promoting Participation of Families with Limited Resources in Early Autism Intervention. *Res. Autism Spectr. Disord.* **2016**, *2*, 87–96. [CrossRef] [PubMed]
11. Peacock, S.; Konrad, S.; Watson, E.; Nickel, D.; Muhajarine, N. Effectiveness of home visiting programs on child outcomes: A systematic review. *BMC Public Health* **2013**, *13*, 17. [CrossRef] [PubMed]
12. Public Health England. Introduction to Logic Models. 2018. Available online: https://www.gov.uk/government/publications/evaluation-in-health-and-well-being-overview/introduction-to-logic-models (accessed on 21 April 2020).
13. Braun, V.; Clarke, V. Using thematic analysis in psychology. *Qual. Res. Psychol.* **2006**, *3*, 77–101. [CrossRef]
14. Robinson, L.; Bond, C.; Oldfield, J. A UK and Ireland survey of educational psychologists' intervention practices for students with autism spectrum disorder. *Educ. Psychol. Pr.* **2017**, *34*, 58–72. [CrossRef]
15. O'Donovan, K.L.; Armitage, S.; Featherstone, J.; McQuillin, L.; Longley, S.; Pollard, N. Group-Based Parent Training Interventions for Parents of Children with Autism Spectrum Disorders: A Literature Review. *Rev. J. Autism Dev. Disord.* **2018**, *6*, 85–95. [CrossRef]
16. Jones, E.A.; Fiani, T.; Stewart, J.L.; Neil, N.; McHugh, S.; Fienup, D.M. Randomized controlled trial of a sibling support group: Mental health outcomes for siblings of children with autism. *Autism* **2020**. [CrossRef] [PubMed]
17. McConkey, R. The rise in the numbers of school pupils with autism: A comparison of the four countries in the United Kingdom. *Support Learn.* **2020**, in press.
18. Cidav, Z.; Munson, J.; Estes, A.M.; Dawson, G.; Rogers, S.; Mandell, D. Cost Offset Associated With Early Start Denver Model for Children With Autism. *J. Am. Acad. Child Adolesc. Psychiatry* **2017**, *56*, 777–783. [CrossRef] [PubMed]

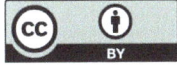

© 2020 by the authors. Licensee MDPI, Basel, Switzerland. This article is an open access article distributed under the terms and conditions of the Creative Commons Attribution (CC BY) license (http://creativecommons.org/licenses/by/4.0/).

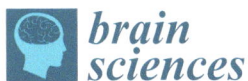

Article

Parental Education and Youth Inhibitory Control in the Adolescent Brain Cognitive Development (ABCD) Study: Blacks' Diminished Returns

Shervin Assari

Department of Family Medicine, Charles R Drew University of Medicine and Science,
Los Angeles, CA 90059, USA; assari@umich.edu; Tel.: +734-232-0445; Fax: +734-615-8739

Received: 18 April 2020; Accepted: 19 May 2020; Published: 21 May 2020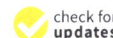

Abstract: Background: Non-Hispanic Black (NHB) youth are at a higher risk of high-risk behaviors compared to non-Hispanic White (NHW) youth. Some of this racial gap is shown to be due to weaker effects of parental educational attainment on reducing the prevalence of behavioral risk factors such as impulsivity, substance use, aggression, obesity, and poor school performance for NHBs, a pattern called Minorities' Diminished Returns. These diminishing returns may be due to lower than expected effects of parental education on inhibitory control. Aim: We compared NHW and NHB youth for the effect of parental educational attainment on youth inhibitory control, a psychological and cognitive construct that closely predicts high-risk behaviors such as the use of drugs, alcohol, and tobacco. Methods: This was a cross-sectional analysis that included 4188 youth from the Adolescent Brain Cognitive Development (ABCD) study. The independent variable was parental educational attainment. The main outcome was youth inhibitory control measured by the stop-signal task (SST), which was validated by parent reports on the Child Behavior Checklist (CBCL). Results: In race/ethnicity-stratified models, high parental educational attainment was associated with a higher level of inhibitory control for NHB than NHW youth. In the pooled sample, race/ethnicity showed a statistically significant interaction with parental educational attainment on youth inhibitory control suggesting that high parental educational attainment has a smaller boosting effect on inhibitory control for NHB than NHW youth. Conclusion: Parental educational attainment boosts inhibitory control for NHW but not NHB youth. To minimize the racial gap in youth brain development, we need to address societal barriers that diminish the returns of family economic and human resources, particularly parental educational attainment, for racial and ethnic minority youth. Social and public policies should address structural and societal barriers such as social stratification, segregation, racism, and discrimination that hinder NHB parents' abilities to effectively mobilize their human resources and secure tangible outcomes for their developing youth.

Keywords: race/ethnicity; ethnicity; socioeconomic status; youth; cognition; brain; inhibitory control

1. Introduction

Inhibitory control (IC), also known as response inhibition, is a cognitive process/executive function—that can be defined as an ability to inhibit impulses in order to increase the chance of appropriate behaviors that are consistent with completing long-term goals [1,2]. An extreme example of a disorder with impaired IC is attention deficit hyperactivity disorder (ADHD) [3]. Low IC is associated with a wide range of outcomes such as obesity, food choices, eating disorders, school performance, peer preferences, externalizing behaviors, aggression, prosocial behaviors, sexual debut, and use of drugs, alcohol, and tobacco [4–12]. Low IC may be one of the reasons why youth from low socioeconomic status (SES) and racial and ethnic minority groups engage in more risky behaviors, compared to high SES and majority youth [1,13–16]. Thus, studies are needed that investigate the additive effects of race/ethnicity and SES on youth IC as a mechanism of disparities and inequalities in high-risk behaviors [1,10,17–19].

Family SES and parental behaviors are shown to be predictors of IC in youth [20–24]. In a study on 147 7–10-year-old children, Cabello et al. investigated the relationship between parental educational attainment and youth IC as well as aggressive behavior. Teachers rated the aggressive behavior of the children using the Teacher Rating Scale (TRS) of the Behavior Assessment System for Children 2 (BASC-2). The youth themselves completed a go/no-go task that assessed their IC. Parents reported their educational attainment. Analysis of the data showed that both lower parental educational attainment and lower IC were predictive of higher aggressive behavior in the youth. Interestingly, authors found evidence suggesting that IC partially mediates the effects of parental educational attainment on aggressive behavior. However, sex moderated this mediation, as IC explained this effect for boys, not girls. Their study suggests the parental educational attainment impacts IC and IC may be why parental educational attainment is associated with youth aggressive behavior, particularly in boys [6].

Compared to non-Hispanic White (NHW) youth, non-Hispanic Black (NHB) youth are at an increased risk of high-risk behaviors that are largely associated with poor IC. For example, NHB youth are more likely than NHW youth to be at risk of engaging in aggressive behavior [25], early sexual debut [26], and becoming school dropouts [27]. As many of these early undesired outcomes are gateways to future economic and health problems later in life [28–31], it is important to study why and how IC is different in NHB and NHW youth. Such knowledge may be helpful in closing, or at least reducing, the existing racial and ethnic economic and health inequalities experienced later in life [28–31].

Given the close overlap between race/ethnicity and SES in the US, there has been an interest in trying to decompose the effects of race/ethnicity and SES on health and behavioral inequalities [32–34]. In theory, both low SES and racial/ethnic minority status generate marginalization and increase exposure to food and housing insecurity, economic adversities, stress, and financial difficulties [35–38]. Thus, one remaining question is whether race/ethnicity and SES have separate, additive, or multiplicative effects on health inequalities [39–42]. While SES provides access to buffers and protections, the SES effects on health and behaviors and their precursors [39–42] may depend on race/ethnicity. In addition, SES may carry the effect of race/ethnicity on health and behavioral outcomes [43].

There are, however, two complementary hypotheses that explain how race/ethnicity and family SES may jointly impact youth health and behavioral outcomes. The first hypothesis, a more traditional one, attributes the racial and ethnic gap in youth outcomes to racial and ethnic differences in family SES (e.g., lower SES in NHBs than NHWs) [43–46]. In this view, family SES is believed to mediate the effects of racial and ethnic minority status on youth outcomes [47–49]. As such, the belief is that enhancing racial and ethnic minorities' family SES and closing the racial and ethnic differences in SES would be the primary strategy for closing racial and ethnic youth inequalities [50,51]. Some policy solutions based on this view is income redistribution, income tax credit, and empowering racial and ethnic minorities to attain and accumulate education, income, and wealth.

The alternative explanation is Minorities' Diminished Returns (MDRs) [52,53], which explains that some of the racial and ethnic inequalities are due to the weaker effects of family SES indicators for NHBs than NHWs. This view is supported by extensive empirical evidence showing that parental education [54], family income [55,56], and marital status [57] generate more outcomes for NHW than NHB youth. However, this literature is mainly focused on self-reported outcomes [54–56,58,59]. For example, high family SES showed smaller preventive effects on impulsivity [55], ADHD [60], depression [58], anxiety [61], aggression [54], poor GPA [54,62,63], and substance use [54] for NHB than NHW youth. That means, while high SES NHW youth show the lowest levels of risk across domains, high SES NHB youth remain at high levels of risk across multiple domains and outcomes.

As shown by the MDRs literature, parental educational attainment [64–66] generates unequal outcomes for diverse racial and ethnic groups. This might be because society may differently allow NHB and NHW parents to mobilize their education and secure high paying jobs, particularly at high levels of education [53,55,61,65,67,68]. As a result of diminishing returns of parental education, compared to their non-HW counterparts, NHB youth with highly educated parents may show worse than expected outcomes that are disproportionate to their family SES [52,53,55,56,59].

2. Aims

To extend the existing knowledge on the role of IC as a mechanism for explaining MDRs for other behavioral outcomes, we studied the interactive and combined effects of race/ethnicity and parental educational attainment on youth outcomes. This study compared NHB and NHW youth for the effects of parental educational attainment, as one of the strongest family SES indicators, on youth IC. We expected weaker effects of parental educational attainment on youth IC for NHB than NHW youth.

3. Methods

3.1. Design and Settings

We performed a secondary analysis of data from the Adolescent Brain Cognitive Development (ABCD) study [69–73], a landmark youth brain development study in the United States. Detailed information on the details of the ABCD study is available elsewhere [69,74].

3.2. Participants and Sampling

Participants of the ABCD study were youth age 9–10 years. Youth in the ABCD study were recruited from multiple cities across states. Overall, there were 21 sites that recruited youth to the ABCD study. The recruitment of the ABCD sample was mainly done through school systems. A detailed description of the ABCD sampling is available here [75]. Four thousand one hundred eighty-eight participants entered our analysis. Eligibility for our analysis had valid data on race/ethnicity, CBCL, task-based IC, parental education, marital status, and being NHB or NHW

3.3. Study Variables

The study variables included race/ethnicity, demographic factors, parental educational attainment, parental marital status, and task-based IC (validated by the Child Behavior Checklist (CBCL)).

3.3.1. Outcome

The study also used the stop-signal task (SST) to measure IC. The SST applied two runs of 180 trials showing images of a black arrow pointing either right or left are displayed on the screen participants' view while in the scanner. They were instructed to click the appropriate button corresponding to the arrow direction as quickly as they can after seeing the image using their dominant hand. Thirty of the 180 trials display neither option, signaling the participant to inhibit answering with either option being randomly dispersed throughout the trials. Successful inhibition of motor response represents a successful trial, while impulsively answering with either wrong answer is considered unsuccessful inhibition. IC was measured as the rate of correct "Stop" trials in the run. This variable was treated as a continuous measure with a higher score indicating a higher level of IC [76–79].

3.3.2. Validation of the IC Using CBCL Domains

We used the Child Behavior Checklist (CBCL) to validate lab(task) based measures of IC. The CBCL, also known as the Achenbach System of Empirically Based Assessment, the study had the following eight outcomes: (1) Anxious and depressed mood, (2) withdrawn and depressed affect, (3) social and interpersonal problems, (4) somatic complaints, (5) thought problems, (6) attention problems, (7) violent and aggressive behaviors, and (8) rule-breaking behaviors [80]. These CBCL sub-scores closely correlate with the Diagnostic and Statistical Manual of Mental Disorders (DSM-IV-TR) based diagnoses [81]. The CBCL instrument uses parental reports to screen for social, behavioral, and emotional problems. The CBCL is commonly used across settings including but not limited to schools, medical settings, mental health facilities, child and family services, Health Management Organizations, and public health agencies [82]. CBCL has been used by thousands of published scholarly articles [82]. As expected, in our study, IC was correlated with behavioral rather than emotional domains of the CBCL, which was an indicator of its validity.

3.3.3. Moderator

Race/ethnicity. Race/ethnicity was self-identified. Race/ethnicity was a categorical variable and coded 1 for NHBs and 0 for NHWs (reference category).

3.3.4. Independent Variable

Parental Educational Attainment. Participants were asked, "What is the highest grade or level of school you have completed or the highest degree you have received?" Responses were 0 = Never attended/Kindergarten only; 1 = 1st grade; 2 = 2nd grade; 3 = 3rd grade; 4 = 4th grade 4; 5 = 5th grade; 6 = 6th grade 6; 7 = 7th grade 7; 8 = 8th grade; 9 = 9th grade; 10 = 10th grade 10; 11 = 11th grade; 12 = 12th grade; 13 = High school graduate; 14 = GED or equivalent Diploma; 15 = Some college; 16 = Associate degree: Occupational; 17 = Associate degree: Academic Program; 18 = Bachelor's degree (ex. BA; 19 = Master's degree (ex. MA; 20 = Professional School degree (ex. MD; 21 = Doctoral degree. This variable was an interval measure with a range between 1 and 21, with a higher score indicating higher educational attainment.

3.3.5. Confounders

Age, sex, and parental marital status were the confounders. Parents reported the age of their youth. Age (years) was calculated as the difference between the date of birth to the date of enrollment to the study. Sex was a dichotomous variable: males = 1, females = 0. Parental marital status was a dichotomous variable. This variable was self-reported by the parent who was interviewed. This variable was coded as married = 1 vs. other = 0.

3.4. Data Analysis

We used the statistical package SPSS to perform our data analysis. Mean (standard deviation (SD)) and frequency (%) were described depending on the variable type. We also performed a Pearson bivariate test to test bivariate associations between study variables. For our multivariable modeling, we performed four linear regression models. Our first two models were performed specifically to race/ethnicity (race-stratified models). *Model 1* was tested in NHW, and *Model 2* was tested in NHB youth. The next two models were performed in the overall sample. *Model 3* was performed without the interaction terms. *Model 4* added an interaction term between race/ethnicity and parental education attainment. Our models used age, sex, and marital status were the covariates. Unstandardized regression coefficient (b), standardized regression coefficient, SE, 95% CI, and *p*-value were reported for each model. *p* values equal to or less than 0.05 were statistically significant.

3.5. Ethical Aspect

The ABCD study received an Institutional Review Board (IRB) approval from the University of California, San Diego (UCSD). Each youth participant provided an assent. Each parent signed an informed consent [74]. As this analysis was performed on fully de-identified data, the study was found to be non-human subject research. Thus, our analysis was exempt from a full IRB review.

4. Results

4.1. Descriptives

As shown in Table 1, 4188, 8–11 years old youth entered to this analysis. From this number, most were NHWs (n = 2985; 71.3%) and the rest were NHBs (n = 1203; 28.7%). Table 1 presents a summary of the descriptive statistics for the pooled sample.

Table 1. Data overall and by race/ethnicity (n = 4188).

	All		NHWs		NHBs	
	n	%	n	%	n	%
Ethnicity						
NHWs	2985	71.3	2985	100.0	-	-
NHBs	1203	28.7	-	-	1203	100.0
Sex						
Male	2026	48.4	1426	47.8	600	49.9
Female	2162	51.6	1559	52.2	603	50.1
Marital Status *						
Other	1103	26.5	399	13.4	704	60.0
Married	3054	73.5	2584	86.6	470	40.0
	Mean	SD	Mean	SD	Mean	SD
Age (Year)	9.45	0.50	9.45	0.50	9.46	0.51
Parental Educational Attainment *	16.90	2.42	17.58	1.99	15.20	2.55
CBCL Anxiety Depressed *	2.62	3.15	2.74	3.19	2.31	3.05
CBCL Withdraw Depressed *	1.00	1.71	0.93	1.63	1.16	1.89
CBCL Somatic Complaints	1.48	1.91	1.51	1.89	1.42	1.98
CBCL Social Problems *	1.58	2.29	1.46	2.22	1.88	2.44
CBCL Thought Problems *	1.66	2.25	1.71	2.22	1.54	2.32
CBCL Rule Breaking *	1.25	1.94	1.07	1.69	1.70	2.40
CBCL Attention Problems *	5.39	5.40	5.24	5.24	5.75	5.77
CBCL Aggressive Behaviors *	3.44	4.58	3.27	4.32	3.85	5.15
14 SST-based IC	0.54	0.11	0.54	0.10	0.54	0.12

Child Behavior Checklist (CBCL); Inhibitory Control (IC); Non-Hispanic Black (NHB); non-Hispanic White (NHW); Stop-Signal Task (SST); Standard Deviation (SD); * $p < 0.05$.

Table 2 shows a correlation matrix of all study variables, including the CBCL reports in the pooled sample and by race/ethnicity. In the pooled sample, NHB status was closely associated with lower parental education and marital status but was not associated with IC. IC was associated with behavioral rather than emotional domains of CBCL measure, which indicated the validity of our IC measure. In the pooled sample, parental educational attainment was not correlated with IC. In NHWs (r = 0.06, $p < 0.05$), but not in NHBs (r = −0.04, $p > 0.05$), parental educational attainment was correlated with IC.

Table 2. Correlations between study variables ($n = 4188$).

	1	2	3	4	5	6	7	8	9	10	11	12	13	14
All														
1 Race (NHBs)	1	−0.02	0.01	−0.48 **	−0.45 **	−0.06 **	0.06 **	−0.02	0.08 **	−0.03 *	0.15 **	0.04 **	0.06 **	0.02
2 Sex (male)		1	0.03	0.01	−0.00	0.01	0.05 **	−0.04 *	0.05 **	0.09 **	0.11 **	0.15 **	0.10 **	−0.11 **
3 Age (Years)			1	−0.01	−0.02	0.01	.042 **	0.02	0.00	0.01	0.02	0.00	0.00	−0.03
4 Family Structure (married)				1	0.37 **	−0.02	−0.11 **	−0.05 **	−0.11 **	−0.03 *	−0.17 **	−0.10 **	−0.11 **	−0.02
5 Parental Educational Attainment (Years)					1	0.00	−0.11 **	−0.04 **	−0.13 **	−0.07 **	−0.18 **	−0.10 **	−0.11 **	0.01
6 Child Behavior Checklist (CBCL) Anxiety Depressed						1	0.57 **	0.48 **	0.61 **	0.60 **	0.40 **	0.56 **	0.56 **	−0.02
7 CBCL Withdraw Depressed							1	0.40 **	0.55 **	0.49 **	0.38 **	0.47 **	0.49 **	−0.01
8 CBCL Somatic Complaints								1	0.43 **	0.45 **	0.29 **	0.44 **	0.39 **	−0.03 *
9 CBCL Social Problems									1	0.61 **	0.56 **	0.70 **	0.68 **	−0.02
10 CBCL Thought Problems										1	0.52 **	0.73 **	0.64 **	−0.06 **
11 CBCL Rule Breaking											1	0.67 **	0.75 **	−0.04 **
12 CBCL Attention Problems												1	0.76 **	−0.05 **
13 CBCL Aggressive Behaviors													1	−0.04 **
14 IC														1
NHWs														
2 Sex (male)		1	0.03	−0.02	−0.03	0.01	0.06 **	−0.05 **	0.04 *	0.08 **	0.10 **	0.15 **	0.10 **	−0.13 **
3 Age (Years)			1	0.01	−0.03	0.03	0.05 **	0.03	−0.00	0.02	0.00	0.00	0.01	−0.06 **
4 Family Structure (married)				1	0.17 **	−0.07 **	−0.12 **	−0.09 **	−0.11 **	−0.07 **	−0.13 **	−0.11 **	−0.10 **	0.04 **
5 Parental Educational Attainment (Years)					1	−0.08 **	−0.12 **	−0.12 **	−0.16 **	−0.13 **	−0.18 **	−0.15 **	−0.14 **	0.06 **
6 CBCL Anxiety Depressed						1	0.57 **	0.47 **	0.59 **	0.57 **	0.39 **	0.53 **	0.55 **	−0.00
7 CBCL Withdraw Depressed							1	0.38 **	0.53 **	0.48 **	0.40 **	0.45 **	0.48 **	−0.03
8 CBCL Somatic Complaints								1	0.42 **	0.43 **	0.30 **	0.44 **	0.38 **	−0.03
9 CBCL Social Problems									1	0.60 **	0.56 **	0.68 **	0.67 **	−0.03
10 CBCL Thought Problems										1	0.51 **	0.72 **	0.61 **	−0.05 **
11 CBCL Rule Breaking											1	0.64 **	0.74 **	−0.04 *
12 CBCL Attention Problems												1	0.73 **	−0.04 *
13 CBCL Aggressive Behaviors													1	−0.03
14 IC														1

Table 2. *Cont.*

	1	2	3	4	5	6	7	8	9	10	11	12	13	14
NHBs														
2 Sex (male)	1													
3 Age (Years)		0.03	1											
4 Family Structure (married)			0.03	1										
			−0.01											
5 Parental Educational Attainment (Years)					0.02									
					0.02									
					0.26 **									
6 CBCL Anxiety Depressed						0.03								
						−0.01								
						−0.01								
						0.07 *								
7 CBCL Withdraw Depressed							0.02							
							0.03							
							−0.06 *							
							−0.05							
							0.59 **							
							1							
8 CBCL Somatic Complaints								−0.01						
								0.01						
								−0.02						
								0.07 *						
								0.51 **						
								0.44 **						
								1						
9 CBCL Social Problems									0.09 **					
									0.01					
									−0.05					
									−0.01					
									0.70 **					
									0.58 **					
									0.46 **					
									1					
10 CBCL Thought Problems										0.12 **				
										0.01				
										−0.03				
										−0.01				
										0.67 **				
										0.52 **				
										0.49 **				
										0.65 **				
										1				
11 CBCL Rule Breaking											0.14 **			
											0.04			
											−0.09 **			
											−0.07 *			
											0.48 **			
											0.34 **			
											0.31 **			
											0.58 **			
											0.57 **			
											1			
12 CBCL Attention Problems												0.17 **		
												−0.00		
												−0.05		
												0.01		
												0.64 **		
												0.51 **		
												0.45 **		
												0.72 **		
												0.75 **		
												0.72 **		
												1		
13 CBCL Aggressive Behaviors													0.12 **	
													−0.00	
													−0.08 **	
													−0.03	
													0.62 **	
													0.50 **	
													0.42 **	
													0.70 **	
													0.69 **	
													0.79 **	
													0.80 **	
													1	
14 IC														−0.06 *
														0.04
														−0.08 **
														−0.04
														−0.04
														0.01
														−0.04
														−0.01
														−0.07 *
														−0.05
														−0.07 *
														−0.04
														1

$p < 0.05$; ** $p < 0.01$.

4.2. Multivariate Analysis (Race-Stratified models)

Table 3 shows the results of two linear regression models in racial/ethnic groups. *Model 3* (NHW) showed protective effects of high parental educational attainment on IC of NHW youth. *Model 4* (NHB) did not have a protective effect of high parental educational attainment on IC for NHB youth.

Table 3. Summary of linear regressions by race/ethnicity ($n = 4183$).

	Model 1 NHWs			Model 2 NHBs		
	Beta	SE	p	Beta	SE	p
Sex (Male)	−0.13	−0.03	<0.001	−0.06	−0.01	0.047
Age	−0.06	−0.01	0.002	0.04	0.01	0.165
Married household	0.03	0.01	0.139	−0.08	−0.02	0.012
Parental Educational Attainment	0.05	0.00	0.003	−0.02	0.00	0.503
Constant		0.60	<0.001		0.48	<0.001

Unstandardized Regression Coefficient (B); Confidence Interval (CI); Standard Error (SE); Non-Hispanic Black (NHB); Outcome: Stop-Signal Task (SST)-based Inhibitory Control (IC).

4.3. Multivariate Analysis (Pooled Sample)

Table 4 shows the results of two linear regression models in the overall (pooled) sample. *Model 1* (Main Effect Model) showed an only marginally significant effect of high parental educational attainment on IC. *Model 2* (Interaction Model) showed a statistically significant interaction term between race/ethnicity and parental educational attainment on IC, suggesting that the boosting effect of high parental educational attainment on IC is significantly weaker for NHB youth relative to NHW youth.

Table 4. Summary of linear regressions overall ($n = 4183$).

	Model 1 Main Effects			Model 2 Interaction Effects		
	Beta	SE	p	Beta	SE	p
Race/Ethnicity (NHBs)	0.02	0.00	0.315	0.35	0.08	0.001
Sex (Male)	−0.11	−0.02	<0.001	−0.10	−0.02	<0.001
Age	−0.02	−0.01	0.118	−0.02	0.00	0.131
Married household	−0.02	0.00	0.300	−0.02	0.00	0.386
Parental Educational Attainment	0.03	0.00	0.097	0.07	0.00	0.001
Parental Educational Attainment × NHBs				−0.31	0.00	0.002
Constant		0.58	<0.001		0.54	<0.001

Unstandardized Regression Coefficient (B); Confidence Interval (CI); Standard Error (SE); Non-Hispanic Black (NHB); Outcome: Stop-Signal Task (SST)-based Inhibitory Control (IC).

5. Discussion

In our race-specific models, high parental educational attainment was associated with higher IC for NHW but not NHB youth. This finding was also supported by a statistical interaction between race/ethnicity and parental educational attainment on youth IC in the pooled sample. Thus, high parental educational attainment has smaller boosting effects on IC for NHB than NHW youth.

Here first, we discuss the observed MDRs. That is why NHB and NHW youth show a different gain in terms of increased IC due to an increase in parental educational attainment. In this section, we report similar literature and also some potential societal mechanisms that may help us understand these MDRs. Then we discuss the results specific to the IC. That is, SES (parental education) boosts IC and, at the same time, race (NHB) may reduce IC. However, the association between race and IC could only be observed for parental reports rather than the lab-based measure of IC. In the end, we list the limitations and strengths of our study. Among the strengths, we discuss why there were different methods of measuring IC (based on the IC neurocognitive task and parent's behavioral ratings).

The observed diminished returns of parental education on IC is in line with the MDRs reported on impulsivity [55], ADHD [60], depression [58], anxiety [61], aggression [54], GPA [54,62,63], and substance use [54]. A large body empirical evidence supports diminishing returns of parental and own educational attainment for NHBs than NHWs [67,83–85]. MDRs are already documented both within individuals and families, and hold across SES resources, age groups, outcomes, and marginalizing identities [52,53]. MDRs are shown for income [55], education [84], employment [86], and marital status [61]. Parental educational attainment results in more gain for NHW than NHB youth [55,56,59], adults [67], and older adults [87]. Also, MDRs not only apply to NHBs [56], or HWs [84,88–90] but also for Asian Americans [91], Native Americans [92], and LGBTQ persons [83].

Various mechanisms may be involved in explaining the MDRs of parental educational attainment or NHB families. NHB families face disproportionately higher levels of financial, environmental, and race-related stress in their daily lives, at all SES levels. According to the social reproduction theory, intergenerational educational outcomes may vary across groups [93]. Chetty showed that the intersection of race/ethnicity and sex alter the likelihood of upward social mobility in the US [94]. Increased exposure to stress is believed to reduce youths' ability to gain from their available SES resources such as education. It is shown that for NHB families, an increase in SES means an increase in experience [95–99] and vulnerability [100] to discrimination. This might be because high SES NHB families are more likely to be surrounded by NHW families, which means a higher level of exposure to discrimination [95,96]. Needless to say, a high level of discrimination means undesired outcomes and reduced gains of SES [98,100,101].

Residential segregation results in differences in NHB and NHW environmental and contextual exposures. Due to segregation, school options are different for high SES NHB and HW families. As a result, children of high SES NHB families attend highly segregated schools with low resources [62,63,102]. That means there are differential effects of SES on education and schooling of NHW and NHB. While high SES NHW youth attend schools in suburban areas with more funding and higher-quality teachers, NHBs should go to schools that are of lower quality [103].

While lower SES of NHBs is one type of disadvantage, MDRs reflect another class of disadvantage [52,53]. While the first one is about a lack of access to SES resources, MDRs are reflective of unequal outcomes despite similar access to SES. Thus, researchers and policymakers should not only address inequality in SES, but they should also address inequality in the returns of SES. Unfortunately, NHB families are at a double disadvantage because they are affected by low SES and low return of the existing SES resources [52,104].

Multilevel economic, psychological, and societal mechanisms may be involved in explaining racial and ethnic gaps in the returns of parental education [52,104]. MDRs may be due to racism across multiple societal institutions and social structures [52,104]. Racial/ethnic prejudice interferes with the processes that are needed to gain benefits from available SES resources [105–107]. MDRs of educational attainment may be in part due to a history of childhood poverty [108]. The current study, however, did not explore societal and contextual processes that could explain such MDRs.

NHB families are more likely to stay in poor neighborhoods despite high SES. Highly educated NHBs are more likely to stay poor than NHWs [66,109]. Similarly, NHB families from high SES backgrounds may remain at risk of environmental exposures than NHWs with similar SES [95,96,98,110–113]. Similarly, high SES NHB youth spend time with peers with higher risk and behavioral problems than NHWs with the same SES [54,91].

The implications of these MDRs are that it is not merely the access to SES, but also the degree to which SES can result in outcomes that should be addressed. Interventions should target the societal, social, environmental, and structure processes that generate MDRs. We argue that the solutions to MDRs-related disparities are different from those due to low SES. While the solution to disparities due to the gap in SES is to increase NHBs' access to SES resources, the remedy to MDRs-related inequalities to empower NHBs so they can more efficiently translate their SES to outcomes. The latter solution requires policies and programs that go beyond access and address structural and environmental factors. For the latter, there is a need to equalize the life conditions of NHBs and NHWs.

6. Implications

The results may still be preliminary and need further evaluation. If these results are replicated by other datasets and samples, then there is a need for an intervention. It can be argued that NHB parents may require some additional help to mobilize their educational resources. NHB parents may benefit from programs that help with the employability of highly educated NHB parents. Schools in urban areas may benefit from additional resources and an enhanced quality of teachers. After school programs are some example solutions that may compensate reduced IC of NHB youth across SES levels. Interventions may also specifically target the developmental needs of NHB youth across all SES levels. Clinicians should be aware that some of the needs of NHB youth remain high across all SES levels. So, clinicians should be informed that some of the benefits and advantages that NHW youth receive from high SES may not be relevant in NHB families. Low attention may also be diagnosed and treated in NHB families across SES levels. Policymakers may also go beyond family SES and address structural factors that hinder NHB families from mobilizing their SES resources, particularly educational attainment, for securing outcomes.

7. Limitations and Strengths

Each study comes with specific types of methodological limitations. As our data were cross-sectional, we cannot draw any causal inferences between race, parental educational attainment, and youth IC. Similarly, this study only tested the MDRs of parental educational attainment. Other research may test if MDRs also hold for other SES indicators such as parental occupational prestige, income, wealth, and neighborhood SES. These investigations are important because associations between various SES indicators depend on race/ethnicity. Finally, this study only described the MDRs and did not explore contextual factors that could potentially explain the observed MDRs.

To list the study strengths, we can refer to the national scope, multi-center nature, large sample size, large sample of NHBs, and focusing on multiplicative rather than additive effects of SES and race. We can also refer to the application of multiple IC measures (the stop-signal task and CBCL) as another strength of the study. It is important to validate the youth IC task performance with the CBCL parent ratings for several reasons. First, in a clinical setting, most clinicians can easily utilize data of CBCL and measure IC using parents' ratings. However, in many clinical and school settings, collecting data on IC using time-consuming tasks may be difficult. This is also applicable to scaling up the study results. While public health programs and interventions may apply self-reported measures of attention as a screening tool, it is unlikely that large programs can access laboratory measures of attention. So, our multiple measures of IC make our results applicable to a large-scale intervention. Finally, any study of racial differences should always cross-validate their measure. We found the IC similarly correlate with clinical presentation (parental report) of IC, so our IC construct was reflecting the same concept and is similarly applicable to NHW and NHB youth. In other terms, our lab-based measure of IC refers to the very same understanding of parents about their youth behavioral and attention problems. So, the results are similarly relevant to NHB and NHW families. This approach helps us rule out that the observed racial differences are simply an artifact and due to racial variation in measurement properties.

8. Conclusions

When compared to NHWs, NHB youth show lower parental educational attainment and parent reported IC. This adversity is compound by another more profound and systemic adversity, which reflects a weaker effect of parental educational attainment and youth IC. As a result of the latter disadvantage, NHB youth show low IC even when they have highly educated parents. That means some of the inequalities in IC remains across all SES levels. In other terms, racial and ethnic inequalities in IC show a spill-over effect in middle-class people. As a result of high IC, NHB youth with highly educated parents may remain at risk of social, emotional, and behavioral problems.

Funding: Shervin Assari is supported by the National Institutes of Health (NIH) grants D084526-03, CA201415 02, DA035811-05, U54MD008149, U54MD007598, and U54CA229974.

Conflicts of Interest: The authors declare no conflict of interest.

References

1. Deater-Deckard, K.; Li, M.; Lee, J.; King-Casas, B.; Kim-Spoon, J. Poverty and Puberty: A Neurocognitive Study of Inhibitory Control in the Transition to Adolescence. *Psychol. Sci.* **2019**, *30*, 1573–1583. [CrossRef] [PubMed]
2. Chikara, R.K.; Lo, W.C.; Ko, L.W. Exploration of Brain Connectivity during Human Inhibitory Control Using Inter-Trial Coherence. *Sensors* **2020**, *20*, 1722. [CrossRef] [PubMed]
3. Neely, K.A.; Wang, P.; Chennavasin, A.P.; Samimy, S.; Tucker, J.; Merida, A.; Perez-Edgar, K.; Huang-Pollock, C. Deficits in inhibitory force control in young adults with ADHD. *Neuropsychologia* **2017**, *99*, 172–178. [CrossRef] [PubMed]
4. Bartholdy, S.; O'Daly, O.G.; Campbell, I.C.; Banaschewski, T.; Barker, G.; Bokde, A.L.W.; Bromberg, U.; Buchel, C.; Quinlan, E.B.; Desrivieres, S.; et al. Neural Correlates of Failed Inhibitory Control as an Early Marker of Disordered Eating in Adolescents. *Biol. Psychiatry* **2019**, *85*, 956–965. [CrossRef]
5. Bessette, K.L.; Karstens, A.J.; Crane, N.A.; Peters, A.T.; Stange, J.P.; Elverman, K.H.; Morimoto, S.S.; Weisenbach, S.L.; Langenecker, S.A. A Lifespan Model of Interference Resolution and Inhibitory Control: Risk for Depression and Changes with Illness Progression. *Neuropsychol. Rev.* **2020**. [CrossRef]
6. Cabello, R.; Gutierrez-Cobo, M.J.; Fernandez-Berrocal, P. Parental Education and Aggressive Behavior in Children: A Moderated-Mediation Model for Inhibitory Control and Gender. *Front. Psychol.* **2017**, *8*, 1181. [CrossRef]
7. Dieter, J.; Hoffmann, S.; Mier, D.; Reinhard, I.; Beutel, M.; Vollstadt-Klein, S.; Kiefer, F.; Mann, K.; Lemenager, T. The role of emotional inhibitory control in specific internet addiction—An fMRI study. *Behav. Brain Res.* **2017**, *324*, 1–14. [CrossRef]
8. Ely, A.V.; Jagannathan, K.; Hager, N.; Ketcherside, A.; Franklin, T.R.; Wetherill, R.R. Double jeopardy: Comorbid obesity and cigarette smoking are linked to neurobiological alterations in inhibitory control during smoking cue exposure. *Addict. Biol.* **2020**, *25*, e12750. [CrossRef]
9. Humphrey, G.; Dumontheil, I. Development of Risk-Taking, Perspective-Taking, and Inhibitory Control During Adolescence. *Dev. Neuropsychol.* **2016**, *41*, 59–76. [CrossRef]
10. Porter, L.; Bailey-Jones, C.; Priudokaite, G.; Allen, S.; Wood, K.; Stiles, K.; Parvin, O.; Javaid, M.; Verbruggen, F.; Lawrence, N.S. From cookies to carrots; the effect of inhibitory control training on children's snack selections. *Appetite* **2018**, *124*, 111–123. [CrossRef]
11. Troller-Renfree, S.V.; Buzzell, G.A.; Bowers, M.E.; Salo, V.C.; Forman-Alberti, A.; Smith, E.; Papp, L.J.; McDermott, J.M.; Pine, D.S.; Henderson, H.A.; et al. Development of inhibitory control during childhood and its relations to early temperament and later social anxiety: Unique insights provided by latent growth modeling and signal detection theory. *J. Child Psychol. Psychiatry* **2019**, *60*, 622–629. [CrossRef] [PubMed]
12. Huijbregts, S.C.; Warren, A.J.; de Sonneville, L.M.; Swaab-Barneveld, H. Hot and cool forms of inhibitory control and externalizing behavior in children of mothers who smoked during pregnancy: An exploratory study. *J. Abnorm. Child Psychol.* **2008**, *36*, 323–333. [CrossRef] [PubMed]
13. Hao, J. Do Children with Better Inhibitory Control Donate More? Differentiating between Early and Middle Childhood and Cool and Hot Inhibitory Control. *Front. Psychol.* **2017**, *8*, 2182. [CrossRef]
14. Hsieh, I.J.; Chen, Y.Y. Determinants of aggressive behavior: Interactive effects of emotional regulation and inhibitory control. *PLoS ONE* **2017**, *12*, e0175651. [CrossRef] [PubMed]
15. Nakamichi, K. Differences in Young Children's Peer Preference by Inhibitory Control and Emotion Regulation. *Psychol. Rep.* **2017**. [CrossRef]
16. Froeliger, B.; McConnell, P.A.; Bell, S.; Sweitzer, M.; Kozink, R.V.; Eichberg, C.; Hallyburton, M.; Kaiser, N.; Gray, K.M.; McClernon, F.J. Association Between Baseline Corticothalamic-Mediated Inhibitory Control and Smoking Relapse Vulnerability. *JAMA Psychiatry* **2017**, *74*, 379–386. [CrossRef]

17. Mora-Gonzalez, J.; Esteban-Cornejo, I.; Solis-Urra, P.; Migueles, J.H.; Cadenas-Sanchez, C.; Molina-Garcia, P.; Rodriguez-Ayllon, M.; Hillman, C.H.; Catena, A.; Pontifex, M.B.; et al. Fitness, physical activity, sedentary time, inhibitory control, and neuroelectric activity in children with overweight or obesity: The ActiveBrains project. *Psychophysiology* **2020**, e13579. [CrossRef]
18. Cueli, M.; Areces, D.; Garcia, T.; Alves, R.A.; Gonzalez-Castro, P. Attention, inhibitory control and early mathematical skills in preschool students. *Psicothema* **2020**, *32*, 237–244. [CrossRef]
19. Zhang, Z.; Wang, Q.; Liu, X.; Song, P.; Yang, B. Differences in Inhibitory Control between Impulsive and Premeditated Aggression in Juvenile Inmates. *Front. Hum. Neurosci.* **2017**, *11*, 373. [CrossRef]
20. Skowron, E.A.; Cipriano-Essel, E.; Gatzke-Kopp, L.M.; Teti, D.M.; Ammerman, R.T. Early adversity, RSA, and inhibitory control: Evidence of children's neurobiological sensitivity to social context. *Dev. Psychobiol.* **2014**, *56*, 964–978. [CrossRef] [PubMed]
21. Swingler, M.M.; Isbell, E.; Zeytinoglu, S.; Calkins, S.D.; Leerkes, E.M. Maternal behavior predicts neural underpinnings of inhibitory control in preschoolers. *Dev. Psychobiol.* **2018**, *60*, 692–706. [CrossRef] [PubMed]
22. Holochwost, S.J.; Volpe, V.V.; Gueron-Sela, N.; Propper, C.B.; Mills-Koonce, W.R. Sociodemographic risk, parenting, and inhibitory control in early childhood: The role of respiratory sinus arrhythmia. *J. Child Psychol. Psychiatry* **2018**, *59*, 973–981. [CrossRef]
23. Bruce, J.; Fisher, P.A.; Graham, A.M.; Moore, W.E.; Peake, S.J.; Mannering, A.M. Patterns of brain activation in foster children and nonmaltreated children during an inhibitory control task. *Dev. Psychopathol.* **2013**, *25*, 931–941. [CrossRef] [PubMed]
24. Zaidman-Zait, A.; Shilo, I. Parental ADHD Symptoms and Inhibitory Control in Relation to Parenting Among Mothers of Children with and Without ADHD. *J. Atten. Disord.* **2018**. [CrossRef]
25. Cotten, N.U.; Resnick, J.; Browne, D.C.; Martin, S.L.; McCarraher, D.R.; Woods, J. Aggression and fighting behavior among African-American adolescents: Individual and family factors. *Am. J. Public Health* **1994**, *84*, 618–622. [CrossRef] [PubMed]
26. Cavazos-Rehg, P.A.; Krauss, M.J.; Spitznagel, E.L.; Schootman, M.; Bucholz, K.K.; Peipert, J.F.; Sanders-Thompson, V.; Cottler, L.B.; Bierut, L.J. Age of sexual debut among US adolescents. *Contraception* **2009**, *80*, 158–162. [CrossRef] [PubMed]
27. Bumpus, J.P.; Umeh, Z.; Harris, A.L. Social Class and Educational Attainment: Do Blacks Benefit Less from Increases in Parents' Social Class Status? *Sociol. Race Ethn.* **2020**, *6*, 233–241. [CrossRef]
28. Cohen, G.L.; Sherman, D.K. Stereotype threat and the social and scientific contexts of the race achievement gap. *Am. Psychol.* **2005**, *60*, 270–271. [CrossRef]
29. Burchinal, M.; McCartney, K.; Steinberg, L.; Crosnoe, R.; Friedman, S.L.; McLoyd, V.; Pianta, R.; Network, N.E.C.C.R. Examining the Black-White achievement gap among low-income children using the NICHD study of early child care and youth development. *Child Dev.* **2011**, *82*, 1404–1420. [CrossRef]
30. Gorey, K.M. Comprehensive School Reform: Meta-Analytic Evidence of Black-White Achievement Gap Narrowing. *Educ. Policy Anal. Arch.* **2009**, *17*, 1–17. [CrossRef]
31. Hair, N.L.; Hanson, J.L.; Wolfe, B.L.; Pollak, S.D. Association of Child Poverty, Brain Development, and Academic Achievement. *JAMA Pediatr.* **2015**, *169*, 822–829. [CrossRef] [PubMed]
32. Valencia, M.L.C.; Tran, B.T.; Lim, M.K.; Choi, K.S.; Oh, J.K. Association Between Socioeconomic Status and Early Initiation of Smoking, Alcohol Drinking, and Sexual Behavior Among Korean Adolescents. *Asia Pac. J. Public Health* **2019**, *31*, 443–453. [CrossRef] [PubMed]
33. Ahmad, A.; Zulaily, N.; Shahril, M.R.; Syed Abdullah, E.F.H.; Ahmed, A. Association between socioeconomic status and obesity among 12-year-old Malaysian adolescents. *PLoS ONE* **2018**, *13*, e0200577. [CrossRef] [PubMed]
34. Merz, E.C.; Tottenham, N.; Noble, K.G. Socioeconomic Status, Amygdala Volume, and Internalizing Symptoms in Children and Adolescents. *J. Clin. Child Adolesc. Psychol.* **2018**, *47*, 312–323. [CrossRef]
35. Dismukes, A.; Shirtcliff, E.; Jones, C.W.; Zeanah, C.; Theall, K.; Drury, S. The development of the cortisol response to dyadic stressors in Black and White infants. *Dev. Psychopathol.* **2018**, *30*, 1995–2008. [CrossRef]
36. Hanson, J.L.; Nacewicz, B.M.; Sutterer, M.J.; Cayo, A.A.; Schaefer, S.M.; Rudolph, K.D.; Shirtcliff, E.A.; Pollak, S.D.; Davidson, R.J. Behavioral problems after early life stress: Contributions of the hippocampus and amygdala. *Biol. Psychiatry* **2015**, *77*, 314–323. [CrossRef]

37. Miller, B.; Taylor, J. Racial and socioeconomic status differences in depressive symptoms among black and white youth: An examination of the mediating effects of family structure, stress and support. *J. Youth Adolesc.* **2012**, *41*, 426–437. [CrossRef]
38. DeSantis, A.S.; Adam, E.K.; Doane, L.D.; Mineka, S.; Zinbarg, R.E.; Craske, M.G. Racial/ethnic differences in cortisol diurnal rhythms in a community sample of adolescents. *J. Adolesc. Health* **2007**, *41*, 3–13. [CrossRef]
39. Alvarado, S.E. The impact of childhood neighborhood disadvantage on adult joblessness and income. *Soc. Sci. Res.* **2018**, *70*, 1–17. [CrossRef]
40. Barreto, S.M.; de Figueiredo, R.C.; Giatti, L. Socioeconomic inequalities in youth smoking in Brazil. *BMJ Open* **2013**, *3*, e003538. [CrossRef]
41. Schreier, H.M.; Chen, E. Socioeconomic status and the health of youth: A multilevel, multidomain approach to conceptualizing pathways. *Psychol. Bull.* **2013**, *139*, 606–654. [CrossRef] [PubMed]
42. Hemovich, V.; Lac, A.; Crano, W.D. Understanding early-onset drug and alcohol outcomes among youth: The role of family structure, social factors, and interpersonal perceptions of use. *Psychol. Health Med.* **2011**, *16*, 249–267. [CrossRef]
43. Kaufman, J.S.; Cooper, R.S.; McGee, D.L. Socioeconomic status and health in blacks and whites: The problem of residual confounding and the resiliency of race. *Epidemiology* **1997**, 621–628. [CrossRef]
44. Bell, C.N.; Sacks, T.K.; Thomas Tobin, C.S.; Thorpe Jr, R.J. Racial Non-equivalence of Socioeconomic Status and Self-rated Health among African Americans and Whites. *SSM Popul. Health* **2020**, *10*, 100561. [CrossRef] [PubMed]
45. Samuel, L.J.; Roth, D.L.; Schwartz, B.S.; Thorpe, R.J.; Glass, T.A. Socioeconomic Status, Race/Ethnicity, and Diurnal Cortisol Trajectories in Middle-Aged and Older Adults. *J. Gerontol. B Psychol. Sci. Soc. Sci.* **2018**, *73*, 468–476. [CrossRef]
46. Fuentes, M.; Hart-Johnson, T.; Green, C.R. The association among neighborhood socioeconomic status, race and chronic pain in black and white older adults. *J. Natl. Med. Assoc.* **2007**, *99*, 1160–1169.
47. Assari, S.; Khoshpouri, P.; Chalian, H. Combined Effects of Race and Socioeconomic Status on Cancer Beliefs, Cognitions, and Emotions. *Healthcare* **2019**, *7*, 17. [CrossRef]
48. Assari, S. Number of Chronic Medical Conditions Fully Mediates the Effects of Race on Mortality; 25-Year Follow-Up of a Nationally Representative Sample of Americans. *J. Racial. Ethn. Health Disparities* **2017**, *4*, 623–631. [CrossRef]
49. Assari, S. Distal, intermediate, and proximal mediators of racial disparities in renal disease mortality in the United States. *J. Nephropathol.* **2016**, *5*, 51–59. [CrossRef]
50. Williams, D.R.; Costa, M.V.; Odunlami, A.O.; Mohammed, S.A. Moving upstream: How interventions that address the social determinants of health can improve health and reduce disparities. *J. Public Health Manag. Pract.* **2008**, *14*, 8–17. [CrossRef]
51. Williams, D.R. Race, socioeconomic status, and health the added effects of racism and discrimination. *Ann. N. Y. Acad. Sci.* **1999**, *896*, 173–188. [CrossRef] [PubMed]
52. Assari, S. Health Disparities due to Diminished Return among Black Americans: Public Policy Solutions. *Soc. Issues Policy Rev.* **2018**, *12*, 112–145. [CrossRef]
53. Assari, S. Unequal Gain of Equal Resources across Racial Groups. *Int. J. Health Policy Manag.* **2017**, *7*, 1–9. [CrossRef] [PubMed]
54. Assari, S.; Caldwell, C.H.; Bazargan, M. Association Between Parental Educational Attainment and Youth Outcomes and Role of Race/Ethnicity. *JAMA Netw. Open* **2019**, *2*, e1916018. [CrossRef]
55. Assari, S.; Caldwell, C.H.; Mincy, R. Family Socioeconomic Status at Birth and Youth Impulsivity at Age 15; Blacks' Diminished Return. *Children* **2018**, *5*, 58. [CrossRef]
56. Assari, S.; Thomas, A.; Caldwell, C.H.; Mincy, R.B. Blacks' Diminished Health Return of Family Structure and Socioeconomic Status; 15 Years of Follow-up of a National Urban Sample of Youth. *J. Urban Health* **2018**, *95*, 21–35. [CrossRef]
57. Assari, S.; Bazargan, M. Being Married Increases Life Expectancy of White but Not Black Americans. *J. Fam. Reprod. Health* **2019**, *13*, 132–140. [CrossRef]
58. Assari, S.; Caldwell, C.H. High Risk of Depression in High-Income African American Boys. *J. Racial Ethn. Health Disparities* **2018**, *5*, 808–819. [CrossRef]

59. Assari, S.; Caldwell, C.H.; Mincy, R.B. Maternal Educational Attainment at Birth Promotes Future Self-Rated Health of White but Not Black Youth: A 15-Year Cohort of a National Sample. *J. Clin. Med.* **2018**, *7*, 93. [CrossRef]
60. Assari, S.; Caldwell, C.H. Family Income at Birth and Risk of Attention Deficit Hyperactivity Disorder at Age 15: Racial Differences. *Children* **2019**, *6*, 10. [CrossRef]
61. Assari, S.; Caldwell, C.H.; Zimmerman, M.A. Family Structure and Subsequent Anxiety Symptoms; Minorities' Diminished Return. *Brain Sci.* **2018**, *8*, 97. [CrossRef] [PubMed]
62. Assari, S. Parental Educational Attainment and Academic Performance of American College Students; Blacks' Diminished Returns. *J. Health Econ. Dev.* **2019**, *1*, 21–31. [PubMed]
63. Assari, S.; Caldwell, C.H. Parental Educational Attainment Differentially Boosts School Performance of American Adolescents: Minorities' Diminished Returns. *J. Family Reprod. Health* **2019**, *13*, 7–13. [CrossRef]
64. Assari, S. Parental Education Attainment and Educational Upward Mobility; Role of Race and Gender. *Behav. Sci.* **2018**, *8*, 107. [CrossRef] [PubMed]
65. Assari, S. Parental Educational Attainment and Mental Well-Being of College Students; Diminished Returns of Blacks. *Brain Sci.* **2018**, *8*, 193. [CrossRef] [PubMed]
66. Assari, S. Parental Education Better Helps White than Black Families Escape Poverty: National Survey of Children's Health. *Economies* **2018**, *6*, 30. [CrossRef]
67. Assari, S. Blacks' Diminished Return of Education Attainment on Subjective Health; Mediating Effect of Income. *Brain Sci.* **2018**, *8*, 176. [CrossRef]
68. Assari, S.; Hani, N. Household Income and Children's Unmet Dental Care Need; Blacks' Diminished Return. *Dent. J.* **2018**, *6*, 17. [CrossRef]
69. Alcohol Research: Current Reviews Editorial Stuff. NIH's Adolescent Brain Cognitive Development (ABCD) Study. *Alcohol. Res.* **2018**, *39*, 97.
70. Casey, B.J.; Cannonier, T.; Conley, M.I.; Cohen, A.O.; Barch, D.M.; Heitzeg, M.M.; Soules, M.E.; Teslovich, T.; Dellarco, D.V.; Garavan, H.; et al. The Adolescent Brain Cognitive Development (ABCD) study: Imaging acquisition across 21 sites. *Dev. Cogn. Neurosci.* **2018**, *32*, 43–54. [CrossRef]
71. Karcher, N.R.; O'Brien, K.J.; Kandala, S.; Barch, D.M. Resting-State Functional Connectivity and Psychotic-like Experiences in Childhood: Results From the Adolescent Brain Cognitive Development Study. *Biol. Psychiatry* **2019**, *86*, 7–15. [CrossRef]
72. Lisdahl, K.M.; Sher, K.J.; Conway, K.P.; Gonzalez, R.; Feldstein Ewing, S.W.; Nixon, S.J.; Tapert, S.; Bartsch, H.; Goldstein, R.Z.; Heitzeg, M. Adolescent brain cognitive development (ABCD) study: Overview of substance use assessment methods. *Dev. Cogn. Neurosci.* **2018**, *32*, 80–96. [CrossRef] [PubMed]
73. Luciana, M.; Bjork, J.M.; Nagel, B.J.; Barch, D.M.; Gonzalez, R.; Nixon, S.J.; Banich, M.T. Adolescent neurocognitive development and impacts of substance use: Overview of the adolescent brain cognitive development (ABCD) baseline neurocognition battery. *Dev. Cogn. Neurosci.* **2018**, *32*, 67–79. [CrossRef] [PubMed]
74. Auchter, A.M.; Hernandez Mejia, M.; Heyser, C.J.; Shilling, P.D.; Jernigan, T.L.; Brown, S.A.; Tapert, S.F.; Dowling, G.J. A description of the ABCD organizational structure and communication framework. *Dev. Cogn. Neurosci.* **2018**, *32*, 8–15. [CrossRef]
75. Garavan, H.; Bartsch, H.; Conway, K.; Decastro, A.; Goldstein, R.Z.; Heeringa, S.; Jernigan, T.; Potter, A.; Thompson, W.; Zahs, D. Recruiting the ABCD sample: Design considerations and procedures. *Dev. Cogn. Neurosci.* **2018**, *32*, 16–22. [CrossRef] [PubMed]
76. Clark, S.V.; King, T.Z.; Turner, J.A. Cerebellar Contributions to Proactive and Reactive Control in the Stop Signal Task: A Systematic Review and Meta-Analysis of Functional Magnetic Resonance Imaging Studies. *Neuropsychol. Rev.* **2020**. [CrossRef] [PubMed]
77. Dupuis, A.; Indralingam, M.; Chevrier, A.; Crosbie, J.; Arnold, P.; Burton, C.L.; Schachar, R. Response Time Adjustment in the Stop Signal Task: Development in Children and Adolescents. *Child Dev.* **2019**, *90*, 263–272. [CrossRef]
78. Hiraoka, K.; Kinoshita, A.; Kunimura, H.; Matsuoka, M. Effect of variability of sequence length of go trials preceding a stop trial on ability of response inhibition in stop-signal task. *Somatosens. Mot. Res.* **2018**, *35*, 95–102. [CrossRef]
79. Carver, A.C.; Livesey, D.J.; Charles, M. Age related changes in inhibitory control as measured by stop signal task performance. *Int. J. Neurosci.* **2001**, *107*, 43–61. [CrossRef]

80. American Psychiatry Association (A.P.A.). *Diagnostic and Statistical Manual of Mental Disorders (DSM-5®)*; American Psychiatric Pubishing: Washington, DC, USA, 2013.
81. Achenbach, T.M.; Rescorla, L. *Manual for the ASEBA School-Age Forms & Profiles: An Integrated System of Multi-Informant Assessment*; Aseba: Burlington, VT, USA, 2001.
82. ASEBA® Web-Link™ ASEBA Overview. 2020. Available online: https://aseba.org/aseba-overview/ (accessed on 5 May 2020).
83. Assari, S. Education Attainment and Obesity Differential Returns Based on Sexual Orientation. *Behav. Sci.* **2019**, *9*, 16. [CrossRef]
84. Assari, S.; Farokhnia, M.; Mistry, R. Education Attainment and Alcohol Binge Drinking: Diminished Returns of Hispanics in Los Angeles. *Behav. Sci.* **2019**, *9*, 9. [CrossRef] [PubMed]
85. Assari, S. Family Income Reduces Risk of Obesity for White but Not Black Children. *Children* **2018**, *5*, 73. [CrossRef] [PubMed]
86. Assari, S. Life Expectancy Gain Due to Employment Status Depends on Race, Gender, Education, and Their Intersections. *J. Racial Ethn. Health Disparities* **2018**, *5*, 375–386. [CrossRef] [PubMed]
87. Assari, S.; Lankarani, M.M. Education and Alcohol Consumption among Older Americans; Black-White Differences. *Front. Public Health* **2016**, *4*, 67. [CrossRef]
88. Shervin, A.; Ritesh, M. Diminished Return of Employment on Ever Smoking Among Hispanic Whites in Los Angeles. *Health Equity* **2019**, *3*, 138–144. [CrossRef]
89. Assari, S. Socioeconomic Determinants of Systolic Blood Pressure; Minorities' Diminished Returns. *J. Health Econ. Dev.* **2019**, *1*, 1–11.
90. Assari, S. Socioeconomic Status and Self-Rated Oral Health; Diminished Return among Hispanic Whites. *Dent. J.* **2018**, *6*, 11. [CrossRef]
91. Assari, S.; Boyce, S.; Bazargan, M.; Caldwell, C.H. Mathematical Performance of American Youth: Diminished Returns of Educational Attainment of Asian-American Parents. *Educ. Sci.* **2020**, *10*, 32. [CrossRef]
92. Assari, S.; Bazargan, M. Protective Effects of Educational Attainment Against Cigarette Smoking; Diminished Returns of American Indians and Alaska Natives in the National Health Interview Survey. *Int. J. Travel Med. Glob. Health* **2019**, *7*, 105–110. [CrossRef]
93. Bowden, M.; Bartkowski, J.; Xu, X.; Lewis, R., Jr. Parental occupation and the gender math gap: Examining the social reproduction of academic advantage among elementary and middle school students. *Soc. Sci.* **2017**, *7*, 6. [CrossRef]
94. Chetty, R.; Hendren, N.; Kline, P.; Saez, E. Where is the land of opportunity? The geography of intergenerational mobility in the United States. *Q. J. Econ.* **2014**, *129*, 1553–1623. [CrossRef]
95. Assari, S.; Gibbons, F.X.; Simons, R. Depression among Black Youth; Interaction of Class and Place. *Brain Sci.* **2018**, *8*, 108. [CrossRef] [PubMed]
96. Assari, S.; Gibbons, F.X.; Simons, R.L. Perceived Discrimination among Black Youth: An 18-Year Longitudinal Study. *Behav. Sci.* **2018**, *8*, 44. [CrossRef] [PubMed]
97. Assari, S. Does School Racial Composition Explain Why High Income Black Youth Perceive More Discrimination? A Gender Analysis. *Brain Sci.* **2018**, *8*, 140. [CrossRef]
98. Assari, S.; Lankarani, M.M.; Caldwell, C.H. Does Discrimination Explain High Risk of Depression among High-Income African American Men? *Behav. Sci.* **2018**, *8*, 40. [CrossRef]
99. Assari, S.; Moghani Lankarani, M. Workplace Racial Composition Explains High Perceived Discrimination of High Socioeconomic Status African American Men. *Brain Sci.* **2018**, *8*, 139. [CrossRef]
100. Assari, S.; Preiser, B.; Lankarani, M.M.; Caldwell, C.H. Subjective Socioeconomic Status Moderates the Association between Discrimination and Depression in African American Youth. *Brain Sci.* **2018**, *8*, 71. [CrossRef]
101. Assari, S.; Caldwell, C.H. Social Determinants of Perceived Discrimination among Black Youth: Intersection of Ethnicity and Gender. *Children* **2018**, *5*, 24. [CrossRef]
102. Boyce, S.; Bazargan, M.; Caldwell, C.H.; Zimmerman, M.A.; Assari, S. Parental Educational Attainment and Social Environment of Urban Public Schools in the U.S.: Blacks' Diminished Returns. *Children* **2020**, *7*, 44. [CrossRef]
103. Jefferson, A.L.; Gibbons, L.E.; Rentz, D.M.; Carvalho, J.O.; Manly, J.; Bennett, D.A.; Jones, R.N. A life course model of cognitive activities, socioeconomic status, education, reading ability, and cognition. *J. Am. Geriatr. Soc.* **2011**, *59*, 1403–1411. [CrossRef]

104. Assari, S.; Cobb, S.; Saqib, M.; Bazargan, M. Diminished Returns of Educational Attainment on Heart Disease among Black Americans. *Open Cardiovasc. Med. J.* **2020**, *14*, 5. [CrossRef]
105. Hudson, D.L.; Bullard, K.M.; Neighbors, H.W.; Geronimus, A.T.; Yang, J.; Jackson, J.S. Are benefits conferred with greater socioeconomic position undermined by racial discrimination among African American men? *J. Mens. Health* **2012**, *9*, 127–136. [CrossRef]
106. Hudson, D.L.; Neighbors, H.W.; Geronimus, A.T.; Jackson, J.S. The relationship between socioeconomic position and depression among a US nationally representative sample of African Americans. *Soc. Psychiatry Psychiatr. Epidemiol.* **2012**, *47*, 373–381. [CrossRef]
107. Hudson, D.; Sacks, T.; Irani, K.; Asher, A. The Price of the Ticket: Health Costs of Upward Mobility among African Americans. *Int. J. Environ. Res. Public Health* **2020**, *17*, 1179. [CrossRef]
108. Bartik, T.J.; Hershbein, B. Degrees of poverty: The relationship between family income background and the returns to education. *SSRN Electron. J.* **2018**. [CrossRef]
109. Assari, S.; Preiser, B.; Kelly, M. Education and Income Predict Future Emotional Well-Being of Whites but Not Blacks: A Ten-Year Cohort. *Brain Sci.* **2018**, *8*, 122. [CrossRef]
110. Assari, S.; Bazargan, M. Second-hand exposure home Second-Hand Smoke Exposure at Home in the United States; Minorities' Diminished Returns. *Int. J. Travel Med. Glob. Health* **2019**, *7*, 135–141. [CrossRef]
111. Assari S, B.M. Unequal Effects of Educational Attainment on Workplace Exposure to Second-Hand Smoke by Race and Ethnicity; Minorities' Diminished Returns in the National Health Interview Survey (NHIS). *J. Med. Res. Innov.* **2019**, *3*, e000179. [CrossRef]
112. Assari, S. Race, Intergenerational Social Mobility and Stressful Life Events. *Behav Sci.* **2018**, *8*, 86. [CrossRef]
113. Assari, S.; Bazargan, M. Unequal Associations between Educational Attainment and Occupational Stress across Racial and Ethnic Groups. *Int. J. Environ. Res. Public Health* **2019**, *16*, 3539. [CrossRef]

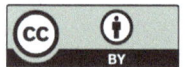

© 2020 by the author. Licensee MDPI, Basel, Switzerland. This article is an open access article distributed under the terms and conditions of the Creative Commons Attribution (CC BY) license (http://creativecommons.org/licenses/by/4.0/).

MDPI
St. Alban-Anlage 66
4052 Basel
Switzerland
Tel. +41 61 683 77 34
Fax +41 61 302 89 18
www.mdpi.com

Brain Sciences Editorial Office
E-mail: brainsci@mdpi.com
www.mdpi.com/journal/brainsci

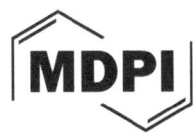

www.ingramcontent.com/pod-product-compliance
Lightning Source LLC
LaVergne TN
LVHW072356090526
838202LV00019B/2557